T3-BUL-820

Springer Series on

REHABILITATION

Volume 1

The Psychology of Disability
Carolyn L. Vash, Ph.D.

Volume 2

Disabled People as Second-Class Citizens
Myron G. Eisenberg, Ph.D., Cynthia Griggins, and Richard J. Duval, Editors

Volume 3

Behavioral Approaches to Rehabilitation: Coping with Change
Elaine Greif, Ph.D. and Ruth G. Matarazzo, Ph.D.

Volume 4

Chronic Illness and Disability through the Life Span: Effects on Self and Family
Myron G. Eisenberg, Ph.D., LaFaye C. Sutkin, Ph.D., and Mary A. Jansen, Ph.D., Editors

Myron G. Eisenberg, Ph.D., is Chief of Psychology Service at the Veterans Administration Medical Center, Hampton, Virginia, Associate Professor in the Departments of Psychiatry and Behavioral Sciences and Physical Medicine and Rehabilitation at the Eastern Virginia Medical School, and Adjunct Faculty Member at The College of William and Mary. He is a Past President and Fellow of the American Psychological Association's (APA) Division of Rehabilitation Psychology, a member of the American Congress of Rehabilitation Medicine's National Sex and Disability Task Force, and a U.S. Contact Person for the International Clearing House on Social and Sexual Intercourse for Disabled Persons, an organization cosponsored by the Rehabilitation International Social Commission and the Swedish Committee for Rehabilitation. Dr. Eisenberg has published widely in the area of rehabilitation and serves as Consulting Editor of *Sex and Disability* (Human Sciences Press) and Associate Editor of *Rehabilitation Psychology* (Springer Publishing Company). He is also a Grant Reviewer for the Paralyzed Veterans of America's Research Technology Foundation.

LaFaye C. Sutkin, Ph.D., is a Health Psychologist at Jerry L. Pettis Memorial Veterans Hospital in Loma Linda, California. Dr. Sutkin works extensively with renal and oncology patients and their families as well as providing services to rehabilitation and nursing home units. She has presented numerous workshops in the areas of health psychology, gerontology, disability, and sexuality and has authored several publications in these and other areas.

Mary A. Jansen, Ph.D., is currently Associate Professional Dean for Professional Affairs at the California School for Professional Psychology, Fresno, California. Prior to that, she was affiliated with the American Psychological Association (APA) in Washington, D.C., where she was Administrative Officer for Professional Practice. Dr. Jansen serves as Editor of *Rehabilitation Psychology* and has sat on committees of several national mental health groups, including the National Mental Liaison Group and the World Federation for Mental Health. She also has served as a consultant to a number of rehabilitation programs and mental health agencies. Dr. Jansen has authored several publications in the areas of rehabilitation, health, and professional psychology.

Chronic Illness and Disability through the Life Span

Effects on Self and Family

Myron G. Eisenberg, Ph.D.
LaFaye C. Sutkin, Ph.D.
Mary A. Jansen, Ph.D.
Editors

Springer Publishing Company
New York

Springer Publishing Company, Inc.
200 Park Avenue South
New York, New York 10003

85 86 87 88 / 10 9 8 7 6 5 4 3 2

Library of Congress Cataloging in Publication Data

Main entry under title:
Chronic illness and disability through the life span.
Includes bibliographies and indexes.
1. Chronic diseases—Psychological aspects. 2. Chronic diseases—Patients—Family relationships. 3. Physically handicapped—Psychology. 4. Adjustment (Psychology) I. Eisenberg, Myron G. II. Sutkin, LaFaye C. III. Jansen, Mary A. [DNLM: 1. Chronic disease—Psychology. 2. Chronic disease—Rehabilitation. 3. Handicapped—Psychology. 4. Rehabilitation—Psychology. 5. Family. W1 SP685SF v.4 / WB 320 C557]
RC108.C47 1984 616 83-20257
ISBN 0-8261-4180-3

Printed in the United States of America

Contents

Part IV Young Adults

Part V Middle Age

Part VI Old Age

Acknowledgments

Appreciation is extended to Beverly J. Smith, Psychology Service, Veterans Administration Medical Center, Hampton, Virginia, for the care taken in preparing the final typed manuscript of this text. Her meticulous attention to detail, promptness, and tact in dealing with the sometimes harassed and harassing senior editor of this volume is deeply appreciated. Special thanks are given to Bill M. Domm, M.D., former Chief-of-Staff, Veterans Administration Medical Center, Hampton, Virginia, for the support, guidance, and encouragement he provided to the senior editor throughout this project. His unswerving dedication to quality patient care has served as a model for providers of health care services.

M. G. E.

Contributors

R. Debra Bendell, Ph.D.
University of Oklahoma Health Sciences Center
Oklahoma City, Oklahoma

Andrew R. Block, Ph.D.
Purdue University—School of Science
Indianapolis, Indiana

Barbara D. Blumberg, Sc.M.
National Cancer Institute
Bethesda, Maryland

Sara L. Boyer, M.S.
Purdue University—School of Science
Indianapolis, Indiana

Carolyn Keith Burr, R.N., M.S.
Florida Atlantic University
Boca Raton, Florida

Marcy Bush, M.A.
Case Western Reserve University
Cleveland, Ohio

Marcia S. Collins-Moore, Ph.D.
McGee Eye Institute
Oklahoma City, Oklahoma

Peggy Crawford, M.S.N.
Rainbow Babies and Childrens Hospital
Cleveland, Ohio

Dennis Drotar, Ph.D.
Case Western Reserve University School of Medicine
Cleveland, Ohio

John M. Eiler, Ph.D.
University of Southern California
Los Angeles, California

Fran Z. Farrell, R.N., M.S.W.
University of Arizona Health Sciences Center
Tucson, Arizona

Robert L. Glueckauf, Ph.D.
University Hospital
London, Ontario

John J. Hutter, Jr., M.D.
University of Arizona Health Sciences Center
Tucson, Arizona

Cheryl Imes, M.A.
Purdue University—School of Science
Indianapolis, Indiana

Henry T. Ireys, Ph.D.
Albert Einstein College of Medicine
Bronx, New York

M. Jane Lewis, M.A.
Kappa Systems, Inc.
Arlington, Virginia

Alexandra L. Quittner, M.A.
University Hospital
London, Ontario

Lynne C. Rustad, Ph.D.
Veterans Administration Medical Center
Cleveland, Ohio

Donald R. Schienle, Ph.D.
Rancho Los Amigos Hospital
Downey, California

Elizabeth J. Susman, R.N., Ph.D.
National Institute of Mental Health
Bethesda, Maryland

J. Kenneth Whitt, Ph.D.
University of North Carolina School of Medicine
Chapel Hill, North Carolina

Judy M. Zarit, Ph.D.
University of Southern California and School of Professional Psychology
Los Angeles, California

Steven H. Zarit, Ph.D.
Ethel Percy Andrus Gerontology Center
Los Angeles, California

1 Introduction

LaFaye C. Sutkin

Recent advances in medical and surgical knowledge and technology have greatly extended the life expectancy of individuals with chronic disabilities, thus providing an ever-increasing number of rehabilitation candidates. In its infancy, rehabilitation psychology often applied a "shotgun approach" to the management of victims of chronic disability. The necessity for prompt action frequently precluded the establishment of an empirical or theoretical basis for intervention. As sophistication (and theoretical and empirical support) develop, however, rehabilitation programs must increasingly recognize the differing needs of the individual and realize that interventions, in order to be maximally effective, must incorporate that knowledge in formulating treatment plans. As Beatrice Wright has recommended (1980), the current direction that rehabilitation must pursue is a focus on the person and the situation. It is, then, in the interest of examining disability within its context that this book was written.

A major dimension in which victims of chronic disability may differ from one another is that of age-group. Clearly, the needs and responsibilities of the adult differ from those of the child or the elderly person; however, the majority of available literature draws support from investigations administered to young adults. There is also an assumption, if implicit, that each disabled person, regardless of age, brings to the situation the same resources. As rehabilitation begins to narrow its focus, age would appear to be an important variable to examine.

Significantly, many personality theorists have examined a series of stages in which development is thought to occur in order to increase their understanding of psychopathology. Much support has been found for the premise that development proceeds by steps rather than smoothly (Erikson, 1963; Havighurst, 1948; Jung, 1933). Throughout these periods of development certain achievements are expected to provide for the emergence of a normal and healthy identity. Each step is believed to contribute uniquely to the developing ego. Normal development is felt to be the result of mastery of the tasks of each life stage *prior* to passage to the subsequent stage.

The hypothesis that the relatively specific effects of an event on a particular life stage will result in equally specific vulnerabilities and, hence, unique psychopathology constitutes the basis of developmental approaches. Moreover, it is implicit in such theories that minimal conditions must exist for the individual to satisfactorily meet the demands of each of these steps. Finally, the ease of passage through later steps is thought to be facilitated by the degree of success in completing preceding stages (Erikson, 1963).

Also implicit in developmental theories is the requirement for physical, emotional, and cognitive tools with which to meet all the demands that any step may impose. Clearly, to the extent that disabling conditions may diminish the physical, emotional, or cognitive capabilities of the individual, they might be expected to disrupt the smooth transition through the current stage. In addition, disabling conditions may impair the capacity of the environment and significant others to provide optimal conditions for a given life stage.

The most immediate effect of a disabling condition is the obstruction of activities normal for that life stage. It should be borne in mind that the tasks of each life stage are also the major activities of that step. For example, if a major task for the school-age child is the development of academic competence, it is not only an important quality for later life, but the major activity of the child. Similarly, if a task for an adult is bearing and rearing children, that activity is of utmost significance, regardless of subsequent life stages.

A further consequence of the disrupting influence of disability on development is failure to acquire essential qualities required for a healthy and complete ego. Moreover, since later development depends, in part, on adequate acquisition of living skills of prior stages, the individual may be handicapped in approaching all the subsequent challenges of life. For example, achievement of a capacity for trust and hope is vital to enable the individual to submit to the rigors of therapy.

In terms of treatment implications, a developmental approach would suggest that interventions be based upon capacities that the individual might reasonably be expected to possess at his life stage, and that treatment demands be avoided that call for more mature capacities. Therapy might also be expected to include efforts to compensate for deficits so that the individual might have the opportunity to master major tasks of his life stage.

Normal development leads to changes in families as well as in the individual. Family members ordinarily have somewhat fixed expectations of age-appropriate behaviors. As a result of those expectations, family members ordinarily adjust their behavior appropriately to interact as the individual passes from one stage to the next. When development fails to proceed normally, family members may be compelled to modify their expectations and alter their behavior when relating to the individual (Kennell & Klaus, 1982).

Several consequences may follow from the demands on the family imposed by disability: (1) The change in the individual may interfere with the accomplishment of the family member's tasks. For example, a severely disabled infant may be an obstacle to its mother's mastery of childrearing, and a disabled adult may interfere with the task of procreation ordinarily appropriate for an adult spouse. (2) The change in the individual's physical capacities may evoke behaviors that are incompatible with the demands of that individual's current psychological development. A spinal injury in a child who should be expanding his independence usually forces his mother to resume caretaking activities that could undermine that budding autonomy. (3) Finally, altered capacities in an individual may leave family members puzzled as to appropriate ways of interacting with the individual. This may be especially true of the injured person whose cognitive capacities are those of middle age, but whose physical capabilities are those of an infant.

The preceding observations suggest that an examination of disabilities within life stages might offer a useful framework for the investigation of the significance of age for the individual and his family who are faced with chronic disability. The organization of this text will follow loosely the stages described by Erik Erikson because Erikson extended the developmental approach to the entire life span and because Erikson's understanding of epigenesis explored normal development as well as the evolution of psychopathology. Erikson speculated that each life stage presents a variety of tasks to be mastered before graduation to the succeeding stage (1963). Erikson maintained that, as a function of uncontrollable events, individual differences, and so on, no individual proceeded with unhampered success to master all the tasks of any stage, but that relative competence in the prior stage was a prerequisite condition to greet the challenges of the next. Although other theorists offer additional challenges for each stage, Erikson's formulations provide a convenient framework in which to view the differing demands of adaptation to disability as a function of the life stage in which the injury or illness first makes its appearance.

Although Erikson did not specifically describe the changing demands placed on families by the developing individual passing from stage to stage, some of these demands are implicit in his discussions. Clearly, the interaction between the individual and family members will be transformed as the individual develops competencies and expresses differing needs.

Before summarizing the relationship between life stages and disabilities that are described in the succeeding chapters, it might be helpful to review Erikson's theory of development. Erikson has described as the major task of infancy the attainment of a sense of basic trust instead of basic mistrust. This is achieved by the perception of the caretaker as consistent and reliable. It is vital that the infant either have needs immediately met or the means for meeting those needs readily available. Successful resolution of the early childhood conflict between autonomy and shame should result in self-control and willpower if the child has experienced firm but reassuring control. The period that Freud has referred to as the Phallic Period brings with it, in addition to gender identity, the possibility of taking initiative rather than being restrained by guilt. The child who has successfully negotiated this stage may go forth with direction and purpose. The major task of the school-age child is the development of a sense of industry, competence, and self-worth. The normal adolescent must question the earlier assurances in order to arrive at a sense of identity that will facilitate a capacity for devotion and fidelity as well as productivity in a social role. During young adulthood, the individual who has satisfactorily established his or her identity must face the challenges of sacrifice and compromise in order to find intimacy in a relationship with another, rather than a life of isolation. In the middle years, to avoid stagnation, the individual must satisfy the mature "need to be needed" through generativity. Finally, the person who has mastered preceding stages with some success may achieve a sense of ego integrity from which he may prepare to face death with the same acceptance with which he faced life in infancy (Erikson, 1963, 1968).

Infancy

For Erikson, the development of basic trust in infancy implies that the infant has learned to rely on the sameness and continuity of outer providers *and* has learned to trust himself and his own capacities. The healthy infant demonstrates this mastery through ease of feeding, depth of sleep, and relaxation of the bowels (Erikson, 1968). The mastery of this stage depends most on the mother; however, absolute quantities of food or love appear to be less significant than the provision of sensitive care to the baby's individual needs with consistency and continuity. The mother must also communicate to the infant a deep sense that there is a meaning in what they are doing. Two steps are apparently necessary for the infant to derive trust from his early experiences: (1) At first, mother must be consistently available to bring comfort, and (2) later, the infant must be satisfied that he can quickly meet his needs by grasping and biting. A great achievement during this period is the realization that mother exists and will return even though she may be out of sight at the moment (Erikson, 1968).

We can see how greatly disability in the infant may disrupt this pattern of normal development when we consider the description of neonatal intensive care units provided by Bendell (Chapter 2). In most cases of chronic disability that begin in infancy, maternal–infant separation is an immediate effect, removing the presence of the consistent and loving caregiver (Klaus & Kennell, 1982). Furthermore, the abnormal environment of the intensive care unit seems hardly suited to provide the sameness of experience that Erikson regarded as so vital to the development of basic trust. As Bendell describes in detail, the ill neonate is subjected to an unusual degree of sensory stimulation and frequently experiences unexplained pain that cannot be readily relieved by food or other maternal caretaking measures. Chaotic events are typical in the care of disabled infants and rob parents of the opportunity to provide their baby with the sense that there is a meaning to all experiences.

Indeed, as Erikson recognized, it is the caregivers, particularly the mother, who are responsible for providing the infant with the assurance that there is a purpose to all things (Erikson, 1963). In the unusual circumstances surrounding chronic disability, the caregivers themselves may be thoroughly puzzled concerning the meaning and purpose of the "defective" infant and his treatment (Young, 1974). And in other ways as well, families may be poorly equipped to supply the developmental requirements of their ill infant. In the case of the hospitalized infant who resides for prolonged intervals in intensive care units, parents may be denied access to their baby. Not only does this interfere with the opportunity to supply the continuous and consistent attention to meet their newborn's needs, their own developmental need to nurture may be thwarted. Even when the baby is at home or parents have unlimited access, the parental grief and depression may result in emotional withdrawal that limits the supply of nurturing behaviors (Butani, 1974). As Collins points out in Chapter 3, more specific disabilities may have specific effects on caregiving. The example is given of the infant whose cleft palate precludes the possibility of ease of feeding (see Chapter 3).

There is some evidence to indicate that those parents who have skillfully traversed developmental stages and are well-adjusted may more readily manage the tragedy of a disabled infant (Butani, 1974; Goldberg, 1977). On the other hand, parents whose development has been incomplete may have additional difficulties. For example, there appears to be a potential for the crisis of a disabled infant to draw the parents closer to one another (Irvin, Kennell, & Klaus, 1982) so that they might support each other. In those couples, however, who have not completed the phase of young adulthood that is concerned with intimacy, the thrust back to intense intimacy might conceivably delay the development of nurturing needs and the expansion of interests and emotional investments that would include the infant under ordinary circumstances. Similarly, when parents are very young, it is possible that true intimacy may not have been fully established, so that the parent is isolated and unable to draw support from a spouse. Undoubtedly, these considerations may have important implications for optimal interventions with troubled parents of ill children. In Chapter 3, Collins has offered treatment recommendations to ease family members through the difficult times of adjusting to disability in an infant.

Early Childhood

Childhood is a period of rapid change in development and abilities. All developmental theorists propose several substages of this period in order to best describe the age and reduce the complexity. Erikson considered three major stages of childhood: (1) early childhood, extending from infancy (about one year) to about three years; (2) childhood, from three years until school age, and (3) the school-age or latency child, who is between six years old and puberty (Erikson, 1963).

Early childhood for the normal child is the period of the toddler, whose task it is, both literally and figuratively, to "stand on one's own feet." It is a time for the infant to begin exercising a choice and making appropriate demands. By active testing, the child begins to learn how to balance the conflict between the desire to hold on and the desire to let go. During this period, that conflict may be clearly seen in efforts to learn bowel control. The child who is provided reassurance and encouragement at the same time he is given firm control against his potential destructiveness may arrive at the succeeding stages with the capacity for self-expression, cooperation, and self-control. On the other hand, the child whose freedom is suppressed or who is left feeling powerless and exposed may also have limited capacity for self-expression and become simply willful. Autonomy, in such a case, is replaced by shame and doubt, so that the individual's activities may be dictated more by constraint than by choice (Erikson, 1968).

With these demands of early childhood in mind, it is easy to predict some of the difficulties that disability may present to the toddler. The child with an orthopedic handicap may be unable to actively explore the world, but the child who is too weak from illness may be similarly inhibited. Many chronic conditions may impose limits as to the choices and activities open to the child. This, combined with the constant presence of adults exerting what must appear to be arbitrary control, leaves the child vulnerable to self-doubt and may provoke the child to willful behavior.

In addition to the physical limitations imposed on the child by his condition and the further limits imposed by treatment, parents and siblings may react to the disabled child in abnormal ways (Moos & Tsu, 1977). In some cases, the child might find his activities restricted as overly protective family members attempt to shield him from further pain or illness. At the same time, aggressive and inappropriate behaviors may be condoned on the premise that such behaviors are understandable, or simply because the parents' sympathy blocks their ability to responsibly control behavior (see Whitt, Chapter 4). Further, when one considers the number of times disabled children must endure the ignominy of being checked over by health professionals who confirm repeatedly that they are defective, it seems a very real possibility that the children will be vulnerable to feelings of shame and doubt.

In Chapter 4, Whitt points to the necessity of recognizing these pitfalls to the rigorous rehabilitation of the disabled child and suggests ways in which some of these effects might be minimized. In Chapter 5, Drotar, Crawford, and Bush suggest that the first consideration in avoiding these pitfalls is to secure the involvement of all concerned family members.

As is true of parents of disabled infants, parents with disabled children may react to the threat produced by the crisis of their child's illness by a retreat to a former, more comfortable stage of their own development (see Chapter 5). For example, the dependency associated with infancy may be triggered by the realistic need of the parents to call on their own families for financial and emotional support, or simply the need to rely on the skill of health care professionals.

It is possible for parents of the disabled child not only to be blocked from bestowing their nurturance on the ill child but to be unable to satisfactorily meet the needs of other children because of the emotional and physical demands of the ill child.

Moreover, even when parents have the emotional energy and opportunity to care for their disabled child, the child's limited capacity and the parents' confusion over what the child may safely do prevent some of the interactions that would foster the important achievements of early childhood. For example, the parent of the cerebral palsied child who has not mastered sufficient muscular control to walk, control his bowels or feed himself independently has difficulty providing the child with opportunities to master exploration and self-control (Mattson, 1972). Even parents of a diabetic child may limit their child's activities in the fear that the child will come to harm from overexertion. The situation is complicated further when a child acquires a disability such as blindness that forces parents to resume caretaking activities of an earlier stage, but has capacities in other spheres that would provide for exploration and expression if allowed the opportunity. Such uneven capabilities are initially a greater challenge, as parents often find it most natural to behave as if the child were consistently dependent once more.

Siblings also face challenges in dealing with a disabled brother or sister. Depending upon the age of the sibling, his cognitive capacities may limit his ability to understand the situation and, ultimately, cope with the changes. The sibling may be deprived of an environment suited to his own development, if attention centers around the disabled child. Moreover, if the sibling is old enough, the anger which may be experienced toward an ill sibling can result in guilt feelings.

Childhood

The preschool period for the normal child, according to Erikson, is a period of "undertaking, planning and attacking" (1968). By the time the healthy child reaches age three, he is typically walking and running without effort. His motor activity has normally developed to the point that his active manipulation of the environment has greater likelihood of success. Because the child now has the cognitive capacity to plan, he also possesses the ability to "go too far" with his plans and experience guilt over imagined outcomes. As a result of the experiences of the preschool period, it is desirable that the child conclude the stage with a moral sense that provides an awareness of limitations and restrictions. At the same time, basic skills necessary to establish goals and have realistic dreams for the future are acquired here. Furthermore, it is during this period of a child's life that sex roles are learned and identification with the same-sex parent is achieved. A child successfully mastering the childhood period may be expected to have direction and purpose (Erikson, 1963, 1968).

In order for the experiences of the child to be positive, parents must again achieve a balance, this time between encouragement of initiative and consistent transmission of a sense of right and wrong. Erikson suggests that consistency is particularly important for the preschool child to avoid the feeling that power is arbitrary. In addition, the cognitive abilities of the child now allow him to distinguish between "what the parents do" and "what they say." It becomes more crucial that parents model the ethics that they attempt to instill in their offspring. Ordinarily, childhood is a time of companionship with the same-sex parent. Through the resulting positive identification with a parent, the child develops his own sense of self-worth (Erikson, 1963).

But for the child with a disability superimposed on the other tasks of this stage, the situation may be very different. Many disabilities will impose direct limits on "undertaking, planning and attacking." Even when physical capacity to run and play is present, prohibitions against natural childhood activities may be imposed, either by the treatment regimen or out of parents' anxieties of possible harm (Tisza, 1962). Prohibitions in these instances may indeed be perceived as arbitrary demonstrations of power. Moreover, as Whitt describes in Chapter 4, the illness may be seen as punishment of actual or imagined misdeeds by the preschool child.

On the other hand, efforts at discipline by sympathetic parents may be curtailed, so that normal limits are not learned. Significant, too, in the child's development is the possibility of almost exclusive care being assumed by the mother. The disabled boy, if he is hospitalized for long periods of time, may have little opportunity to build a close relationship with his father. Although the disabled girl may have more physical contact with her mother, real companionship is difficult to achieve in a sterile hospital environment. In both cases, children may encounter difficulty in establishing their gender identification.

For parents, too, the onset of their preschool child's disability interrupts the evolving relationship they have with him. Not only may contact be restricted by hospitalization, parents may feel that much of their responsibility for parenting has been usurped by the various professionals attending the child's care. In the interest of sparing their own emotional resources, some parents surrender all of their parenting responsibilities to health care staff (Spinetta, 1978). On the other hand, a parent may become overprotective with a child who has suddenly become more physically dependent. This denies the child the increased responsibilities of childhood. Often, overprotectiveness and permissiveness occur because parents no longer have clear expectations for a preschooler with greatly reduced capacities. The families of chronically ill preschoolers face complex challenges when they attempt to facilitate as nearly normal an existence for their child as can be arranged. Facilitation of the child's developing initiative must be accomplished along with provision of physical care. Finally, throughout the process of accommodation to their child's altered needs, parents must cope with their own needs in the face of the crisis.

The School-age Child

School age begins at the time a child enters school and extends until the beginning of puberty. It is a period that is crucial for the development of industry and productivity. Erikson maintained that a sense of inferiority could be expected to evolve in children who fail to master this stage of development (1963). While the preschool child attains his goals through plans and attack, the school-age child begins to learn that he can gain approval for producing things. In this stage, children become aware of their skills and work toward refining them. Simultaneously, they develop the capacity for sustained effort that results in work completion. The capacity to experience pleasure in work completion becomes essential to the individual when he is challenged to become a provider. Self-image during school age is a function of the degree of skill the child perceives himself to possess. For the first time in his life, the opinion of peers takes on greater significance than the opinion of family in making a self-appraisal. Failure of the child to master the demands of this period results in a lack of confidence. If the child makes an unfavorable comparison between his abilities and those of his peers, poor self-esteem develops. Dissatisfaction with his skills discourages the school-age child and causes him to shift back into the family interactions where skills seem less important. Since the child's perception of his abilities as adequate is of paramount importance for optimum development, the capacity of teachers and parents to recognize what the child can do and to offer encouragement for special efforts is vital. A further contribution to development demanded by parents of school-age children is "letting go" comfortably. Since the child in his school years needs to become more autonomous and move into relationships with teachers and peers, those same parents from whom so much nurturance was recently required must now surrender some of their involvement with their child. Parents and teachers cannot, however, provide all the necessary environmental conditions for the school-age child. He or she must experience the interactions with peers and find acceptance among them in order to establish a sense of adequacy and competence. Only with a firm self-acceptance can a child develop the sense of industry (Erikson, 1968).

The onset of disability may erect several obstacles to the adequate mastery of the demands of this stage. One of the first obstacles can be the loss of a valued skill. If the "tools" by which these skills are managed sustain damage through illness or injury, that skill is disrupted. For example, if the successful schoolyard athlete becomes paralyzed or weakened, he loses the skill that may have gained him peer acceptance. If the best reader in the class becomes blind, she will have to cede that status while she "starts over" in Braille. Even children whose illnesses do not directly impair their skills suffer setbacks relative to their peers, and they may feel discouraged at the chore of catching up after prolonged absences (Spinetta & Deasy, 1980).

In addition, social interactions with peers may be curtailed as a result of a disability or because peers fail to accept a child who is "damaged" and, therefore, different than they. Also, the danger of drawing back into the family is great for a disabled schoolchild (see Chapter 4). The very real requirements for care may increase the amount of time the child spends with his family, but the comfort of an accepting family can be seductive for the child who is less certain of peer acceptance. It may become increasingly inviting to stay at home with family members and avoid the competition of peer interactions. Whatever the causes of a disabled child's isolation from peers, the failure to establish a place for himself among peers creates a potential for reduced self-confidence.

Moreover, the risk of pulling the disabled child back into the family is also the greatest new challenge confronting the family of the school-age child. Concern for the child's well-being can easily supplant the willingness to surrender the youngster to his peers and to encourage productivity. Sympathetic parents find it extremely difficult to allow their chronically ill child to experience failures; but in the absence of failures, a child is unable to correctly evaluate his potential. All the challenges faced by younger children must be met by families of the school-age child, but the parents of a seven-year-old epileptic boy must learn to submit their youngster to the mercy of his peers and to demand maximum productivity.

Adolescence

The major tasks of adolescence, if mastered, enable the individual to develop occupational goals with the skills that were discovered and developed earlier. The individual must emerge from adolescence with a sense of who he is and what he believes. In addition, it is during adolescence that a clear sexual identity is established. The desired achievement of adolescence is the development of a distinct identity that will provide the individual with the capacity for devotion and fidelity.

To meet this goal, a child must be given the freedom by his parents to replace the morality developed in childhood with adult ethics that reflect his own identity. The development of identity requires an opportunity for self-expression. The drive of most adolescents for self-expression is sufficiently strong that they will resist with all their might if anyone attempts to thwart them. Erikson (1963) feels that the demands of adolescence are so intense that complete attention to their fulfillment is necessary. That is, it is particularly important that the challenges of earlier stages be sufficiently met to allow the adolescent to put them aside.

Just as the adolescent needs some freedom from parental prohibitions, he needs to feel a part of a group of peers on whom he can project his developing identity and see it reflected. Similarly, adolescents require the opportunity to fall in love so that they may see their egos reflected and clarified and test their capacity for a lasting relationship (Erikson, 1968).

Clearly, any disability that undermines the achievements of earlier stages disturbs the moratorium on those tasks that are so important to the adolescent. The adolescent who develops cancer may have to reexamine issues of basic trust, be uncertain of peer acceptance and need to revise appraisal of skills (Moore, Holton, & Marten, 1960). The incapacitation by an illness such as cancer may bind the adolescent more closely to family members and delay his opportunity to develop independent ethics. Self-expression, so precious to the adolescent, is difficult to achieve when parents have the major responsibility for basic needs, when weakness and pain restrict activities, and when the individual is uncertain of skills and abilities. Peer group membership may also be disrupted by physical and emotional changes in the individual or by the treatment program. Moreover, changes in physical appearance, such as loss of hair and weight loss, may so change the adolescent's body image that romantic relationships are not developed during adolescence. In Chapter 6, Blumberg, Lewis, & Susman, using adolescent cancer patients as examples, propose an effective treatment model to minimize these obstacles to normal development.

Families of disabled adolescents also face all of the pain and all of the pitfalls that confront any parent with a disabled child. It may be particularly difficult, however, for the parent of a severely disabled adolescent to supply the requisite physical care and, simultaneously, devise an emancipating environment that permits the youth to express himself, establish rewarding peer interactions, and develop independent values and ethics (Kellerman & Katz, 1977).

Young Adulthood

In young adults, the skills mastered throughout childhood and adolescence must be integrated into a commitment to vocational goals and an intimate relationship. Erikson has characterized the mastery of young adulthood in the following way:

> The utopia [of this period] should include: (1) mutuality of orgasm (2) with a loved partner (3) of the opposite sex (4) with whom one is able and willing to share mutual trust and (5) with whom one is able and willing to regulate the cycles of (a) work, (b) procreation and (c) recreation (6) so as to secure to the offspring, too, all the stages of a satisfactory relationship [Erikson, 1963, p. 266].

Attainment of this utopian state requires the strength to maintain a commitment when sacrifices and compromises are demanded. The individual who has not derived from previous stages adequate measures of trust, autonomy, initiative, industry, and identity may be reluctant or unable to make a genuinely intimate commitment out of fear of personal loss subtracted from a fragile ego (Erikson, 1963).

It is redundant, perhaps, but important to remember that membership in young adulthood is not entirely dependent upon chronologic age. The disabled individual has, by the age of young adulthood, had several chances to fail in the demands of earlier stages; therefore, careful assessment of psychological maturity is necessary before the assumption of young adulthood may be made. In addition, in the period immediately following the onset of disability, the individual may have returned to former stages in order to allow himself the opportunity to slowly and safely adjust to his situation.

Moreover, a return to former developmental stages may be precipitated by the need to accommodate to actual changes induced by disability. For example, a young man's previously formed identity may be subjected to major alteration (1) if his former capacity for self-expression is blocked, (2) if he has had to revise his appraisal of his abilities, (3) if his sexual identity has been modified, or (4) if his sense of autonomy has been undermined. Indeed, the onset of disability may lead the individual to challenge the assumptions of trust that were established in infancy. A review of Erikson's summary of successful passage reveals the many roadblocks that may result from disability.

A disability that interferes with sexual function clearly limits the opportunity for orgasm. Disfiguring disabilities may inhibit a young woman in her search for a loved partner, just as limited mobility may block her access to eligible young men. Young adults who have recently acquired a disability often have difficulty trusting in the affection of an able-bodied suitor (Hahn, 1981). Furthermore, for the individual who is handicapped, work (even in the home) may be limited, procreation impossible, and recreational activities markedly restricted (Roessler, Cook, & Lillard, 1977). The possibility of providing an environment suitable to the rearing of children may be difficult for a newly injured young adult to imagine. The potential for isolation is great unless active intervention on the part of family members, friends, and health care personnel is undertaken. Glueckauf and Quittner have provided useful advice in Chapter 8 for facilitating support systems in interventions with disabled adults.

The first difficulty faced by family members of young adults is often that of defining the family. As Ireys and Burr point out in Chapter 9, most young adults have left their family of origin (the family of their parents and siblings) but have not yet established a family of commitment (usually a spouse and any children they may have). For young men and women who become disabled before they have established a meaningful relationship there may be no option but to return to the family of origin. The crisis produced by grief over the injury or illness may be compounded by the adjustments necessary to readmit an independent offspring to the nest. For those parents who have arrived at the end of their childrearing phase and begun the adaptation to new roles, the thrust backward into earlier roles as nurturers and caretakers may disrupt their own development.

On the other hand, where the adjustment to the "flown nest" is less complete, the parents of severely physically dependent young adults may lapse enthusiastically into earlier patterns of interaction, providing not only for physical needs, but attempting to supply all of the emotional needs as well. The phrase "You can't go home again" may develop particularly poignant significance for disabled young adults. Misguided but well-intentioned concern and sympathy may result in overprotectiveness that shields the disabled adult from experiences appropriate to his or her age. The return of a son or daughter to a physically dependent state can allow parents to overlook the adult needs of their offspring for sexual expression. Significant effort is sometimes required to move a disabled adult out of the house and into social activities that compel them to confront stage-appropriate challenges.

Somewhat different challenges confront the families of commitment of young adults. In the case of young adults, it is most likely that the new family will represent a recent relationship with levels of commitment and preparation for sacrifice that are variable. A young spouse faced with a disabled partner may lack the developmental capacity to accept additional responsibilities while his capacity for intimacy is still developing. The task of integrating two lives may be interrupted and replaced with the task of accepting a substantially less balanced relationship. Because of the limitations imposed on the disabled partner, the opportunity for sharing experiences may be significantly affected (see Chapter 9).

Even when the young spouse finds sufficient commitment to sustain the relationship, several adjustments remain to be made. Physical limitations that constrain sexual activity affect both partners—not just the disabled individual. The concern over loss of one expression of intimacy and the inability to bear children must be faced by the able-bodied spouse as well. Moreover, most chronic illnesses and disabilities create the necessity for role changes and a renegotiation of the marriage contract to provide satisfaction for both partners. Ireys and Burr (Chapter 9) recommend that community and social resources be considered when there is danger that the disabled spouse may become more of a child than a partner to the able-bodied spouse. For example, when infantilizing services such as bowel and bladder care may be attended to by others, a wife may more easily perceive her husband as a sexual partner. In order to see a disabled spouse as any kind of partner, it is important to reestablish a climate that is accepting of disagreements. Only when the able-bodied spouse discovers that it is the body only that is fragile can balance in the relationship be restored and adult roles maintained. It is all too easy for the individual's problems rather than the individual to become the focus of the most intense emotions in the relationship.

Middle Years

Managing the accomplishments of the middle years, in Erikson's view, requires the achievement of a committed relationship in the previous stage that has provided the individual with enough confidence and free energy to be interested in the next generation. The goal of this period is termed *generativity* and refers to the capacity and willingness to create and guide a new generation, supplying them with all their developmental needs. This period involves an expansion of the interests and pursuits of the preceding stages. While the provision of nurturance and guidance to offspring is the personal focus of the middle years, the middle-aged adult is also expected to make a contribution to the development of the communities' new generation through civic activities and public concern. Mastery of this stage requires faith in oneself and the human race and cannot be accomplished merely by giving birth to offspring. Failure to expand one's interests and master the middle years leaves the individual with a state of personal impoverishment that Erikson describes as stagnation. Pseudo-intimacy and self-indulgence may be benchmarks of failure (Erikson, 1963).

When disability strikes the adult in middle years, several disruptions of normal development may occur. Among the first costs to be counted, particularly for the disabled man, is the loss or reduction of the capacity to develop vocationally. When disability requires retirement, the individual must surrender his economic role in the family and, often, a significant dimension of his self-esteem. Block, Boyer, and Imes suggest in Chapter 10 that even minimal physical disability in a chronically ill individual may lead to a perception that career advancement is no longer possible. Once a disabled adult returns home, further limitations in ability may begin to emerge. Disability often demands that the adult switch roles abruptly from the nurturer to the nurtured. Childrearing chores may be difficult or impossible. Even serving as a role-model for one's own children may seem an overwhelming responsibility for the disabled adult whose own identity has just been shattered. Alterations in sexual functioning may interrupt plans to create a new generation, as well as affect the role of the individual in relation to the spouse. The image of a frightened, insecure, self-absorbed adult with a newly acquired disability stands in sharp contrast to the ideal product of normal development. The free energy that is described as necessary to the generative adult simply cannot be expected to exist in the adult who is in the process of adjusting to chronic disability, and the absence of that energy can result in self-indulgence and temporary stagnation.

Spouses, too, must make significant adjustments in role and life-style when a partner becomes disabled. Rustad (Chapter 11) points out that the changes demanded by disability are sometimes so great as to be seen as a violation of an implied marital contract. Wives may have to assume greater responsibility for breadwinning at the same time that they may also be forced to accept total responsibility for childrearing. Wives may also feel that they have acquired an additional child for whom they must care, just as they experience the loss of a help-mate. Furthermore, changes in the disabled spouses' sexual functioning require adaptations on the part of his wife in order to reestablish her own sexual expression. In addition, the end of childbearing possibilities may represent a major loss for her. Although existing literature provides less information regarding the plight of husbands who must cope with disabled wives, Rustad speculates that husbands are faced with additional responsibilities at home. Frequently, the wife's disability may greatly increase her husband's responsibility for the emotional and physical well-being of their children. As a result of these increased demands, an able-bodied husband may suffer impediments to his own career development. Although fewer disabilities disrupt women's capacity to serve as sexual partners, a lack of responsiveness or significant disfigurement undoubtedly have an effect on their husbands' sexual expression.

Spouses with disabled partners may not only feel that they have acquired an additional child, they may also begin treating their husband or wife as they might another child. The confusing experience of caring for a physically helpless adult may be resolved by evoking the entire pattern of behaviors that are familiar in caring for a helpless child. Often, overprotectiveness is a part of this pattern and is felt in the avoidance of any expression of angry or helpless feelings by the able-bodied spouse. The result is emotional isolation from formerly intimate partners.

The children of disabled middle-aged adults also face shifts in roles and potential disruption of their own developmental stages. The child who is accustomed to being cared for is likely to experience difficulty in adjusting to the demand of giving care to a helpless adult. Younger children may lack the capacity to understand why their mothers are unable to respond to their needs. It may be difficult, too, for children to adjust to a disfigured or physically incapacitated role-model. Older children may understand the illness, but feel anxiety regarding their vulnerability. Older children are sometimes detained in the home to care for a disabled parent at precisely the time when they should be responding to their own need to separate and develop their independent identities. For these reasons, Rustad recommends (Chapter 11) that families be included in therapy with the disabled middle-aged adult in order to facilitate each family member's adjustment to the disability.

Old Age

The final period of life is least clearly delineated by Erikson, perhaps because he believed relatively few individuals achieved mastery of this stage of development. Nonetheless, several important achievements are ascribed to old age. The successful outcome of the period is thought to be *ego integrity*, which is defined as an adaptation to the triumphs and disappointments of life (Erikson, 1963). Failure to master this stage results in a sense of despair. The elements that are considered important in contributing to ego identity include (1) assurance of meaning and a belief in a natural order to life, (2) respect for the human ego, (3) faith in one's own life-style, and (4) an acceptance of the life cycle, including one's own imminent death. Fear of death and despair over one's life may be avoided by mastery of this and previous stages of development (Erikson, 1963).

In Chapter 12, Schienle and Eiler offer statistical evidence of the prevalence of disability in the elderly population. Paradoxically, relatively sparse literature expressly addresses the issues of rehabilitation in old age. Examination of the tasks of old age, however, suggests that the issues differ dramatically from those of earlier periods of development. Vocational concerns are generally not relevant, and offspring no longer require care. The majority of elderly adults, however, are still living with spouses with whom they share their lives. The occurrence of disability has the potential of disrupting that shared life, since the able-bodied spouse may be unable to meet the increased demands occasioned by the disability. It is often the onset of a physical disability or cognitive impairment that forces elderly adults to place their spouse outside the home. Those elderly adults who are living alone must also face the likelihood of being uprooted when they become disabled. Placement is usually to an adult child's home or to a nursing home. In either case, the assurance of meaning that has been established may be disturbed by the change in their life. The accommodation to other adults may necessitate the surrender of the elderly adult's life-style and force him or her to yield defense of his or her existence. When cognitive impairment is involved in the disability, the wisdom that might be expected at the end of a well-lived life may be rendered unavailable to progeny. Even when that wisdom is present, the realities of the convalescent setting may preclude the opportunity to share with a willing audience. Dependency for physical care may disturb integrity and produce despair.

Despair may also be the consequence of disability for the able-bodied spouse. The husband of an elderly woman with Altzheimer's disease will almost certainly have his living patterns disturbed. If he is unable to care for his wife, he must face the separation of his life's companion. If he is unable to provide for his own care in his wife's absence, he must also adjust to new living arrangements, but usually in a location different from hers. Even if he is able to provide for the care of his wife and maintain his home, he must accept the changes in roles, as he assumes more of his wife's responsibilities and gives up the hope of sharing his thoughts and memories with her.

Often, adult children and grandchildren are affected by the onset of disability in elderly parents. When the parent is no longer independent, the offspring may be compelled to adjust his or her life-style to accommodate one or both parents. The consumption of time and energy involved in their care may deprive other family members and lead to family conflicts. Often, the increased demands on the caretakers diminish the opportunity for social activities that might offer emotional support.

A more complex and less tangible problem confronting adult children of the disabled elderly is that of accepting changes, particularly cognitive impairment, in their parents. Even adult children experience a need for continuity and constancy in their parents, possibly explaining the greater subjective burden reported by caretakers whose parents have undergone significant personality changes. (Hendricks & Hendricks, 1977). Zarit and Zarit describe in Chapter 13 a number of family interventions that have been found effective in reducing the crises that accompany the onset of disability in old age.

Summary

The chapters that follow address the issues of disability as they uniquely affect individuals in each life stage. In addition, separate attention is given to the problems which must be solved by involved family members at each period of life. Each chapter provides a review of available research and illuminating literature applicable to that section. The authors have illustrated their discussions with examples from their clinical experiences, and each chapter contains recommendations for treatment that might serve to prevent avoidable disruptions in development and facilitate optimal adjustment for the disabled victims and their families. It is encouraging to note that so many disabled individuals have avoided the pitfalls presented by disability and continue to live useful lives. An effort has been made to examine those successfully rehabilitated individuals and discover what factors contributed to their triumph over chronic illness and disability.

References

Butani, P. Reactions of mothers to the birth of an anomalous infant: A review of the literature. *Maternal–Child Nursing Journal*, 1974, *3*(1), 59–76.

Erikson, E. H. *Childhood and society*. New York: Norton, 1963.

Erikson, E. H. *Identity and crisis*. New York: Norton, 1968.

Goldberg, H. K. Social competence in infancy: A model of parent–infant interaction. *Merrill–Palmer Quarterly*, 1977, *23*(3), 163–178.

Hahn, H. The social component of sexuality and disability: Some problems and proposals. *Sexuality and Disability*, 1981, *14*, 220–233.

Havinghurst, R. *Developmental tasks and education* (3rd ed.). New York: David McKay, 1948.

Hendricks, J., & Hendricks, C. D. Family life and living arrangements. In *Aging in mass society*. Cambridge, Mass.: Winthrop, 1977.

Irvin, N. A., Kennell, J. H., & Klaus, M. H. Caring for parents with a congenital malformation. In M. H. Klaus & J. H. Kennell (Eds.), *Maternal–infant bonding*. St. Louis: Mosby, 1982.

Jung, C. G. *Modern man in search of a soul*. New York: Harcourt, Brace & World, 1933.

Kellerman, J. & Katz, E. The adolescent with cancer: Theoretical clinical and research issues. *Journal of Pediatric Psychology*, 1977, *2* (3), 127–131.

Kennell, J. H., & Klaus, M. H. Caring for the parents of premature or sick infants. In M. H. Klaus & J. H. Kennell (Eds.), Parent-infant bonding. St. Louis: Mosby, 1982.

Mattsson, A., & Agle, D. P. Group therapy with parents of hemophiliacs: Therapeutic process and observations of parental adaptations to chronic illness in children. *Journal of the American Academy of Child Psychiatry*, 1972, *11*, 558–571.

Moore, D., Holton, C., & Marten, G. Psychological problems in the management of adolescents with malignancy. *Clinical Pediatrics*, 1960, *8*, 464–473.

Moos, R. H., & Tsu, V. D. The crisis of physical illness: An overview. In R. H. Moos (Ed.), *Coping with physical illness*. New York: Plenum Publishing Company, 1977.

Roessler, R., Cook, D., & Lillard, D. Effects of systematic counseling on work adjustment clients. *Journal of Counseling Psychology*, 1977, *24*, 313, 317.

Spinetta, J. J. Communication patterns in families dealing with life-threatening illness. In O. J. Z. Sahler (Ed.), *The child and death*. St. Louis: C. V. Mosby, 1978.

Spinetta, J. J. & Deasy, P. M. Coping with childhood cancer: Professional and family communication patterns. In M. G. Eisenberg, J. Falconer, and L. Sutkin (Eds.), *Communications in a health care setting*, Springfield, Ill.: Charles C. Thomas, 1980.

Tisza, V. B. Management of the parents of the chronically ill child. *Journal of Orthopsychiatry*, 1962, *32*, 53.

Wright, B. Person and situation: Adjusting the rehabilitation focus. *Archives of Physical Medicine and Rehabilitation*, 1980, *61*, 59–63.

Young, R. K. Chronic sorrow: Parents' response to the birth of a child with a defect. *The American Journal of Maternal–Child Nursing*, 1974, 3(1), 59–76.

I

Infancy

2 Psychological Problems of Infancy

R. Debra Bendell

Introduction

The birth of a medically at-risk infant who is ill instead of a healthy, normal newborn is demanding and traumatic for the new parents. Expectations of normality are reinforced by the communication media and advertisements. Prepared childbirth classes do not emphasize the possibilities of less than optimum outcomes of pregnancy nor the reality of neonatal intensive care units.

Prenatal attachment begins long before the onset of labor and delivery. Many women develop affectionate feelings toward their unborn infant prior to or following the onset of fetal movement. This fetal embodiment engenders fantasies regarding the infant, and names are often chosen. The family begins to reorganize and prepare for the arrival of the new member. The first year of life, however, remains an age where the risk of mortality and morbidity is high (National Center for Health Statistics, 1978; Shapiro, McCormick, & Starfield, 1980.)

In the early 1960s scientific advancements and technologic innovations were first widely applied to the management of medically high-risk infants through a system of regionalized neonatal intensive care units (NICUs.) These units are organized as tertiary care facilities and are located primarily in teaching/research hospitals in urban areas. The establishment of regionalized care has effected better survival rates, but it has also resulted in a multiplicity of iatrogenic complications. An abnormal postnatal environment, ususual sensory stimulation, maternal/infant separation, and interrupted family integration are but a few such complications. These factors, often occurring in combination, result in the premature and low-birth-weight infant being labeled high-risk.

The intrauterine period might correctly be considered the most significant months of life. At no other life stage can the normal progression

Special thanks to Camille Landry-Gaters, research assistant.

of growth and development be so drastically disrupted and the eventual capabilities of the human be so easily impaired. The well-being of the fetus is dependent on the degree to which the maternal host deprives, protects, or nurtures it. Infectious, chemical, radiological, immunological, and psychological forces all dramatically influence the well-being and growth of the infant. This chapter will examine prenatal, perinatal, and neonatal variables which have impact upon the mental and physical well-being of an infant and cause illness.

Premature Labor

A variable of great import relates to the length of gestation. Premature labor occurs when frequent uterine contractions result in progressive cervical dilation and/or effacement prior to the completion of the thirty-seventh week of gestation. Normal gestation lasts from 38 to 42 weeks. Premature labor may be the result of maternal, placental, or fetal disorders. Whatever the cause, and the etiology is often unknown or obscure, the delivery of an immature neonate is a medical and psychological crisis for the newborn as well as for the family.

The increasing intact survival of small preterm infants poses a dilemma. When should labor be halted and when should it be allowed to progress? There is no optimal strategy for management. Risks of acute fetal distress, sepsis, and respiratory distress syndrome are major areas of concern.

Small for Gestational Age

Fetal undergrowth or intrauterine growth retardation, often called dysmaturity, is another high-risk category of infant. Optimal weight for the lowest perinatal mortality is 3,500 to 4,000 grams (Korones, 1976.) Weights below the tenth percentile curve are considered small for gestational age (SGA.) At first glance these infants appear prematurely born; however, clinical estimation of gestational age is based on a systematic evaluation of neuromuscular and physical maturity. Assessment of posture and reflexes, appearance of skin, genitalia, length, weight, ear formation, and head circumference are completed shortly after birth and scored on a standardized instrument (Dubowitz, Dubowitz, & Goldberg, 1963).

SGA babies are frequently found to have developmental delays and deficits and continual growth retardation, although they may rank above the tenth percentile for growth and may, therefore, not be "retarded" or "damaged" (Fitzhardinge & Murkestad, 1981). Such problems may manifest later in life as learning disabilities or behavioral disorders.

Large for Gestational Age

Birth weight above 4,000 grams is another high-risk factor. Its most frequent cause is maternal diabetes. The hormonal and chemical imbalance of diabetes mellitus crosses the placenta, placing an additional burden on fetal homeostatic mechanisms. Diabetic pregnancies may be marked by secondary complications of infection, diabetic ketoacidosis, or hypoglycemic shock. Meticulous and continuous medical attention is necessary for the fetus to survive. Infants of diabetic mothers are subject to hypocalcemia, hypoglycemia, hyperbilirubinemia, and other metabolic disorders. There is also an enhanced susceptibility to respiratory distress syndrome and thrombosis of vessels. The perinatal mortality of the large-for-gestational-age infant has been reduced due to better metabolic control, utilizing insulin to maintain plasma glucose levels as close to normal as possible. Both biochemical and biophysical monitoring are used to ascertain fetal well-being (Coustan, 1980).

Infection

More than 14 percent of all pregnancies are complicated by a maternal infection (Alford & Pass, 1981). These infections can result in insidious disease which may not be manifest for many years after delivery or may result in acute disease in the neonatal period. By far the most common infection of pregnancy is cytomegalovirus (CMV). Ocular abnormalities (Frenkel, Keys, & Hefferen, 1980), neurological abnormalities, including sensorineural hearing loss (Kairam & DeVivo, 1981), and hepatic inflammation and injury (Hanshaw & Dudgeon, 1978) are sequellae of CMV. Other infections affecting newborns include rubella, toxoplasmosis, herpes simplex, hepatitis, congenital syphilis, and gonorrhea.

Respiratory Disorders

The most significant respiratory disorders affecting premature infants are hyaline membrane disease and the respiratory distress syndrome of the newborn (Fawcett & Gluck, 1977). Treatment of these disorders requires that the infant be mechanically assisted to ventilate properly to prevent hypoxia and acidosis. The alveoli can usually be held open by continuous positive transpulmonary pressure (CPAP); however, the most seriously affected infants need mechanical ventilation. Overall survival rates are better than 85 percent (Whung, Stark, & Hegyi, 1976). An infant who fights against the ventilator efforts of the respirator can develop a pneumothorax. In such cases, curare or its equivalent must be used to paralyze the infant (Brady & Gregory, 1979). Several complications are possible, including cerebral hemorrhage (Pope, Armstrong, & Fitzhardinge, 1976). Although mortality is an occasional complication, most cases can be resolved with varying degrees of risk and morbidity to the pulmonary and cerebral function of the infant.

Asphyxia

The major causes of serious hypoxemia in the perinatal period are: (1) disturbance of gas exchange across the placenta with respiratory failure at the time of birth; (2) postnatal respiratory insufficiency, secondary to respiratory distress syndrome or recurrent apneic spells; and (3) cardiovascular diseases. The most prevalent form of hypoxemia constitutes an interruption of the maternal or fetal circulation to the placenta with an arrest of respiratory gas exchange (Sheldon, 1977).

An indicator of the amount of trauma the infant has suffered is the time it takes regular breathing to return during the resuscitative process. In most cases, eight minutes is the upper limit of anoxia tolerated (Adamson, Mueller-Heubach, & Meyers, 1964; James & Lanman 1976).

Another indicator of a precipitous or prolonged labor with a difficult extraction is reflected in Apgar scores (Apgar, Holoday, James, Weisbrot, & Berrien, 1958). The Apgar score is the most universal criterion for assessment in the first five minutes of life for the neonate. It measures at one and five minutes after birth the functions necessary to sustain life in five categories: color, respiratory and cardiac effort, body tone, and responsiveness to aversive stimuli. The score is influenced by perinatal events such as hypoxia, prolonged labor, and drugs or anesthesia given to the mother. As an initial screening level the Apgar scores are invaluable. Drogl, Kennedy, and Berendes (1966) documented a fourfold increase in neurological abnormalities at one year in infants with low Apgar scores (at the five minute evaluation), compared to those with high scores.

Congenital Anomalies

Congenital anomalies can result in a wide range of psychological and developmental difficulties for infants in addition to their medical complications. Conditions may result in massive impairment or life-threatening illness. Infants with these diseases are affected by the hospitalization, medical procedures, separation, and iatrogenic complications that have impact on other high-risk neonates.

Non-life-threatening conditions, such as cleft palate, gastroschisis, and other visible anomalies can also result in adaptational difficulties for infants (Abrahamson & Shandling, 1972). Problems with feeding and elimination, the obvious and visible differences of a child with such syndromes, and the need for medical and surgical intervention may predispose these infants to a maladaptive relationship with their families (Solnit & Stark, 1961).

While the presence of one or more minor defects in an adult may be of no great importance, the presence of two or three seemingly minor anomalies in a neonate justifies a careful diagnostic workup in search of possible significant internal defects. A single major defect (e.g., a missing umbilical artery or clinodactyly) requires careful diagnosis and study for possible systemic involvement (Broman, 1979). Major categories of congenital diseases and anomalies are outlined in Table 2.1

Table 2.1 Chronic Conditions of Childhood Often Associated with Maladaptive Behaviors

Type	*Clinical Disorder*
Developmental	Cerebral palsy, mental retardation, epilepsies, childhood autism, hearing and visual impairment, multiple handicaps
Malformative	Myelomeningocele, hydrocephaly, orthopedic deformations
Myopathies	Muscular dystrophies, central core disorders, myasthenia gravis
Attentional deficit disorders	Minimal brain dysfunction, visual-percerptual-motor dysfunction
Growth	Dwarfism, primary and secondary growth retardation
Musculoskeletal	Scoliosis-lordosis, arthrogryposis multiplex congenita
Respiratory	Cystic fibrosis, BPD, pulmonary hypoplasia
Cardiovascular	Congenital heart disease
Digestive	Chronic hepatitis, peptic ulcer, short gut syndrome
Genitourinary	Chronic renal disease
Hematologic-lymphatic	Sickle cell anemia, hemolytic anemia, thrombocytopenic purpura, leukemia, lymphoma
Endocrine	Hyperthyroidism, hypothyroidism, adrenogenital syndrome, parathyroid disease, diabetes insipidus, gonadal dysgenesis
Multiple	Immune deficiency disorders
Metabolic	"Inborn errors" of metabolism
Cytogenic syndromes	

Adapted from Denhoff, E., & Feldman, S. A. Behavior perspectives in children with chronic disabilities: a pediatric viewpoint. *The Journal of Developmental and Behavioral Pediatrics,* Vol. 2, No. 3, September 1981.

Iatrogenic Factors

Many of the procedures commonly utilized to save the lives of high-risk infants carry with them associated risks of physical and emotional complications. Iatrogenic complications range from infections to hemorrhage to organ damage and may include psychological sequelae due to separation and other factors.

Respirators and oxygen therapy are invasive procedures commonly necessarily used in neonatal medicine. Abnormal pressure upon immature lungs can cause several complications (see above), the most serious of which is a spontaneous pneumothorax, a painful leak of air from the lungs into the thoracic cavity.

All therapies are inherently stressful as a result of mechanical or environmental factors. As in other areas of medicine, however, risks and complications of diagnosis and therapy are inversely related to volume of patient treated; thus, better outcomes occur in large, regionalized centers.

Ethical Issues

Once it is apparent that an infant cannot survive, issues surface regarding the efficacy of painful medical procedures, extensive hospitalizations, and family hardship, and consideration may be given to the refusal of certain types of therapy (Hemphill & Freeman, 1977). Duff and Campbell (1973) have reported that 14 percent of the deaths recorded in the special care nursery of the Yale-New Haven Hospital over an eighteen-month period in the early 1970s were associated with refusal, discontinuation, or withdrawal of treatment. Usually some form of partnership between the medical professional and the family is employed.

In these situations the medical professional presents therapeutic alternatives and makes recommendations to help the family become involved in the decision-making process. With regard to the decisions, several alternatives have been proposed.

McCormick (1977) has suggested broad guidelines based on the quality of the human life to be preserved and feels that one of the vital qualities that must be considered is the capacity or the potential capacity for human relationships. Nonmaleficence, described as the principle "first do no harm," has been espoused by Reich (1978). This principle encompasses a viewpoint of doing nothing directly intended to shorten an infant's life.

A second aspect is that the dying process should not be unnecessarily prolonged when it is unequivocally and irreversibly taking place. Much of the dilemma in these decisions arises from the uncertainty of prognosis in many infants. It is, therefore, reasonable to depend upon judgments of a senior medical officer, the attending neonatologist.

The impact of multiple anomalies, expectations for anomalies incompatible with survival, and severe central nervous system defects are best understood from a perspective of the "right to die" (Duff & Campbell, 1973).

Other aspects of ethics are financial and include moral cost ceilings, measurement of net costs in dollars, and issues of utilization of limited resources. In 1973, NICU hospitalization costs for infants under 1,200 grams at birth averaged $9,586. Yet as a result of high in-hospital mortality, a total of $38,344 in hospital costs was expended per survivor. Thus, costs must be considered cross-sectionally (Kramer, 1976).

To the uninsured couple contemplating the NICU for their infant, their severely abnormal survivor of an NICU may represent a cost picture that includes, in addition to the substantial hospitalization cost and normal expenditures, the cost of custodial care or of forgone earnings if the child is cared for by a parent. In addition, the possibility of special educational needs and extraordinary medical attention must be considered.

The parents of the very ill or very premature baby usually worry more about intellectual functioning ("Will she be slow and/or brain-damaged") than about other issues. This emphasis frequently leads to unresolved anxiety, as the extent and nature of impairment are usually impossible to predict with accuracy in the immediate neonatal period. Development has to be assessed after recovery from illness and with the passage of time.

Numerous factors may contribute to the development of brain damage in the high-risk infant. Neurologic defects seem to be largely secondary to ischemia or hemorrhage in the periventricular area. Infants born prior to 32 weeks are at highest risk, especially if they are subject to asphyxia, RDS, or decrease in cerebral blood flow.

The etiology of other intellectual deficits is less clear-cut. Hypoxic-ischemic injury obviously plays a major role, as do inadequate intrauterine and postnatal nutrition. We still do not know the long-term effects associated with the abnormal environmental conditions imposed upon the high-risk infant during a long-term stay in an NICU. Several researchers have demonstrated a strong association between child intelligence and social factors, as measured by mother's education. When considering whether to institute or continue *extraordinary* treatment measures, however, major consideration must be given to the likelihood of normal human activities and relationships.

Postnatal Factors

Treatment issues must include a contrast between the healthy and the ill neonate (see Table 2.2).

Competencies of the Healthy Neonate

The healthy newborn infant has the capabilities to initiate an early relationship with its father. The infant will respond preferentially to its mother's voice (Eisenberg, 1969).

An infant will turn its head toward the spoken word in the first hour of life (Klaus & Kennell, 1982). At the age of six days an infant has the ability to reliably differentiate the scent of its own mother's breast pads from those of other women (MacFarlane, Smith, & Garrow, 1978) and will follow and show visual preference (Goren, Sorty, & Wu, 1975; Korner & Thoman, 1970; Robson, 1967).

Newborns even move in time with the structure of speech (Conden & Sander, 1974). As the adult speaker pauses for breath or accents a syllable, the infant almost imperceptibly raises an eyebrow or lowers a foot. Neither tapping sounds nor disconnected vowel sounds show the same degree of correspondence with neonatal movements as does natural, rhythmical speech.

Cassel and Saunder (1975) have demonstrated another aspect of newborn perceptual abilities. On day seven, when the mother interacts with the neonate while wearing a mask and does not verbalize during a feeding period, the infant takes significantly less milk and has disruptions of the next sleep cycle. The neonate thus indicates upset upon unusual maternal appearance and behavior in early life.

A crying neonate becomes quiet and visually alert when lifted to the caregiver's shoulder (Korner & Thoman, 1970). This movement temporarily soothes even a hungry infant and increases visual attentiveness in the already alert baby and arouses the sleepy infant. Neither being in an upright position nor receiving physical contact alone have the identical effect (Gregg, Haffner, & Korner, 1976).

The newborn can also initiate interaction by a range of cries that are spectrographically distinct and audibly different to the mother (Formby, 1967; Morsbach & Bunting, 1979). Wolff (1969) has distinguished four types of neonate cries: signaling hunger, anger, frustration, and pain. The newborn's cry affects blood flow to the breasts in the mothers. Formby (1967) examined blood flow in sixty-three mothers utilizing thermal photography. The infant's cry caused a change in blood flow to the breasts that might induce the mother to nurse.

Researchers such as Bowlby (1958), Ainsworth and Bell (1970), and Ainsworth, Bell and Slayton (1974) have catalogued infant behaviors into

Table 2.2 Healthy versus At-risk Neonatal Characteristics

*Characteristics and Competencies of the Healthy Neonate**	*Characteristics and Deficits of the At-risk Neonate*
Can look at parents and maintain eye-to-eye contact within first hour after birth	May be too groggy or lack ability to focus appropriately.
Can recognize threat and turn away in avoidance	Lacks ability to recognize or avoid threats
Can reach toward desired object (successfully or unsuccessfully)	Lacks ability to reach
May imitate facial expressions	Often cannot interact socially
Actively seeks appropriate level of stimulus and responds to overstimulation by shutting it out	Unable to control input and acceptance of stimuli
Has reflexes appropriate for age	
Can elicit desired attention/assistance via cries, smiles, etc.	
Attends longer to stimuli of moderate complexity	May prefer less complex stimulation
Progressively greater distinctions between waking and sleeping states	Less distinction between waking and sleeping states
May show some apneic episodes, which decline in frequency with advancing age and CNS maturity	Apneic episodes may be of greater frequency and duratiuon
Lung function good	May require artificial respiration
Plasma bilirubin less than 12 mg/dl; good liver function in first 3–4 days of life (levels may be higher in non-white infants)	May exhibit high plasma bilirubin levels; liver may be immature
Appropriate development of vision, hearing, smell	May have developmental deficits in sensory systems
Can suck strongly, long, and frequently enough to satisfy hunger and nonnutritive sucking needs	Sucking reflex frequently absent or insufficient to ensure adequate nutrition from breast or regular bottle
Can lift head while in prone position	May or may not be too weak to lift head (some healthy preterm infants exhibit more movement than term babies as their muscle: weight ratio is higher).
Molds body to that of caretaker; "cuddly"	Weak cry, does not "mold" or exhibit "cuddliness"
Increased self-regulation of attention states, moods	Frequently cannot regulate attention states
Habituates to stimuli; shows appropriate shift in heart rate	May not habituate, or may do so more slowly; often shows retardation in tachycardia/bradycardia shift
Can focus on and visually track objects 8–10 inches from face as they move across field of vision	May not possess tracking ability
Controls temperature well (after 24–36 hours)	Lacks ability to regulate body temperature; at increased risk of hypothermia

*Under optimal conditions: Apgar score greater than 8 at 1 and 5 minutes, minimal maternal medication, nontraumatic birth and labor of less than 24 hours' duration; no midforceps extraction.

executive or signal. Executive behaviors, those that tend to maintain physical contact between mother and infant, are rooting, grasping, and postural adjustment. Signal behaviors (those that increase proximity and interaction) consist of crying, smiling, grimacing, and imitation. Imitation of visually presented behaviors such as protruding a lip or sticking out a tongue also occur in neonates (Meltzoff & Moore, 1975).

Another important aspect of the healthy neonate's behavioral repertoire is the heightened state of arousal and alertness in the hour after birth (Brazelton, School, & Robey, 1966.) In this time period the newborn will visually follow the mother over an arc of 180 degrees. Klaus and Kennel (1982) seem almost apologetic in their discussions of intense reaction to the documented findings of the importance of parent–infant contact in the postnatal period.

It is necessary to emphasize that the process of attachment to a baby starts during early pregnancy and continues throughout pregnancy. The human mother has an increased potential to attend and bond to her infant in the time period immediately following birth (Salk, 1970); however, the locus of control moves to a different orientation in a high-risk pregnancy and delivery (Bendell, 1981). What would be optimally a quiet, joyful, family-centered event becomes a high-technology, stressful occasion in which parents play a passive role.

The ill and preterm infant is deprived of the opportunities for reciprocal interaction which occur during the celebration of a normal birth. Feelings of maternal failure are processed during the experience (Sosa & Cupoli, 1981), as are initial responses of shock, disbelief, and grief (Klaus & Kennell, 1972). The importance of the infant's birth is diminished by the apparatus of survival, transfer to an NICU, and implementation of medical procedures.

Budin (1907), the author of the first text on neonatology, noted: "Unfortunately, . . . a certain number of mothers abandon the babies whose needs they have not had to meet and in whom they have lost all interest. The life of the little one has been saved, it is true; but at the cost of its mother."

The cost to the mother is still high today. Although most neonatal intensive care units allow unlimited parental and grandparent visits, mothers are encouraged to breastfeed by the provision of a special room and the necessary apparatus for expressing and storing their milk, and hospital practice today encourages involvement, no matter how much support and early contact a parent has, as Field (1977) has stated: "An intensive care nursery, after all, . . . denotes a place of treatment for life and death conditions." Certainly the environment conducive to modern medical management and reduced neonatal mortality and morbidity is not conducive to feelings of love and security for the infant.

The most important etiologic factor in any subsequent behavioral disturbance is the variable parental reaction to the infant's illness (Carey, Donald, & Capelli, 1977). There is evidence that even objectively trivial medical problems, or simply the threat of neonatal illness that has been prompted by any real or perceived abnormality in the antenatal or perinatal period, may be associated with behavior disturbance (Sherman, 1980).

Green and Solnit (1964) defined the "vulnerable child syndrome," involving children who were expected to die from real or imagined conditions or illness. Such a syndrome may also be the result of a perceived or neurotic expectation of risk on the part of their parents. In either case, such a child is later found to have disturbances in psychosocial development. Pathological separation difficulties and sleep and feeding disturbances are often manifest in infancy. School phobia, infantilization, hypochondriacal complaints, and school underachievement are frequent findings in older children.

Management of the vulnerable child syndrome consists of an authoritative statement by the health care providers of physical soundness and favorable prognosis following thorough physical examination and other necessary diagnostic procedures. This should be followed by counseling and other intervention with the family unit aimed at clarification of real and perceived vulnerability. Families must be assisted in discontinuing patterns of infantilization and overprotectiveness.

Secondary prevention of the vulnerable child syndrome may be accomplished by acquainting medical personnel with the potential for this complication following the treatment of a high-risk infant. Such awareness may result in more accurate representation of risk factors and a reduction in unnecessary and pathological parental anxiety (Carey et al., 1977.)

Nor is the neonatal intensive care unit an environment conducive to optimal development (Als, Lester, & Brazelton, 1979; Cornell & Gottfried, 1976; Laursen, Merkatz, & Tejani, 1977). Data collected in a study at the University of Southern California Medical Center Women's Hospital, Los Angeles County, indicated that infants in NICUs do not lack visual, auditory, and tactile stimulation, but rather only infrequently receive coordinated sensory experiences (Gottfried, Wallace-Lande, Sherman-Brown, King, Coen, & Hodgman, 1981). The overall noise level in an NICU is comparable to light auto traffic and, at times, reaches that of large machinery. Bright white fluorescent lighting is monotonous throughout the twenty-four-hour period. Treatment includes incessant, vigorous ventilation and oxygenation, noisy, mechanized monitoring, and the use of drug therapies, such as theophylline with its documented side effects of central nervous system stimulation.

Artificial recreation of the intrauterine environment may be inappropriate, since the transition from intrauterine environment to extrauterine life triggers functions of the respiratory, cardiac, and digestive systems incompatible with antenatal experience. The preterm infant, especially, is an artifact of modern medicine. The more physiologically vulnerable an infant is, the more the demands of survival consume energy which might otherwise be expended in interaction with the environment (DiVitto & Goldberg, 1979) and on work toward the normal tasks of development.

Procedures which might otherwise be considered abusive, such as drug injections, forced feedings, intubation, and blood drawing, are required for survival. Certainly there is little in this environment to teach the infant a positive anticipation of social encounters.

Field (1979) reviewed approximately twenty-three studies on supplemental stimulation and concluded that "early supplemental stimulation may have some enduring effects on development." She further observed that provision of more "tender loving care" and attention to the infants by the intensive care medical team has a positive effect upon parental perceptions of the experience.

Tactile kinesthetic stimulation, ranging from non-nutritive sucking (Field, 1979) to stroking, handling, and rocking for 260 minutes a day (Hasselmeyer, 1964) also proved beneficial to infants.

Oscillating waterbeds produced mixed results. Korner et al (1970) documented a lower incidence of apnea, but observed no increase in weight gain. Barnard (1982) documented greater weight gain among infants with waterbeds. Barnard's findings are obscured because of the additional stimulation variable of a recorded heartbeat.

Contingent stimulation related to cues from the infant are an aid to infant development and enhance parent–infant interactions. Klaus and Kennell (1982) suggest that mothers should fondle and talk to their infants as they would under normal life circumstances. Field (1981) compared gaze behavior differences and found that infants showed the least gaze aversion with the moderately active mother. This is an important finding because there are relationships between early interaction behavior such as gazing and later social behavior (Bakeman & Brown, 1980; Sigman & Parmelee, 1974). These factors correlate positively with later intelligence quotients (Fagan, 1980).

One salient feature of enhancing parent–infant interaction is educative in nature. The Brazelton Neonatal Behavioral Assessment Scale (1973) has been widely utilized as a tool to educate parents regarding their neonate's capacities (Bendell, 1981; Brazelton, 1981; Field, 1981). The Brazelton scale delineates the infant's adaptive and coping strategies and capacities as he gains control of and interacts with social stimuli. All investigators discovered that the study of an infant in the presence of the parents altered the nature of the investigation such that an intervention had been introduced.

The most extensive investigation of this artifact utilized an adaptation of the Brazelton scale called the Mother's Assessment of the Behavior of Her Infant Scale with a group of teenaged, lower socioeconomic status black mothers (Widmayer & Field, 1981). The results of this intervention were positive over an extended time period. At one month of age, the experimental group performed more optimally on the Brazelton Scale interactive process items than did control-group infants. At four months, fine motor adaptation, as measured on the Denver Developmental Screening Test, was superior and, at one year, the infants in the experimental groups received higher scores on the Bayley Scales of Infant Development. Thus, it is seen that a facilitation of early parent–infant interactions seems to contribute to early cognitive development.

Nonetheless, the encouraging findings of these investigations should not detract from the overwhelming evidence that, even under optimal circumstances, the intensive care environment is hazardous to the infant and his family.

References

Abrahamson, J., & Shandling, B. Esophageal atresia in the underweight baby: a challenge. *Journal of Pediatric Surgery*, 1972, *7*, 608.

Adamson, S., Mueller-Heubach, E., & Meyers, R. Production of fetal asphyxia in the rhesus monkey by administration of catecholamines to the mother. *American Journal of Obstetrics and Gynecology*, 1964, *109*, 248–262.

Ainsworth, M., & Bell, S. Attachment, exploration and separation: Illustrated by the behavior of one-year olds in a strange situation. *Child Development*, 1970, *41*, 49–67.

Ainsworth, M., Bell, S., & Slayton, D. The integration of a child into a social world. In M. Richards, (Ed.), *Attachment, exploration, and separation*. New York: Cambridge University Press, 1974.

Alford, C., & Pass, R. Epidemiology of chronic congenital and perinatal infections of man. In S. Plotkin, & S. Starr (Eds.), *Clinics in perinatology*. Philadelphia: Saunders, 1981.

Als, H., Lester, B., & Brazelton, T. Dynamics of the behavioral organization of the premature infant: A theoretical perspective. In T. Field, A. Sostek, S. Goldberg, & H. Shuman (Eds.), *Infants born at risk*. Jamaica, N.Y.: Spectrum Publications, 1979.

Apgar, V., Holoday, D., James, L., Weisbrot, L., & Berrien, C. Evaluations of the newborn infant—2nd report. *Journal of the American Medical Association*, 1958, *168*, 1985–1988.

Bakeman, R., & Brown, J. Early interaction. *Child Development*, 1980, *51*, 437–447.

Barnard, K. Caring for the parents of premature or sick infants. In M. Klaus & J. Kennel (Eds.), *Parent–infant bonding*. St. Louis: Mosby, 1982.

Bendell, D. Enhancing parental development with medically-at-risk infants.

Presentation made at the Annual Convention of the American Psychological Association, Los Angeles, 1981.

Bowlby, J. *Attachment and loss* (Vol I). New York: Basic Books, 1958.

Broman, N. Perinatal anoxia and cognitive development in early childhood. In T. Field (Ed.), *Infants born at risk*. Jamaica, N.Y.: Spectrum Publications, 1979.

Brady, J., & Gregory, G. Assisted ventilation. In M. Klaus, & A. Fanaroff, (Eds.), *Care of the high-/risk neonate*. Philadelphia: Saunders, 1979.

Brazelton, T. Neonatal behavioral assessment scale. *Spastics International Medical Publications, Monograph #50*. London: William Heinemann, 1973.

Brazelton, T. Assessment as a method for enhancing infant development. *Bulletin for the National Center for Clinical Infant Programs*, Vol. I, September 1981.

Brazelton, T., School, M., & Robey, J. Visual responses in the newborn. *Pediatrics*, 1966, *37*, 284–290.

Budin, P. *The nursling*. London: Coxton, 1907.

Carey, M., Donald, J., & Capelli, A. Mothers' reactions to their newborn infants. *Journal of the American Academy of Child Psychiatry*, 1977, *20*, 16–31.

Cassel, Z., & Sander, L. Neonatal recognition processes and attachment: The masking experiment. Presented at the Society for Research in Child Development, Denver, Colorado, 1975.

Condon, W., & Sander, L. Neonate movement is synchronized with adult speech: Interactional participation and language acquisition. *Science*, 1974, *183*, 99–101.

Cornell, E., & Gottfried, A. *Child Development*, 1976, *47*, 32.

Coustan, D. Management of diabetic pregnant women. In R. Berkowitz (Ed.), *Clinics in perinatology—symposium on high risk pregnancy*. Philadelphia: Saunders, 1980.

DiVitto, B., & Goldberg, S. The effects of newborn medical status on early parent-infant interaction. In T. Field (Ed.), *Infants born at risk*. New York: Spectrum Publications, 1979.

Drogl, J., Kennedy, C., & Berendes, H. The five minute APGAR scores and 4 year psychological performance. *Developmental Medicine and Child Neurology*, 1966, *8*, 144.

Dubowitz, L., Dubowitz, V., and Goldberg, C. Clinical assessment of gestational age in the newborn infant. *Journal of Pediatrics*, 1963, *77*, 1.

Duff, R., & Cambell, A. Moral and ethical dilemmas in the special care nursery. *New England Journal of Medicine*, 1973, *287*, 890–894.

Eisenberg, R. Auditory behavior in the human neonate; functional properties of sound and their ontogenic implications. *Ear, Nose, Throat, Audiology*, 1969, *9*, 34.

Fagan, J. Infant memory. Paper presented at Symposium on High Risk Infants, Miami, 1980.

Fawcett, W., & Gluck, L. Respiratory distress syndrome in the tiny baby. *Clinics in Perinatology*, 1977, *4* (2).

Field, T. Effects of early separation, interactive deficits and experimental manipulations on infant–mother face-to-face interaction. *Child Development*, 1977, *3*, 539–540.

Field, T. Interaction patterns of preterm and term infants. In T. Field, A. Sostek, S. Goldberg, & H. Shuman (Eds.), *Infants born at risk*. Jamaica, N.Y.: Spectrum Press, 1979.

Field, T. Gaze behavior of normal and high risk infants during early interaction. *Journal of American Academy of Child Psychology*, 1981, *20*, (2).

Field, T., Stringer, S., Ignatoff, E., & Anderson-Shanklin, G. Effects of non-nutritive sucking on pre-term infants. Unpublished manuscript.

Fitzhardinge, P., & Murkestad, T. Growth and development in children recovering from bronchopulmonary dysplasia. *Journal of Pediatrics*, 1981, *100*(3), 597–602.

Frenkel, L., Keys, M., & Hefferen, S. Unusual eye abnormalities associated with congenital cytomegalovirus infection. *Pediatrics*, 1980, *66*, 763.

Formby, D. Maternal recognition of infant's cry. *Developmental Medicine and Child Neurology*, 1967, *9*, 293.

Goren, C., Sorty, M., & Wu, P. Visual following and pattern discrimination of face-like stimuli by newborn infants. *Pediatrics*, 1975, *56*, 544.

Gottfried, A., Wallace-Lande, P., Sherman-Brown, S., King, J., Coen, C., & Hodgman, J., Physical and social environment of newborn infants in special care units. *Science*, 1981, *214* (6).

Green, M., & Solnit, A. Reactions to the threatened loss of a child: a vulnerable child syndrome. *Pediatrics, 34*, 1964, 58–66.

Hanshaw, J., & Dudgeon, J. (Eds.), *Viral diseases of the fetus and newborn*. Philadelphia: Saunders, 1978.

Hasselmeyer, E. The premature neonate's response to handling. *American Nursing Association*, 1964, *1*, 15–24.

Hemphill, M., & Freeman, J. Ethical aspects of care of the newborn with serious neurological disease. *Clinics in Perinatology*, 1977, *4* (1).

James, L., & Lanman, J. (Eds.). History of oxygen therapy and retrolental fibroplasia. *Pediatrics*, 1976, *57* (Supplement), 59.

Kairam, R., & DeVivo, D. Neurological manifestations of congenital infection. *Clinics in perinatology*, 1981, *8*.

Klaus, M., & Kennell, J. *Parent–infant bonding* (2nd ed.). St. Louis: C. V. Mosby, 1982.

Korner, A., & Thoman, E. Visual alertness in neonates as evoked by maternal care. *Journal of Experimental Child Psychology*, 1970, *10*, 67.

Korones, S. *High risk newborn infants*. St. Louis: Mosby, 1976.

Kramer, M. Ethical issues in neonatal intensive care: an econimic perspective. In A. Jansen & M. Garland (Eds.), *Ethics of newborn intensive care*. Berkeley: Institute of Governmental Studies, 1976.

Laursen, N., Merkatz, I., & Tejani, M. Inhibition of premature labor: a multicenter comparison of ritodrine and ethanol. *American Journal of Obstetrics and Gynecology*, 1977, *127*, 837.

MacFarlane, J., Smith, D., & Garrow, D. The relationship between mother and neonate. In S. Kitzinger & J. Davis (Eds.), *The place of birth*. New York: Oxford University Press, 1978.

McCormick, A. Retinopathy of prematurity. *Current Problems in Pediatrics*, 1977, *7*, 1–28.

Meltzoff, A., & Moore, M. Neonate imitation: A test of existence and mechanism.

Paper presented at the Society for Research in Child Development, Denver, Colorado, 1975.

Morsbach, G., & Bunting, C. Maternal recognition of their neonate's cries. *Developmental Medicine and Child Neurology*, 1979, *21*, 178.

National Center for Health Statistics: *Facts of life and death*. Publication #79–1222, Department of Health, Education and Welfare. Pittsburgh, 1978.

Pope, K., Armstrong, D., & Fitzhardinge, P. Central nervous system pathology associated with mask ventilation in very low birth weight infants: a new etiology for intracerebellar hemorrhages. *Pediatrics*, 1976, *58*, 473.

Reich, W. Quality of life. In W. Reich (Ed.), *The encyclopedia of bioethics*. New York: Free Press, 1978.

Robson, K. The role of eye-to-eye contact in maternal–infant attachment. *Child Psychology and Psychiatry*, 1967, *8*, 13.

Salk, L. The critical nature of the post-partum period in the human for the establishment of the mother–infant bond: a controlled study. *Diseases of the Nervous System*, 1970, *31*, 110.

Schechner, S. "For the 1980's: How small is too small?" In P. Auld (Ed.), *Clinics in perinatology*. Philadelphia: Saunders, Vol. 7, No. 1, 1980.

Shapiro, S., McCormick, M., & Starfield, B. Relevance of correlates of infant mortality for significant morbidity at one year of age. *American Journal of Obstetrics and Gynecology*, 1980, *136*, 363.

Sheldon, R. Management of perinatal asphyxia and shock. *Pediatric Annals of Respiratory Therapy*, April 1977.

Sherman, M. Psychiatry in the neonatal intensive care unit. *Clinical Perinatology*, 1980, 7(1), 33–46.

Sigman, M., & Parmelee, A. Visual preferences of 4 month old premature and full-term infants. *Child Development*, 1974, *45*, 959–965.

Solnit, A., & Stark, M. Mourning the birth of a defective child. *Psychoanalytic Study of the Child*, 1961, *16*, 523.

Sosa, S., & Cupoli, M. Birthing process: Effects on the parents. In *Clinics in Perinatology*, Vol. 8, No. 1, February, 1981.

Whung, J., Stark, R., & Hegyi, T. CSP: A major breakthrough. *Pediatrics*, 1976, *58*, 783.

Widmayer, S., & Field, T. Effects of Brazelton demonstrations for mothers on the development of preterm infants. *Pediatrics*, 1981, *67*, 5.

Wolff, P. The natural history of crying and other vocalizations in early infancy. In B. Foss (Ed.), *Determinants of infant behavior*. London: Methuen, 1969.

3 Birth and Diagnosis: A Family Crisis

Marcia S. Collins-Moore

The birth and diagnosis of an anomalous or chronically ill infant typically provokes a crisis for the family. Numerous investigators agree that the experience and atmosphere of crisis is not unique to any specific disease entity or handicap, but is instead characteristic of family reactions to congenital anomalies. Expectations and hopes for a healthy, normal infant are shattered. Parents and other family members are confronted with a traumatic and unexpected situation which upsets the equilibrium of the family and causes at least temporary disorganization.

The "patient" in this situation includes not only the affected infant but also the parents, siblings, and extended family (Goldberg, 1980; Irvin, Kennell, & Klaus, 1982; Kennell & Klaus, 1982). The infant may be at risk physically and require specialized medical care. However, the "patient group" also may be at risk because of the complex and multifaceted adjustments required to successfully cope with the psychosocial, practical, and financial impact of the initial crisis.

This chapter describes reactions of family members to the birth and diagnosis of an anomalous or chronically ill infant. Observations and research regarding common psychosocial responses in the family serve as the basis for review of clinical interventions and care for family members. Selected references to pertinent research and interventions with parents of premature infants are included since the premature infant may be critically ill, and premature birth is also a crisis producing event (see Kennell and Klaus, 1982, for an in-depth review). Although primary attention is focused on experiences during the neonatal period, the impact of diagnosis during the first year of the infant's life is addressed because the presence of illness or anomaly may not be apparent at birth. Furthermore, it is not unusual for the diagnoses of a multihandicapped infant to extend beyond the neonatal period. Reactions to stillbirth and neonatal death, although conceptually related, are beyond the scope of the present chapter.

Literature Review

Observers from diverse frames of reference have reported parental reactions to the birth and diagnosis of a defective infant. Physicians, psychologists, social workers, nurses, clinical geneticists, rehabilitation counselors, and parents have contributed to the literature. Although much has been written about the impact on parents, limited attention has been given to the impact on siblings. Observations of reactions by grandparents and extended family are practically nonexistent.

Much of the literature is characterized by descriptive studies based on clinical observations or interviews with small samples of parents, primarily mothers. Retrospective accounts abound, but these are limited by potential inaccuracy in recalling past events and the influence of perceptions which change with time. The interval of time between birth and the interviews is not always specified. Also, the terms *handicapped, anomalous,* and *sick* or *chronically ill* have been used often in a generic sense although the reactions to only one anomaly or illness may have been under consideration.

Despite the limitations of the literature, the expected variations in parents because of background and personality variables, and a wide variety of infant illnesses and anomalies, common psychosocial reactions have been reported. Primarily descriptive accounts of the reactions of family members will be summarized in the literature review, followed by consideration of empirical findings based on theoretical rationale.

Parental Reactions

The first observations of the parents of anomalous, sick, and/or premature infants in the United States were made during the 1950s and 1960s. At that time parents were completely separated from their infants, who were placed in nurseries which "limited parental visiting to only 30 to 60 minutes, once or twice a week for older children" (Kennell & Klaus, 1982, p. 154). More recent trends in neonatal intensive care units provide for extensive visitations and encourage interactions between these infants and their parents. The general pattern of parents' reactions to birth and diagnosis of their infant's defect or illness, however, appears to be very much the same today as in the 1950s and 1960s.

Parents typically expect their infant to be at least normal and hopefully superior. Klaus and Kennell (1982; Kennell & Klaus, 1982) indicate that after quickening, the sensations of fetal movement, a woman often will begin to fantasize about the infant. Expectant mothers in the West attribute human personality characteristics and dream of the unborn infant, forming a mental image which often includes specific hair color, sex, and other features. According to a psychoanalytic perspective, the image of the expected baby is a "composite of representations of the self and love objects from the past (mother, husband, father, siblings)" (Solnit & Stark, 1961, p. 524).

During pregnancy expectant parents experience what has been called a normal crisis involving profound endocrine as well as somatic and psychological changes for the woman (Benfield, Leib, & Reutor, 1976) and concomitant psychological changes for the man. The successful delivery of an infant usually brings a sense of stress reduction. The birth of an anomalous or sick infant, however, marks a transition into a period of heightened stress and anxiety rather than the end of a normal crisis. The parents are plunged into an unexpected crisis at a time when their physical and emotional resources are depleted.

Diagnosis of an anomaly or illness within the first few days or months of the infant's life also precipitates a crisis for the parents. In this case the parent(s) may suspect the defect and experience an exacerbation of anxiety because of a prolonged or gradual diagnosis (Solnit & Stark, 1961).

A Catalogue of Common Responses. The parental reactions which appear to be experienced most consistently following the birth or diagnosis are shock, denial, grief, guilt, inadequacy, anger, and depression. It has been suggested that these and other reactions such as withdrawal, bitterness, resentment, and rejection are experienced to one degree or another by all parents, whether or not they realize and acknowledge it (Love, 1970; Pozanski, 1973; Yu, 1972).

The initial shock has been described as a period of pure emotion in coping with the dashed dream of a perfect child and as nature's way to buffer the traumatic experience (Scott, Jan, & Freeman, 1977).

After the initial shock, parents often try to deny that the anomaly or illness signifies permanent loss. Disbelief and denial may be especially strong after diagnosis of "silent" conditions such as phenylketonuria, which presents few if any clinical symptoms initially. This hope that the infant will "outgrow it" or "get better," or that "a cure will be found" may be a stage in parental adjustment or a lifelong attitude (O'Brien, 1976; Pozanski, 1973). Olshansky (1962) argued that some parental denial is necessary to ease "chronic sorrow" and may even be adaptive to some extent. Similarly, Shokier (1979) described denial as a protective device prompted by self-preservation and therefore not altogether maladaptive. When denial persists beyond the initial adjustment phase, however, it is generally believed to interfere with good medical management and psychological adaptation by both parents and child (O'Brien, 1976; Pozanski, 1973; Vernon, 1979).

Grief or mourning is apparently experienced universally by parents, and yet descriptions of grief reactions differ significantly. Grief has been described as an initial expression of sorrow or loss, a characteristic pattern of behavior as distinguished from anger and guilt responses or from defense mechanisms (Butani, 1974), a stage of crisis adjustment (Egg, 1964), and a theoretical framework from which to interpret all parental reactions (Collins, 1982; Irvin et al., 1982; Mitsos, 1972; Moses, 1974; Solnit & Stark, 1961; Tenbrinck & Brewer, 1976). Regardless of the observer's description, the grief reaction is perceived as a response to loss. Parents grieve for their loss of the "perfect child," for the missing or defective part of the infant, for a perceived loss of personal self-esteem, for loss of the illusion of invulnerability (It can't happen to me), and at times, loss of the baby itself (Butani, 1974; Cohen, 1964; Shokier, 1979; Solnit & Stark, 1961). Grieving also may be attributed to parental perceptions of ongoing losses in their lives due to the continuous burden or additional responsibilities and stress inherent in caring for a handicapped or sick infant.

Parents of infants with a genetic disorder may experience "multiple" grief. They grieve not only for the affected infant, but also for the yet unborn children who may be similarly affected, and for themselves as inadequate, "defective" procreators. If the infant is born with a genetic disorder which is also life threatening such as cystic fibrosis or Tay-Sachs disease, parents also grieve for the possible or probable death of the infant.

In addition to multiple grief, parents of infants with a genetic abnormality are subject to feelings of guilt, with the defective infant as living confirmation of their biological inadequacy (Waechter, 1977). Even without a genetic etiology, strong feelings of guilt are common.

Guilt has been interpreted as an extreme on a continuum of pathological reactions to the birth of a handicapped child (Solnit & Stark, 1961). However, it is more often accepted as a normal and natural parental reaction (Love, 1970; Moses, 1974). In giving birth to an anomalous or sick infant, parents may feel guilty due to their failure to live up to "ideal" expectations of themselves and society for producing a normal, if not perfect child (Greer, 1975; Shokier, 1979). Likewise, when the infant acquires an illness or a handicap through injury or disease, parents often experience guilt from their perceived failure to meet societal and personal expectations of a parent as the protector who somehow should have prevented it (Featherstone, 1981; Moses, 1974; O'Brien, 1976; Schulman, 1976).

Brazelton (1981a), Carreto (1981), Vernon (1979), and others believe that as a parent searches for a "cause" for their infant's misfortune, they inevitably feel responsible and, therefore, guilty. Since parents frequently perceive an infant as an extension of themselves, they may feel that the defect is a divine punishment for their omission or commission of some imagined or real behavior in the past (Butani, 1974; Cohen, 1964; Jordan, 1963; Love, 1970; Vernon, 1979). Similarly, they may feel that the infant's anomaly or illness may have been caused directly or indirectly by some assumed unworthiness or defect in themselves or their spouse. Guilt may be associated with feelings of revulsion and rejection of the infant (Ayrault, 1964; Pozanski, 1973). It also may be attributed to a recurrent parental love–hate conflict regarding the child, characterized by anger, hostility, and other negative feelings and thoughts including death wishes (Olshansky, 1966; Pozanski, 1973; Wendt, 1977). Guilt may stem, however, not from hostility, but from love and affection, and from the desire to see the handicap or illness undone. According to a psychodynamic interpretation, the sense of guilt may be conscious or unconscious and may be manifested in parental behaviors such as blaming oneself or others, denial, shopping around for a cure, rejection, and overprotection (Blank, 1973; Love, 1970; Ross, 1964; Stewart, 1978).

The conscious and unconscious guilt experienced by parents is closely associated with feelings of inadequacy and inferiority. A serious defect in an infant tends to be experienced by a parent as his or her own defect, which contributes to feelings of responsibility and guilt (Greer, 1975; Ross, 1964). When a genetic disease or abnormality is diagnosed, the parents' reality-based sense of biological inadequacy and guilt compounded by a sense of helplessness in governing their own lives and influencing events can contribute to further erosion of self-esteem (Bocian & Kaback, 1978; Waechter, 1977). Feelings of shame, defensiveness, loss of self-respect, and increased ambivalence are among some of the more typical reactions. Self-esteem may be threatened by the destruction of the fantasy of immortality through one's children (Gordeuk, 1976). Parents also may feel personal inadequacy due to doubts regarding their ability to give and do for the infant what is needed (Irvin et al., 1982; MacKeith, 1973). Feelings of guilt and inadequacy lead to or accompany depression (MacKeith, 1973; Moses, 1974) and may be associated with anger, since anger may be expressed in terms of self-pity and guilt (Butani, 1974).

Parental anger may be directed initially at the infant as the obvious source of the frustration of hopes and expectations built before the anomaly or illness was diagnosed. Parents often are unaware of the anger, however, because society frowns on such a primitive reaction (Butani, 1974; Cohen, 1964). Therefore, anger may be displaced from the infant to the physician, diagnostician, spouse, another family member, fate, or even God (Butani, 1974; Gordeuk, 1976). Anger periodically is generated by feelings of helplessness and frustration in interacting with the infant, and by extra burdens and relentless demands experienced by the parents

(O'Brien, 1976; Pozanski, 1973). Anger turned inward may be expressed as depression by the parents (Moses, 1974).

Depression has been equated to the grief experienced by parents and identified as one phase or characteristic of a grief or mourning process. Symptoms of depression such as deep sadness, low energy level, and apathy may be present in varying degrees. The depressed parent is perenially sad and commonly needs to expiate guilt by hovering over the infant (Irvin et al., 1982; Stewart, 1978; Wendt, 1977). Depressed parents have been described as the parents who are most apt to isolate themselves from other members of the extended family unit. Feelings of great loss persist. The depression may be reactive or it may be preparatory for resignation to, and hopefully the acceptance of, the infant and the handicap or illness (Mitsos, 1972; Moses, 1974; Tenbrinck & Brewer, 1976).

It is notable that love is rarely mentioned within the array of parental reactions to the birth and diagnosis of a defective infant. Review of the literature suggests that the turbulent negative reactions interfere with feelings and expressions of love and nurturing, especially when strong feelings of revulsion and rejection are apparent (Ayrault, 1964; Butani, 1974; Gath, 1977; Pozanski, 1973). Fortunately, as MacKeith (1973) points out, any revulsion is usually accompanied by a wish to protect the helpless infant. MacKeith also makes the interesting point that parents "fall in love" (1973, p. 524) with a normal baby so that the child is felt to be part of them regardless of what happens to him or her. If an anomaly is evident at birth, however, there is no time for this to happen. As Wills (1979) has observed with regard to blind infants, most parents do "fall in love" with their babies to a greater or lesser extent, but it may take longer to do so.

Impact on Family and Siblings

The family's ability to negotiate the initial crisis and adjust to the presence of a defective infant in the family is largely dependent on the parents. As Trevino (1979) reasoned, for example, since children may be considered extensions of their parents, a sibling's ability to accept the defective infant is greatly influenced by, and perhaps a function, if not a reflection, of parental reactions. As the parents are able to accept the infant, so will he be accepted within the family.

Several intraparental variables have been identified as significant to the parental reactions. These same variables have been cited as mediating the family's reactions to and acceptance of the infant.

Intraparental Factors. The general mental health and emotional maturity of the parent when the diagnosis is made are of vital importance. Persons who have achieved a relatively satisfying adjustment and who have learned to bear frustration, fulfill their mastery needs, trust in human relations, and feel free from excessive guilt or fear seem to (1) react more moderately, and (2) resolve their problematic emotional reactions more easily (Butani, 1974; Jordan, 1963; Goldberg, 1980; Waechter, 1977; Yu, 1972).

The parents' culture and society are also of great significance. The parents' attitudes usually are based on the accepted values of the social environment with regard to, for example, physical achievements and behavioral characteristics (Goffman, 1963; Waechter, 1970, 1977).

The parents' attitude toward the specific illness or anomaly is another mediating variable that is culturally and personally determined. It is common for parents to identify with the baby and imagine how their world would be if they were, for example, blind. But it is important to remember that a child who is born blind does not know what normal sight is. He has not lost anything because he never had it, and in his infancy and early years he will not be particularly aware that he is any different from the rest of the family unless he is made to feel that way (O'Brien, 1976; Scott et al., 1977).

Numerous observers agree that religion and religious values influence parental reactions; however, research is limited and the findings are contradictory. It appears that Catholic mothers of mentally retarded infants are equally or more accepting of the handicapped infant than non-Catholic mothers (Zuk, Miller, Bartram, & Kling, 1961). In a study of mothers of cerebral palsied children, however, Boles (1959) found that Catholic mothers of handicapped and nonhandicapped children verbalized more guilt and anxiety and were more socially withdrawn than non-Catholic mothers. Zuk and associates (1961) interpreted these results as evidence for less acceptance of handicapped infants by Catholic mothers.

Socioeconomic status (SES), including parents' income and occupational level, is also significant. Investigators working with mothers of deaf and retarded infants have found that the higher the social and occupational level of the family, the higher the expectations for comparable achievement by their children and the greater their disappointment with a child who is incapable of realizing their hopes (Meadow, 1968; Meadow & Meadow, 1971; Pozanski, 1973). Although acceptance appears to be lower as SES increases, there is compelling evidence that premature and sick infants from lower SES families are more physically and developmentally at risk than those from middle-class families.

Educational level, which is closely associated with SES, also seems to be related to parental acceptance or rejection. Parents with higher educational achievements may have more guilt feelings and experience more difficulty in accepting a mentally retarded infant, whereas parents with somewhat lower educational achievements seem less concerned (Jordan, 1963; Meadow & Meadow, 1971).

Family constellation factors including age of the parent and birth order and sex of the defective infant may create family problems. Impact on the parents may be greater if the infant is first born or a "premium child"—one born after years of effort to conceive, after multiple spontaneous abortions, or to an older, newly married couple (Bocian & Kaback, 1978). The handicapped first born son of a young couple may create more intense emotional responses than a first born daughter or a later born son. Teenage mothers are at risk because of numerous developmental and social factors. Older mothers also seem to be at risk since not only does the incidence of handicapping conditions in newborns increase with mothers over age 40, but the child may not have been as planned or welcomed. Older parents also may worry more about providing for the child's needs (Collins, 1982; Freud, 1982; Meadow & Meadow, 1971).

A physical impairment in the parent similar to that of the infant apparently eases the parental adjustment. Emotional reactions tend to be less severe and more quickly resolved (Meadow, 1968). Similarly, previous experience with children and adults with an illness or handicap similar to their infant's seems to positively affect emotional reactions (Meadow & Meadow, 1971; O'Brien, 1976; Scott et al., 1977).

Intrafamilial Factors. With diagnosis of an infant's chronic illness or handicap, parents may see their lives altered instantly and permanently. During this time of emotional turmoil the nuclear family is most vulnerable and in need of support. Unfortunately, they find "few built in supports such as those available in other crises such as the death of a relative or a community disaster" (Irvin et al., 1982, p. 237). Disequilibrium is experienced by the entire family system, negatively affecting the support which customarily eases parents' role transition (Farrell, 1977). Extended family and friends feel awkward and uncertain about how to respond, and often are silent. Immediately following the birth or diagnosis, parents are likely to experience intense loneliness.

Grandparents may be unavailable at first as they cope with their own personal crisis at having an anomalous or chronically ill infant in their family. They, too, experience loss. Berns (1980) observed that "Rare are the grandparents who do not themselves experience ambivalence: love for all their grandchildren and yet personal disappointment or rejection of the handicapped grandchild" (p. 238). Although a gamut of reactions from ostracizing to assuming total care of the infant has been reported, grandparents have been found to be the most supportive family members (Walker, Thomas, & Russell, 1971). Maternal grandmothers appear to be especially responsive.

The repercussions of the initial crisis on the nuclear family are many, subtle, and extensive. If the infant remains hospitalized, and especially if his condition is life threatening, normal family life may be suspended until his physical condition is stabilized. The atmosphere of crisis, adjustments to the mother's homecoming without the baby, and visits to the hospital inevitably affect family routine.

When the infant is discharged from the hospital, family life is further affected as parents adjust to assuming caretaking responsibilities. Although the regimen of care for each infant differs according to the specific illness or anomaly, stress for the parents is apparent, with an increase in tension and expressed concerns (Klaus & Kennell, 1982; Pinelli, 1981; Waechter, 1977). For example, very real and practical feeding problems exist for parents of infants with phenylketonuria or cleft palate. As the parents' self-confidence and comfort with the infant increase, family life may then resume a more normal status with the exceptions made necessary by special requirements of the infant.

With a chronic illness, as the infant's physical condition varies, so will the parents' reactions and ability to relate to the infant, to each other, and to other children in the family. Brazelton (1981b) has observed that the grief reaction is close to the surface during the first few months of a premature or defective infant's life, "ready to be mobilized by any setback" (p. 172). If the infant must be rehospitalized, the reality of the defect is confirmed, parent grief is reactivated, and complexities of the situation for the whole family must be confronted and reexamined. With anomalies such as spina bifida and hydrocephalus, the first year of the infant's life may be especially difficult, with repeated hospitalizations for treatment and surgery (Schulman, 1976).

The organization of the family and the ways in which family members relate to each other are at least temporarily altered by the presence of a defective infant in the family. The impact of the initial crisis and gradual adjustment on the marriage and siblings are of special concern.

With respect to the marriage, a supportive marital relationship is a source of strength for both parents during the crisis of the defective infant's birth or diagnosis. The crisis has "the potential for bringing the parents closer as a result of the mutual support and communication required for adaptation" (Irvin et al., 1982, p. 237). Gath (1977) found that despite their grief, parents of almost half of the Down's syndrome infants in her study felt drawn closer together and believed their marriage had been strengthened by the shared tragedy. On the other hand, the quality of the marital relationships showed more severe tension, high hostility, or marked lack of warmth between husband and wife among these parents than among a control group of parents with normal infants. Similarly, Walker and colleagues (1971) reported that although the majority of parents of spina bifida infants felt their marital relationship had not been affected, 56 percent of parents who perceived a change felt that there had been deterioration as opposed to improvement in the marriage.

In a review of studies with a population of parents with a diversity of anomalous infants, Irvin and associates (1982) reported that the baby's birth estranged the parents in many families. Problems were attributed to (1) increased isolation between parents because of ongoing demands of the infant's care, particularly if the parents did not share the caretaking tasks, and (2) progression through stages of adaptation at different rates, labeled "asynchronous" adaptation. It was observed that "asynchronous" parents usually did not share their feelings with each other, and a temporary emotional separation resulted.

A temporary emotional as well as physical separation is often experienced by a child when a sibling is born. The mother is physically absent during birth in the hospital and emotionally distant immediately thereafter. Consequently, the father assumes an important role in the child's experience of the birth of a sibling. The father can provide continuity in his children's emotional lives at the time surrounding the birth. He can be particularly helpful when the mother is temporarily absent and assume a central role in maintaining family stability (Legg, Sherick, & Wadland, 1974; Trause & Irvin, 1982). "The more adequately the father is coping and mastering psychological conflict and anxiety related to the pregnancy and delivery, the more he will be able to deal adequately with his older child's anxiety, queries, and needs" (Legg et al., 1974, p. 21).

When the father is confronted with the trauma of birth or diagnosis of an anomalous or sick infant, however, he too may become emotionally and physically unavailable to the normal child. His preoccupation with the well-being of his wife and defective infant in addition to his own emotional turmoil leave little energy or attention for the other child. His limited involvement with the older child has potentially damaging effects in that the child's level of adjustment to the temporary separation from mother and degree of acceptance shown the new sibling appear to be directly related to the father's prior and contemporary involvement in the child's life (Legg et al., 1974).

Children must contend with added burdens when their sibling is born defective. Their reactions to the crisis will be affected by their parents' reactions, the quality of the family relationships, and their developmental level. The toddler or preschool child is aware of his parents' sadness and worry but may not understand what is wrong. The young child needs the parent in the midst of the atmosphere of crisis but is likely to become the forgotten family member (Trause & Irvin, 1982). Older children also may be in need and yet ignored. It is possible that the older child who is developmentally mature enough to appreciate the meaning of a defective infant to the family may mourn the loss of the "expected" baby. While the mother and infant are hospitalized, however, the older child may be left in charge of arranging meals and carrying out normal household duties (Walker et al., 1971), with minimal attention to emotional needs.

If siblings have inadequate information and limited opportunities to discuss their concerns and feelings, they may be expected to develop understanding based on fantasies and suppositions. Young children are subject to "magical thinking," which may result in feeling that they are to blame in some way for the infant's condition. Their ambivalent feelings about a new child in the family and perhaps a wish that the child had never been born may seem sufficient to have caused the baby's problems (Bocian & Kaback, 1978; Trause & Irvin, 1982). Older siblings may wonder why the baby is defective and sometimes begin feeling guilty that they are normal.

Trause and Irvin (1982) believe that children cope better when they remain part of the household and experience the situation with the parents rather than being sent away to extended family or friends. They advise that parents need to discuss the newborn's problems with the siblings, including (1) what is wrong with the baby and (2) how the parents feel and why. The sibling's developmental level should guide the parents' explanations. Young children need to be reassured, perhaps repeatedly, that they are not to blame for the baby's problems and that the illness or anomaly will not happen to them or to their parents. All siblings should be encouraged to talk honestly to their parents about their feelings and be observed for potential adverse reactions due to the trauma which the family has suffered.

External Factors. The impact of the defective infant's birth or diagnosis on the family unit and individual family members is significantly influenced by the external factors which characterize the parents' support system. Parents and families in crisis need both expressive (social/emotional) and instrumental (technical/educational) support from significant others in their environment. Aside from the compassionate involvement of relatives and friends, support from hospital staff is of primary importance. After the birth of an impaired infant, the attitudes of health professionals profoundly affect the reactions of the parents. Parents seem to accept their own negative feelings more readily if professional personnel encourage the expression of these feelings and if such feelings appear to be accepted. A lack of understanding by hospital staff will intensify the parents' perceptual and emotional distortions. Also, the avoidance of responses to or contact with the infant by hospital staff communicates to the parents that their baby is not acceptable to others and adds to feelings of grief, guilt, and loss of personal worth (Blank, 1973; Butani, 1974; Gordeuk, 1976; Irvin et al., 1982; Meadow & Meadow, 1971).

Empirical Findings

Empirical investigations of the reactions of family members to the birth and diagnosis of an anomalous or sick infant consist primarily of various studies focusing on the process of mourning and others focusing on the process of attachment. The mourning metaphor and attachment issues originally were investigated by Solnit and Stark (1961), whose creative work has become the foundation of most therapeutic approaches to the parents of sick and anomalous infants.

Solnit and Stark (1961) based their analyses on material from pediatric, psychiatric, and casework contacts with mothers and their retarded children. They described the birth of a "defective" or "deviant" infant as an experiment created by nature in which "one could observe more directly the 'sudden' loss of the baby that was expected; and the 'sudden' birth of a feared, threatening, and anger-evoking child" (Solnit & Stark, 1961, p. 525). From their case studies of parents, they determined that the infant is a complete distortion of the dreamed-of or planned-for infant. Therefore, the parents must mourn the loss of this infant before they can become attached to the living "blighted" child. "There is no time for working through the loss of the desired child before there is the demand to invest the new and handicapped child as love object" (Solnit & Stark, 1961, p. 526). Solnit and Stark (1961) concluded that the process probably cannot be as effective when the handicapped child survives.

Theoretical Perspective: A Mourning Process

Several models of the mourning process have been utilized to interpret parental reactions to the birth and diagnosis of a defective infant. Authors have either presented an acknowledged model of grief and mourning to explain their clinical observations and impressions, or they have developed their own theoretical models. However, very few empirical investigations have been conducted. Therefore, minimal references to supportive research are available.

The mourning process has been conceptualized in terms of a sequence of three to five stages, each having characteristic emotions and symptoms. A progression of emotions from initial shock and denial through some form of reorganization and acceptance is generally acknowledged. The expression of emotions during the more turbulent, active mourning period between shock and acceptance is less clearly delineated.

Reaching some resolution of their grief following the initial crisis has been considered essential for both parents within a family. There is general consensus in the literature that parents must resolve their emotional reactions before they are able to look realistically at the infant and provide appropriately for the needs of the infant, each other, and the family unit. How parents deal with the mourning process significantly influences (1) their relationship with the infant, (2) patterns of family interactions within the nuclear and extended family, and (3) patterns of social relationships outside the family unit (Ende, 1972; Irvin et al., 1982; Marshall, 1980; Mitsos, 1972; Ross, 1964; Shokier, 1979).

What resolution may represent optimal adjustment for the parents during the infant's first year of life? The normal period of time for resolution of the mourning process is six months to one year according to the death and dying literature. Therefore, it would seem natural to expect the emotional reactions to be apparent or easily aroused during infancy. Some partial resolution, with progress beyond the initial shock and denial, are considered essential so that parents can participate in decision making relevant to medical treatment and risk the initial interactions with the infant which are essential for attachment. As discussed in the literature review, however, numerous characteristics of the parent, the infant, and the family's support system affect the occurrence, intensity, and/or duration of the emotional reactions. Since the presence of the infant may be a "constant reminder of the grief and loss" (Pozanski, 1973, p. 323) and since there is no finality or discrete end point possible as in adjustment to terminal illness or death (Mitsos, 1972), Olshansky's (1962) "chronic sorrow" with ongoing and recurrent expression of emotions analogous to mourning may be present at some level throughout infancy and perhaps throughout the child's life.

Normal mourning reactions evolving toward some form of resolution during the first year must be distinguished from maladaptive responses by parents. Kennell and Klaus (1982) identified the following abnormal or pathological reactions of parents with an infant in an intensive care nursery: pronounced avoidance (no visits), marked denial when there are problems, absence of affective responses, constant accusation of staff, and consistent lack of maternal behavior. According to Marshall (1980), maladaptive reactions may include absence of reaction to the diagnosis, severe depression more than a few weeks after the diagnosis, persistent psychiatric symptoms, suicide attempts, or suicidal ideation. Other abnormal reactions may be total preoccupation with the infant to the exclusion and neglect of spouse and siblings, inability to say anything good about the infant, refusal to take the infant out in public, lasting loss of patterns of social interaction, obsessive sexual dysfunction, or impending breakup of a marriage based on the infant's presence in the family.

Parents who are experiencing intense grief and mourning or maladaptive, pathological reactions are emotionally unavailable to their infants. Their turbulent negative reactions interfere with feelings and expressions of love and nurturing.

Attachment

A parent's "falling in love" with his or her infant is apparently delayed or inhibited during the crisis precipitated by the birth and diagnosis of an anomaly or illness. "Falling in love" is part of attachment: the fundamental process of the first year of life according to Robson (1972). The bidirectional process of attachment involving reciprocal interactions between infant and parent is influenced by a number of factors. Those factors unique to the attachment process between parents and critically ill or anomalous infants are related to characteristics of the infant and to separation during the neonatal period.

Characteristics of the defective infant which have been identified as significant to the attachment process include the infant's appearance, properties of the anomaly or illness, and the ability of the infant to respond to and interact with the parent.

The appearance of the infant has a significant impact on the parent. Solnit and Stark (1961) determined that one early task for the parent is to reconcile the idealized image of the "expected" baby and the appearance of the "actual" baby. A number of investigators agree that the greater the discrepancy between the "expected" and "actual" baby, the more difficult is resolution and acceptance for the parent.

Waechter (1977) found that of the infants born with a visible abnormality, parents of facially disfigured children responded most profoundly, particularly to infants with bilateral cleft lip. Similarly, Wills (1979) indicated that when a baby's eyes are absent and only sunken eyelids meet the mother's gaze, a loving relationship is impeded until artificial eyes can be fitted.

Another property of the anomaly or illness which influences the attachment process is the etiology of the defect—whether or not it is genetic (Cohen, 1964; Jordan, 1963; Waechter, 1977). The parent's perception of the severity of the infant's anomaly/physical condition and the extent to which the defect may be corrected are significant (Marshall, 1980; Pozanski, 1973; Solnit & Stark, 1961; Stewart, 1978; Tisza & Gumpertz, 1962). The question of a life-threatening status affects the parents' ability and willingness to invest emotionally in the infant (Irvin et al., 1982; Newman, 1980; Waechter, 1977). Other variables include the presence of mental deficiency or blindness (Irvin et al., 1982; Pozanski, 1973; Scott et al., 1977; Waechter, 1977). Finally, defects involving the infant's genitalia are disturbing, particularly when gender is not obvious at birth (Irvin et al., 1982; Waechter, 1977).

The ability of the infant to respond and interact with the parent can positively or negatively affect the attachment process. According to Klaus and Kennell (1982),

> The infant's appearance, coupled with his broad array of sensory and motor abilities, evokes responses from the mother and father and provides several channels of communication that are most helpful in the process of attachment and the initiation of a series of reciprocal interactions [p. 63].

In contrast, when parents are "confronted with an infant of limited competence the potential risks of interactive failures are high" (Goldberg, 1977, p. 174). Since critically ill and high-risk premature infants as well as those with severe sensory or intellectual deficits are restricted in normal social interchanges, impediments in attachment are likely to occur.

A classic example of an infant's inability to initiate contact and respond in a normal interactive pattern occurs with congenitally blind infants. Parents of blind infants are denied the eye-to-eye contact which Robson (1967) has identified as an innate releaser of maternal caretaking responses. As Fraiberg (1974) has demonstrated, the parent is denied the signs of discrimination, recognition, preference, and valuation that are normally read through visual responses of an infant. Also, the large vocabulary of facial expressions typical of a sighted infant is restricted. Parents do not know to look to the blind baby's hands for subtle indications of affect, wish, and choice, and the difficulties they encounter in interpreting the needs of their infants lead to a sense of estrangement and incompetence. Parents need to be taught how to interpret their baby's signals and to interact effectively (Heidelise, Tronick & Brazelton, 1980; Fraiberg, 1974).

An infant's ability to respond to and interact with the parent may be limited by not only the biological deficit, but also by the constraints of numerous physical interventions required to maintain life in an intensive care nursery. Various tubes, wires for monitors, and bandages may cover the infant in the isolette. Furthermore, the environment of the intensive care nursery is not conducive to the development of affectional bonds. In what Kennell and Klaus described as the "brightly lit, stainless steel and glass citadel" (1982, p. 195) of the intensive care nursery, parents play an unnaturally passive role and "are treated as guests with privileges to visit which may be withdrawn at any time" (Freud, 1982). Miller (1978) suggested that the circumstances of life in an intensive care nursery can disrupt, and perhaps sometimes sabotage, the attachment process.

More important than the environment is the physical separation of infant from parents. Freud (1982) noted that normally the baby is caregiver to the parent as much as the parent is to the baby. Therefore, separation is traumatic for both parent and infant. Extensive separation for medical treatment during the neonatal period interferes with three important components of parent–infant interaction: its timing and duration, the senses involved, and its caretaking nature (Barnett, Leiderman, Grobstein, & Klaus, 1970). Until recently, limited visitations, sensory contact restricted to observation through plexiglass and touching through portholes of an incubator, and delay of caretaking activities by the parents were common occurrences. Although most intensive care nurseries now allow unlimited parent and grandparent visitation and parents are encouraged to fondle their infants, many normal caretaking activities continue to be delayed of necessity (Klaus & Kennell, 1982).

It is generally agreed that any prolonged parent–infant separation delays or inhibits the attachment process. The circumstances of early separation, however, need not damage the ultimate development of an optimal attachment between parent and infant. Nevertheless, an overrepresentation of premature, sick, and anomalous infants in populations of abused and neglected infants has been attributed to separation interfering with the attachment process (Fanaroff, Kennell, & Klaus, 1972; Klaus & Kennell, 1970). In contrast, Egeland and Vaughn (1981) argued that separation immediately following birth is not associated with abuse, neglect, or other forms of mistreatment. They suggested that disorders of parenting may be attributed instead to personality characteristics of the mother which were present prior to birth of her infant and which negatively influenced her intitial bonding and subsequent mothering, or to the difficulties in caring for premature and sick infants. Other risk factors for potential abuse by parents of an anomalous infant include extreme isolation from family and friends and a history of abuse in the childhood of either parent (Fost, 1982).

The unresolved question of the role of neonatal separation in subsequent parenting disorders does not diminish the need to foster the infant–parent relationship. Early intervention to assist and support the attachment process should begin to take place while the initial crisis of birth or diagnosis is being negotiated, the operations performed, the diets started.

Treatment Issues

The helping professionals who serve families in the midst of the crisis of birth and diagnosis and throughout the subsequent period of initial adjustment can profoundly affect the eventual outcome for each member of the family. With consistent services available to support their needs, the parents and other family members generally are able to expend the emotional energy to participate in the infant's habilitation. Without support and guidance, the family is increasingly at-risk as they struggle through the process from shock to adaptive behavior and assume caretaking responsibilities for the defective infant. Some families are able to negotiate the mourning and attachment processes with minimal intervention while others are not. In all situations, however, every family trying to cope with the crisis is in need of some form of therapeutic intervention.

In discussing treatment issues, it must be remembered that the circumstances of the birth and diagnosis will differ for each family. The anomaly or illness may be apparent at birth and require immediate and specialized treatment in a neonatal intensive care nursery. If so, parents and infant may be separated within the same hospital or by a distance of blocks within the same city to miles away in a separate city. Neonatal intensive care may be unnecessary, but corrective surgery required during the neonatal period. The impairment or illness may not be suspected and diagnosed until days, weeks, or months after birth.

Likewise, the personnel providing services to a family will be unique to the hospital or clinic. Ideally, a team of professionals would be able to respond to all of the patient group—infant, parents, siblings, and grandparents. For example, a neonatal team would include the neonatologist, consulting physician regarding the infant's special illness or anomaly, a nurse, social worker, psychologist, or psychiatrist, and other professionals as needed. Each team member would have full knowledge and understanding of the specific illness or impairment and its psychosocial implications for the infant and family. However, many variations from the ideal exist.

Regardless of the specific circumstances and personnel, the goal of treatment remains consistent: habilitation of the infant and family in the broadest sense. Interventions need to be supportive and preventive, with attention to both the expressive and instrumental needs of family members. A general overview of treatment issues and alternative intervention strategies to attain the goal will be reviewed in the next few pages.

Tasks of Helping Professionals

Six tasks were identified by Kennell and Klaus (1982) for health professionals working with parents in a neonatal intensive care nursery. Variants of these same tasks seem to apply equally well to helping professionals who work with parents during and after the birth or diagnosis of sick or anomalous infants in general. The following tasks are an expanded and revised version of the tasks enumerated by Kennell and Klaus (1982, pp. 192–194). Implicit in the tasks are the concomitant tasks which parents and/or other family members need to accomplish in order to assimilate the defective infant into the family.

Helping professionals need to (1) help both parents adapt their idealized image of the "expected" infant to the "actual" infant; (2) help relieve the parents' guilt about producing a defective infant; (3) help the parents begin to build or to maintain a close affectional tie to their infant, developing a mutual interaction so that they will be attuned to their baby's special needs as he or she grows; (4) teach the parents how to care for their infant while he or she is hospitalized so that after the infant's discharge, they will be competent and relaxed in caretaking activities; (5) encourage the entire family to work together during the crisis of the birth and diagnosis, helping the parents to discuss their emotional reactions and difficulties with one another as they attempt to arrive at satisfactory solutions; (6) encourage parents to talk to siblings about the infant and be aware of their needs for attention and reassurance during the crisis; (7) help meet the special needs of individual families; and (8) assist families in the transition that occurs after the infant's discharge, including follow-up support and assistance as well as information about available community resources.

Accomplishing these tasks begins with informing both parents after the birth or diagnosis.

Communicating Information

Issues of when, what, how, and by whom the initial information should be given to parents about the infant's illness or anomaly have been topics of debate and periodic research since the 1950s. The general consensus is to communicate direct and simple information in a sensitive and caring manner to both parents, in privacy, and soon after the birth or diagnosis. Information should be conveyed by the infant's primary physician. Seeing the baby with a visible defect generally dispels fearful fantasies and relieves parents' anxieties.

Shokier (1979), a clinical geneticist involved in management of families of defective newborns, recommends that the guiding principal of when to tell is "to avoid rejection of the baby or its condition by first establishing the mother–infant bonding. This will be possible in most but not all cases" (p. 209). Shokier has developed a timeline for informing the parents of their baby's anomaly (or suspicion thereof) according to the ostensible nature and outlook of the disorder. For example, parents of an infant with an apparent, lethal grotesque (e.g., anencephaly) or acceptable looking (e.g., trisomy E) lesion should be informed as soon after birth as possible and before seeing the baby, whereas parents of an infant with a nonlethal, apparent (e.g., cleft lip and palate) or concealed (e.g., TE fistula) lesion requiring medical management may be told after they have seen, held, and fed (if possible) the baby, within one or two days after birth.

Kennell and Klaus (1982) agree that when possible, as with Down's syndrome, it is desirable to allow the process of parental bonding to begin before informing parents unless the family suspects there is a problem. When an infant is being treated in a neonatal intensive care nursery, however, the parents should be informed about the appearance of the baby and the life support system before seeing him. Furthermore, parents should be shown the normality of the infant as well as the disorder to help them perceive the infant as a person and promote attachment (Brazelton, 1981a, b; Irvin et al., 1982; Shokier, 1979).

Initial and subsequent information should be adequate—neither overload nor ignorance, without medical jargon, interpreted clearly, and repeated often. The adjustment reactions of shock and denial may be expected to interfere with the parents' understanding and recall of information during the acute phase of the crisis and perhaps for the first three to four months of the baby's life. Therefore, patient repetition of information is necessary. However, a parent's continuous denial with inability to process information after numerous repetitions is cause for concern.

Kennell and Klaus (1982) recommend that during initial treatment of a critically ill infant in a neonatal intensive care nursery, parents need a brief report about the infant's condition every 15 to 20 minutes. The information is intended to help parents cope with the anticipatory grief which they experience, regardless of the severity of the infant's illness, when infants are admitted to a neonatal intensive-care nursery (Benfield et al., 1976) Frequent information, even when the medical status is unchanged, can help parents maintain more accurate reality testing and prevent excessive fantasy or denial. After the first few hours, Kennell and Klaus (1982) inform parents of a critically ill baby about the medical status one to two times daily.

As the diagnosis and/or treatment progress, Brazelton (1981a), Freud (1982), Kennell and Klaus (1982), and others recommend informing the parents about their infant's behavior and medical status. This information as well as an explanation that the baby needs and is waiting for the parent's touch and contact personifies the infant and reduces phobic reactions of withdrawal and rejection.

Allowing parents to guide the professional regarding what they want to know and are ready to hear is essential. Detailed or lengthy information about anatomical and functional implications of the illness or anomaly is contraindicated during the initial shock because parents are rarely able to absorb it. Also, parents have difficulty absorbing information about several major problems in their baby all at one time. Individual parents respond to the crisis in their own unique ways and are ready for different information at different times. Therefore, assessing their present concerns enables the helping person to intervene in a timely fashion, progressing at the parent's pace.

A final recommendation regarding information is to avoid sharing concerns about *possible* neurological sequelae if parents have not raised the issue. Although some disagreement remains, clinicians generally agree that mental retardation should not be discussed until the diagnosis is verified.

Communicating information as discussed above is a source of support for parents, can allay fears, maintain reality testing, foster attachment, and assist parents in participating in decision making relative to their infant's medical treatment. Parents should be encouraged to ask questions, speak openly, and learn about the illness or anomaly. The same principles may be applied to communicating with grandparents, older siblings, and others who may visit the infant in the hospital and thereafter.

Inpatient Environmental Considerations

With a congenital anomaly or illness both mother and infant may be hospitalized for several days postpartum, especially if the mother delivered by caesarean section. The traumatic recognition of a congenital defect sets the mother apart from other mothers who are rejoicing with their families. She is shocked and distraught and cannot share in their joy. If her baby is transferred to a neonatal intensive care unit for treatment, the baby will not be brought to her, nor may she be able to go to him for feedings and other activities which mothers of normal infants enjoy. Her intense loneliness is exacerbated by the juxtaposition of their joy and her pain. She needs privacy in her grief. Therefore, Bocian and Kaback (1978) and others recommend that mothers of anomalous and sick newborns have private rooms, away from mothers of normal infants.

In order to reduce separation and facilitate interactions between parents and infants, several interventions have been developed to bring the family unit into the same inpatient environment. Kennell and Klaus (1982) present the most comprehensive review of both tried and innovative approaches to date. These include opening the intensive care nursery to parents, transporting the mother to be near her small infant who requires care in an intensive care nursery, and maternal day care of the hospitalized infant.

Freud (1982) has emphasized the parents' need for both a territory and a role when visiting the infant in the intensive care nursery. He suggests personalizing the area around the infant's isolette and providing a space for a chair where the parent can be close and comfortable. The parents' role would be defined in terms of fondling the infant and slowly assuming caretaking responsibilities. He believes that if parents are given both a territory and a role, the incidence of parent visitation would increase markedly. Both of these elements are provided for in the following interventions.

Rooming-in is another alternative, with mothers and infants permitted to live together. Mothers assume a primary role in caretaking activities. Various models of rooming-in have been developed, including a twenty-bed special infant care unit in High Wycombe, England, where "No matter how seriously ill they may be, some 70% of the babies have their mothers with them from the first few hours of life" (Kennell & Klaus, 1982, p. 177). Fathers are allowed to stay overnight and young siblings may visit as frequently as the family wishes. Six of the parents' rooms open into the nursery so that parents can easily see or care for their infants.

A final intervention which has been utilized in an effort to normalize the interaction between parents and hospitalized infants is called "nesting" by Kennell and Klaus (1982). A mother is admitted into the hospital several days prior to the baby's discharge in order to assume full caretaking responsibility of the infant under supervision. The father is given unlimited visiting privileges, a comfortable chair, and a cot.

Vermillion, Ballantine, and Grosfeld (1979) reported a successful intervention in a pediatric surgical service analogous to the care by parent interventions of rooming-in and nesting. In the Parent Care Unit described by Vermillion and associates, families have a private room similar to motel accommodations and enjoy recreational and dining activities in a group area. The parent provides all of the care the infant will require in the home setting. This may include administration of medicines, appliance care, mixing formulas, feeding, and any other special procedures that may be prescribed. Instruction for parents occurs daily. When diagnostic studies are necessary, the parent must accompany the infant patient for the medical procedure.

Caretaking Activities

Assuming responsibility for taking care of a sick or anomalous infant is a frightening prospect for most parents. Parents whose infants will require special care in the home setting need to learn procedures and feel competent prior to the infant's discharge. Before caretaking can begin, parents generally need to have extended contact with the infant: time to look, to touch, and to fondle the baby. Eventually the parents may be taught/encouraged to begin nonmedical tasks such as changing diapers and cleaning the baby. As parents gain confidence, new responsibilities may be added. Regardless of the task, parents are not to be asked to assume responsibility if any potential for failure exists (Brazelton, 1981b; Freud, 1982; Kennell & Klaus, 1982). Failure in initial attempts to care for the baby may reinforce the parents' feelings of inadequacy and delay interactions necessary for both parents and infant to form an attachment.

Pinelli's (1981) research with mothers of infants with congenital heart disease suggested the need to teach them how to differentiate between the normal needs of newborns and the needs specific to the infant's illness or anomaly. Inability to distinguish between these needs may produce lack of confidence and increased concern in assuming care in the home setting. Therefore, attention to the deviancy alone is inadequate. Normal infant behavior also must be learned and acknowledged for comfort in caretaking.

This finding lends support to Brazelton's (1981b) recommendation to play with the infant in front of the parents to demonstrate the baby's intact behavioral responses. The baby may thereby be perceived as more of a total person to the parents, able to interact and respond in his own uniqueness.

Parents whose infants do not require neonatal inpatient care do not benefit from learning about their baby's special needs under the guidance of supportive professionals. These parents need outreach services from the hospital or clinic making the diagnosis, or referral to a community agency able to serve the family. For example, parents of hearing or visually impaired children are potentially in need of long-term, specialized medical, educational, and psychosocial intervention beginning in early infancy.

Encouraging and assisting parents in caretaking activities facilitates attachment and resolution of emotional reactions experienced by parents during initial crisis adjustment. Prolonged contact with the baby allows parents to become acquainted with all of his or her features, both normal and deviant. The contact provides opportunities for parents to realign their images of the "expected" baby with the "actual" one (Irvin et al., 1982). Combining contact with a positive responsible role which fits parents' expectations for parenting promotes feelings of comfort and competence in the parent–infant relationship.

Supportive Counseling

Supportive counseling following the birth and diagnosis of a defective infant is therapeutic for the parents and the family. Prolonged discussions with a helping professional assist them to cope more effectively with the traumatic experience. Counseling enables parents to acquire information, express and review their thoughts and feelings, explore existing coping mechanisms and learn new ones, and begin to make rational decisions and plans regarding the management of the baby and the family.

Group and individual counseling techniques have been utilized with parents during periods of hospitalization for the infant and for follow-up support thereafter. In recent years, neonatal intensive care nurseries have formed groups of parents who meet together once or twice a week for one- or two-hour discussions. Groups generally continue for six to ten weeks. Use of films, lectures, structured discussions, and open-ended discussions have been reported in clinical literature (Erdman, 1977; Meier, 1978;

Minde, Shosenberg, Marton, Thompson, Ripley, and Burns, 1980). Professionally led group meetings have included veteran parents who have lived through a parallel experience and other parents currently experiencing the same crisis.

Meier (1978) found that parents felt more support and preferred talking to other parents currently in crisis more than those who had experienced a similar crisis in the past. She also suggested that two groups would be beneficial for parents: a crisis group which focuses on expressing feelings and issues of coping, followed by a discharge planning group which focuses on caretaking tasks, decision making, and future planning.

Minde and colleagues (1980) reported that parents of premature infants who participated in group meetings with a nurse coordinator and veteran mother visited their hospitalized infants significantly more than a control group; rated themselves more competent in infant care; touched, looked, and talked with their infants in the *en face* position more; and continued to show more involvement and concern with their babies three months after their hospital discharge.

Parent–parent support systems in which new and veteran parents are matched also have been developed in intensive care nurseries. For example, visiting parent teams of veteran parents have provided nonprofessional outreach support and counsel to parents separated from their infants who have been transferred to a neonatal intensive care nursery away from the local hospital where the mother remains (Eager & Exoo, 1980).

Numerous approaches to individual counseling with parents and couples have been reported in clinical literature. Irvin and associates (1982) provide an exemplary outline of topics for the first counseling sessions to guide consideration of parents' reactions. Topics include parental feelings, parental perception of the infant's illness or anomaly, parent reaction to the baby, parental coping, parents' relationship to one another, and the family's attitude toward others. To this list may be added reactions of siblings and care for them during the crisis. Assessment of these issues facilitates planning for future counseling sessions. With genetic anomalies, Shokier (1979) also addresses genetic risk in future pregnancies.

Parents need time to adjust, with guidance and support to help them anticipate their emotional reactions and understand that what they are experiencing is normal and natural. Through an ongoing, supportive counseling relationship the family's coping mechanism may be assured, diagnostic information interpreted, and emotional and environmental support provided during the crisis of birth and diagnosis.

After discharge from the hospital, support and assistance should continue through frequently scheduled appointments, including, if possible, home visits. Follow-up during the early months and years is necessary to facilitate ongoing habilitation of the infant and family. If continued hospital support systems are unavailable, the family should be assisted in identifying available community resources for instrumental and affective support.

Future Trends

Green (cited in Irvin et al., 1982) has indicated that health care providers may be on the threshold of a major reorganization of hospital, home, and office care of infants with major disabilities. He envisions a specially trained FACT, or Family Crisis Team, providing care in the immediate newborn period to families with anomalous, premature, stillborn, or critically ill infants. He also foresees regional centers with neonatal intensive care nurseries, early intervention programs, centers for handicapped infants, or parent care pavilions where heavy emphasis will be placed on parent participation.

In building new neonatal intensive care nurseries, design of facilities such as the rooming-in unit in High Wycombe, England (Kennell & Klaus, 1982), or the Parent Care Unit in Indianapolis, Indiana (Vermilion et al., 1979), should be provided. Such family-oriented facilities which allow privacy and promote more normal interactions and parent participation in caretaking activities should prove cost effective both financially and psychosocially.

Other services on the horizon for sick and anomalous infants and their families may include more extensive home-based intervention programs for parent education and respite aid. These programs should be available through developmental clinics associated with pediatric hospitals providing multidisciplinary teams to diagnose and treat defective infants and their families.

References

Ayrault, E. V. *You can raise your handicapped child*. New York: Putnam's Sons, 1964.

Barnett, C. R., Leiderman, P. H., Grobstein, R., & Klaus, M. H. Neonatal separation: the maternal side of interactional deprivation. *Pediatrics*, 1970, *45*, 197–205.

Benfield, D. G., Leib, S. A., & Reutor, J. Grief response of parents following referral of the critically ill newborn. *New England Journal of Medicine*, 1976, *294*, 975–978.

Berns, J. H. Grandparents of the handicapped. *Social Work*, 1980, *25*, 238–239.

Blank, H. R. Psychic consequences of congenital lack and acquired loss of body parts. In "Psychic consequences of loss and replacement of body parts." *Journal of the American Psychoanalytic Association*, 1973, *22*, 170–181.

Bocian, M. E., & Kaback, M. M. Crisis counseling: The newborn infant with a chromosomal anomaly. *Pediatric Clinics of North America*, 1978, *25*(3), 643–650.

Boles, G. Personality factors in mothers of cerebral palsied children. *Genetic Psychology Monographs*, 1959, *59*, 159–218.

Brazelton, T. B. *Development of attachment during pregnancy and early infancy*. Seminar presented at the C.V. Ramana Saturday Seminar, Oklahoma City, Oklahoma, November 21, 1981. (a)

Brazelton, T. B. *On becoming a family*. New York: Dell Publishing Co., 1981. (b)

Butani, P. Reactions of mothers to the birth of an anomalous infant: A review of the literature. *Maternal–Child Nursing Journal*, 1974, *3*(1), 59–76.

Carreto, V. Maternal responses to an infant with cleft lip and palate: A review of literature. *Maternal–Child Nursing Journal*, 1981, *10*(3), 197–205.

Cohen, P. C. The impact of the handicapped child on the family. *New Outlook for the Blind*, 1964, *58*(1), 11–15.

Collins, M. S. Parental reactions to a visually handicapped child: A mourning process. Unpublished dissertation, The University of Texas, 1982.

Eager, M., & Exoo, R. Unequaled support. *Maternal–Child Nursing Journal*, 1980, *5*, 35–36.

Egeland, B., & Vaughn, B. Failure of "bond formation" as a cause of abuse, neglect, and maltreatment. *American Journal of Orthopsychiatry*, 1981, *51*(1), 78–84.

Egg, M. *When a child is different*. New York: John Day Co., 1964.

Ende, M. L. Three congenitally blind infants and their mothers. *Maternal-Child Nursing Journal*, 1972, *1*(1), 55–65.

Erdman, D. Parent-to-parent support: The best for those with sick newborns. *Maternal–Child Nursing Journal*, 1977, September/October, 291–292.

Fanaroff, A., Kennell, J., & Klaus, M. Follow-up of low birthweight infants: the predictive value of maternal visiting patterns. *Pediatrics*, 1972, *49*, 287–290.

Farrell, H. M. Crisis intervention following the birth of a handicapped infant. *Journal of Psychiatric Nursing and Mental Health Service*, 1977, *15*, 32–36.

Featherstone, H. *A difference in the family*. New York: Penguin Books, 1981.

Fost, N. Counseling families who have a child with a severe congenital anomaly. *Pediatrics*, 1982, *67*, 321–324.

Fraiberg, S. Blind infants and their mothers: An examination of the sign system. In M. Lewis & L. A. Rosenblum (Eds.), *The effect of the infant on its caregiver*. New York: Wiley, 1974.

Freud, E. *Psychological aspects of neonatal intensive care: the mother's and the baby's needs*. MASUA Lecture presented at the University of Oklahoma Health Sciences Center, Oklahoma City, Oklahoma, April 1, 1982.

Gath, A. The impact of an abnormal child upon the parents. *British Journal of Psychiatry*, 1977, *130*, 405–410.

Goffman, I. *Stigma*. Englewood Cliffs, N.J.: Prentice-Hall, 1963.

Goldberg, H. K. Hearing impairment: A family crisis. *Social Work in Health Care,* 1980, *5*(1), 33–40.
Goldberg, S. Social competence in infancy: A model of parent–infant interaction. *Merrill-Palmer Quarterly,* 1977, *23*(3), 163–178.
Gordeuk, A. Motherhood and a less than perfect child: A literary review. *Maternal–Child Nursing Journal,* 1976, *5*(2), 57–68.
Greer, B. G. On being the parent of a handicapped child. *Exceptional Children,* 1975, *41*(8), 519–521.
Heidelise, A., Tronick, E., & Brazelton, T. B. Affective reciprocity and the development of autonomy. *Journal of the American Academy of Child Psychiatry,* 1980, *19,* 22–40.
Irvin, N. A., Kennell, J. H., & Klaus, M. H. Caring for parents of an infant with a congenital malformation. In M. H. Klaus & J. H. Kennell (Eds.), *Parent–infant bonding.* St. Louis: Mosby, 1982, 227–258.
Jordan, T. E. Physical disability in children and family adjustment. *Rehabilitation Literature,* 1963, *24,* 330–336.
Kennell, J. H., & Klaus, M. H. Caring for the parents of premature or sick infants. In M. H. Klaus & J. H. Kennell (Eds.), *Parent–infant bonding.* St. Louis: Mosby, 1982, 151–226.
Klaus, M. H., & Kennell, J. H. Labor, birth and bonding. In M. H. Klaus & J. H. Kennell (Eds.), *Parent–infant bonding.* St. Louis: Mosby, 1982, 22–98.
Klaus, M., & Kennell, J. Mothers separated from their newborn infants. *Pediatric Clinic of North America,* 1970, *17,* 1015–1037.
Legg, C., Sherick, I., & Wadland, W. Reaction of preschool children to the birth of a sibling. *Child Psychiatry and Human Development,* 1974, *5*(1), 3–39.
Love, H. D. *Parental attitudes toward exeptional children.* Springfield, Ill.: Charles C. Thomas, 1970.
MacKeith, R. The feelings and behavior of parents of handicapped children. *Developmental Medicine and Child Neurology,* 1973, *15,* 524–527.
Marshall, I. The grief process. Paper presented at the International Seminar of Preschool Blind Children, Austin, Texas, March, 1980.
Meadow, K. P. Parental response to the medical diagnosis of congenital deafness. *Journal of Health and Social Behavior,* 1968, *9,* 299–309.
Meadow, K. P., & Meadow, L. Changing role perceptions for parents of handicapped children. *Exceptional Children,* 1971, *38*(1), 21–27.
Meier, P. P. A crisis group for parents of high risk infants. *Maternal–Child Nursing Journal,* 1978, *7*(1), 21–30.
Miller, C. Working with parents of high-risk infants. *American Journal of Nursing,* 1978, July, 1228–1230.
Minde, K., Shosenberg, N., Marton, P., Thompson, J., Ripley, J., & Burns, S. Self-help groups in a premature nursery—a controlled evaluation. *The Journal of Pediatrics,* 1980, *196*(5), 933–940.
Mitsos, S. B. The grieving process of parents of atypical children. *Journal of Rehabilitation,* 1972, *38*(2), 5–7.
Moses, K. *The mourning theory and family dynamics: A presentation for the parents and families of impaired children.* A videotape for Regional Resource Center VII, Peoria, Ill., 1974.

Newman, L. F. Parents' perception of their low-birth weight infants. *Paediatrician*, 1980, *9*, 182–190.

O'Brien, R. *Alive . . . aware . . . a person: A developmental model for early childhood services with special definition for visually impaired children and their parents*. Rockville, Md.: Montgomery County Public Schools, 1976.

Olshansky, S. Chronic sorrow: A response to having a mentally defective child. *Social Casework*, 1962, *43*, 190–193.

Olshansky, S. Parent responses to a mentally defective child. *Mental Retardation*, 1966, *4*(4), 21–23.

Pinelli, J. M. A comparison of mothers' concerns regarding the caretaking tasks of newborns with congenital heart disease before and after assuming their care. *Journal of Advanced Nursing*, 1981, *6*, 261–270.

Pozanski, E. A. Emotional issues in raising handicapped children. *Rehabilitation Literature*, 1973, *34*, 322–326.

Robson, K. S. Development of object relations during the first year of life. *Seminars in Psychiatry*, 1972, *4*(4), 301–316.

Robson, K. S. The role of eye-to-eye contact in maternal–infant attachment. *Journal of Child Psychology and Psychiatry*, 1967, *8*, 13–25.

Ross, A. O. *The exceptional child in the family*. New York: Grune & Stratton, 1964.

Schulman, J. L. *Coping with tragedy: Successfully facing the problem of a seriously ill child*. Chicago: Follett Publishing Company, 1976.

Scott, E. P., Jan, J. E., & Freeman, R. D. *Can't your child see?* Baltimore, Md.: University Park Press, 1977.

Sherman, M. Psychiatry in the neonatal intensive care unit. *Clinics in Perinatology*, 1980, *7*(1), 33–47.

Shokier, M. H. K. Managing the family of the abnormal newborn. *Birth Defects: Original Article Series*, 1979, *15*(5C), 199–222.

Solnit, A. J., & Stark, M. H. Mourning and the birth of a defective child. *Psychoanalytic Study of the Child*, 1961, *16*, 523–537.

Stewart, J. C. *Counseling parents of exceptional children*. Columbus, Ohio: Charles E. Merrill Publishing Company, 1978.

Tenbrinck, M. S., & Brewer, P. W. The stages of grief experienced by parents of handicapped children. *Arizona Medicine*, 1976, *33*(9), 712–714.

Tisza, V. B., & Gumpertz, E. The parents' reaction to the birth and early care of children with cleft palate. *Pediatrics*, 1962, *30*, 86–90.

Trause, M. A., & Irvin, N. A. Care of the sibling. In M. H. Klaus & J. H. Kennell (Eds.), *Parent–infant bonding*. St. Louis: Mosby, 1982, 110–129.

Trevino, F. Siblings of handicapped children: Identifying those at risk. *Social Casework*, 1979, *60*, 488–493.

Vernon, M. Parental reactions to birth-defective children. *Postgraduate Medicine*, 1979, *65*(2), 183–189.

Vermilion, B. D., Ballantine, T. V. N., & Grosfeld, J. L. The effective use of the parent care unit for infants on the surgical service. *Journal of Pediatric Surgery*, 1979, *14*(3), 321–324.

Waechter, E. H. Bonding problems of infants with congenital anomalies. *Nursing Forum*, 1977, *16*(3, 4), 298–318.

Waechter, E. H. The birth of an exceptional child. *Nursing Forum*, 1970, *10*(11), 202–216.

Walker, J. H., Thomas, M., & Russell, I. T. Spina bifida and the parents. *Developmental Medicine and Child Neurology*, 1971, *13*, 462–476.

Wendt, J. A. On being the parent of a handicapped child. *The New York Times Magazine*, 1977, March 21, 10–14.

Wills, D. M. The ordinary devoted mother and her blind baby. *Psychoanalytic Study of the Child*, 1979, *34*, 31–49.

Yu, M. The causes for stresses to families with deaf-blind children. Paper presented at the Southwest Regional Meeting of the American Orthopsychiatric Association, Galveston, Texas, 1972.

Zuk, G. H., Miller, R. L., Bartram, J. B., & Kling, F. Maternal acceptance of retarded children: A questionnaire study of attitudes and religious background. *Child Development*, 1961, *32*(3), 525–540.

II

Children

4 Children's Adaptation to Chronic Illness and Handicapping Conditions

J. Kenneth Whitt

Recent advances in medical technology, promising therapeutic regimes, and new transplantation procedures have improved mortality rates for many childhood diseases. Extended life with a chronic illness or physical handicap, however, is not without repercussion to the child's cognitive, emotional, and social development. Children's reactions to treatment demands, diminished quality of life, prolonged uncertainty, and disruptions of the family system persist as challenges to the pediatric health care system (Haggerty, Roghmann, & Pless, 1975).

Defining the impact of chronic physical illness or handicap on young, school-age children is a complex biopsychosocial task. The child's capacity for coping with these stressful realities is intertwined with transactions among medical, family, and social support networks. Pediatric and psychiatric reviews by Nagera (1978), Prugh and Eckhard (1974), Prugh, Staub, Sands, Kirschbaum, and Lenihan (1953), and Vernon, Foley, Sipowicz, and Schulman (1965), among others, document multiple developmental and familial parameters which influence a child's adaptation and the family equilibrium. From these perspectives, deleterious individual adjustment depends largely upon the child's pre-illness stage of cognitive and affective development, previous coping capacities, prevailing parent–child relationships, current family homeostasis, and the psychological meaning of a specific illness. Other writers, while acknowledging the utility of a psychopathological model for comprehending disorders of coping, present the equally cogent view that illness or impairment introduces a constellation of adaptational tasks and challenges which, if successfully negotiated, may promote psychological growth (cf. Lipowski, 1970).

The author gratefully acknowledges comments on an earlier draft by Melissa R. Johnson, Morton J. Schwartz, Lon E. Ussery, and James A. Whitt.

The inability of clinicians to reliably predict child and family adjustment lends credence to these observations—the developmental resilience of many children is truly remarkable. Children often seem invulnerable to the stressful onset of disease, physical deterioration, lengthy hospitalizations, continued and often painful treatment procedures, disruptions in family and school routines, and even threat to life (Rutter, 1979). What factors determine the impact of chronic illness on a child? Why does this challenge to the maturational process impede or derail development in some children, yet strengthen the developmental momentum of others? What skills and coping styles facilitate adaptation? What roles do the family, the social support network, and the health care system play in the child's adjustment? What comprehensive pediatric care programs benefit childhood adaptation? How might professionals predict at diagnosis the effects of illness on a child, thus justifying subsequent allocation of limited psychological support resources among families?

The present chapter explores these questions by first reviewing the normal developmental tasks of childhood and describing illness onset from the young child's point of view. Then a conceptual framework of childhood adaptation to chronic illness will be summarized along with four areas of clinical research: (1) stage-specific childhood reactions to illness and treatment procedures; (2) children's comprehension of illness; (3) the effects of change in interaction patterns between children with chronic illness and their network of family and social support; and (4) long-term childhood adaptation to chronic illness. Finally, implications for the pediatric health care system and future directions will be discussed.

Developmental Context of the Diagnosis

The normal developmental challenges and tasks of young school-age children set the stage on which chronic illness plays out its drama. Leaps and pauses in physical growth, cognitive and linguistic abilities, affective maturation, personality style, and relationships with extended family, peer, and social systems influence the child's capacity for adaptation. The growth of competence is a powerful developmental force. Unless thwarted by emotional insecurity, lagging physical maturation, or environmental demands for precocious coping, children are not content to attain a stable equilibrium with the world. Effectance motivation (cf. Piaget, 1963/1947; White, 1959) fuels the child's active progression along developmental lines including cognitive mastery of environmental incongruities, attainment of social relationships, and development of self-concept, identity, and a role in society. Prodded by the growth of body and mind, enticed by greater independence and new prerogatives, challenged by broadening fields of personal interaction, and lured by fresh social opportunities, the child strives to expand and exercise his or her competence in the mastery of the novel—neither too easy nor too difficult—challenges which characterize each stage of childhood (Breger, 1974; Lidz, 1976). However, the pace of development is also set by the need for emotional security. As Lidz (1976) summarizes, confronting novel tasks also brings insecurity, inability to master new challenges creates frustration, and greater independence requires renunciation of the comforts of dependency.

It is the opposing forces of anxiety versus security on one hand, and growth of competence versus inertia on the other which define the developmental risk besetting the child with chronic illness. That is, normally integrated development is characterized by secure and competent self-identifications which develop from relationships in which the child *actively* encounters other persons and situations, where his or her actions and communications have a meaningful and predictable effect (cf. Breger, 1974). Anxious and more dissociative development seems to follow experiences which are *passively* endured, traumas which occur to but are not mastered by the child.

Before pursuing the implications of this concept, a brief look at the cognitive, intrapsychic, and interpersonal characteristics of childhood development is in order. While a comprehensive review is beyond the scope of the present chapter, Table 4.1 highlights key stages from selected theoretical lines of childhood development. (The interested reader is referred for further elaboration to summary volumes by Breger, 1974, Engel, 1962, and Lidz, 1976, or original writings from developmental theorists including Piaget, Freud, Sullivan, and Erickson.)

While tracing differing perspectives of the developmental process, the theories outlined hold in common several basic tenets: (1) the life cycle unfolds in stages rather than at a steady pace; (2) there is an invariant order to the stages of development; (3) no stage can be successfully skipped; (4) each successive stage qualitatively alters the child's capacities for interaction with and adaptation to the environment, as contrasted to merely reflecting accruing experiential history; and (5) each stage is the result of a transformation—the evolution of a more complex, differentiated, and integrated version of the development phenomenon that preceded it (Breger, 1974). Temporary fixation at a stage of development and regression to an earlier stage may occur as expediencies to regain stability when too rapid developmental progression or external threat upsets equilibrium and increases the child's fearfulness and anxiety. If the fixation or regression becomes permanent, subsequent development may cease or be limited by repetitive attempts to cope with tasks of prior stages. Failure to master the essential challenges of a developmental stage leaves the child unprepared to accept the next phase and its developmental problems and opportunities.

Table 4.1. Theoretical Stages of Childhood Development by Chronological Age

	Approximate Chronological Age of Child (Years)													
Developmental Perspective	0	1	2	3	4	5	6	7	8	9	10	11	12	13–19
Cognitive stage (cf. Piaget)	Sensorimotor			Preoperations						Concrete operations				Formal operations
Intrapsychic stage (cf. Freud)	Oral			Anal			Phallic			Latency				Genital
Psychosocial crisis (cf. Erickson)	Basic trust vs. mistrust			Autonomy vs. shame & doubt			Initiative vs. guilt			Industry vs. inferiority				Identity vs. identity confusion
Interpersonal context of development	Maternal person			Parental persons			Nuclear family			Neighborhood, same-sex peers, school				Peer group
Stage-specific vulnerability	Abandonment			Loss of control			Bodily injury			Loss of group approval				Self-concept distortion

Cognitive Development

Cognitive development, for example, proceeds from the undifferentiated state of sensations and reflexes at birth; to an infantile physical (sensory and motor) interaction with the environment; to a crude form of symbolic (intuitive) thinking; to a more precise, yet still literal and concrete mode of thought; to, finally, the ability to manipulate logical abstractions (Ginsburg & Opper, 1969). Piaget (1952/1936; 1963/1947) described these principal intellectual stages as the sensorimotor stage, covering the first eighteen to twenty-four months of a child's life; the stage of preoperational thinking from about one-and-one-half to six years; concrete operations from six or seven years to eleven years; and formal operations, which spans early adolescence through adulthood. (Stages of childhood development are somewhat related to chronological age; however, due to the uniqueness of maturational time tables and individual children's experiential histories, all age norms must be considered approximate.)

The often imperceptible steps between these stages represent giant leaps forward in a child's capacity to understand new and more complex concepts of illness and health care phenomena (Papalia & Olds, 1975). Preoperational children's growing acquisition of language, competence with deferred imitation and symbolic play, and use of complex classificatory strategies, however, make it easy to overestimate their conceptual abilities. The preschool child's thought remains empirical rather than logical in nature and is dominated by the static, perceptual characteristics of events (Ginsburg & Opper, 1969). Egocentrism characterizes thought during this stage. The viewpoint of the child is not differentiated from the perspectives of other people. Time is present-centered, consisting of a series of succeeding "nows." The tendency of the preoperational child to center (or focus) on a single aspect of a situation, while neglecting other important features, often leads to patently illogical conclusions. For these children, reality is as it is perceived, a form of reasoning which, along with belief that the world is purposive (everything has a reason or cause, nothing is arbitrary or by chance), explains the preschooler's penchant toward phenomenalistic causality—the belief that when two events occur in succession, the first "causes" the second (Papalia & Olds, 1975).

The onset of concrete operational thinking ushers in the initial manifestations of logical thought. In contrast to the younger preoperational child whose attention centers on a single, static perception of an experience, the concrete operational child accomplishes a more balanced "decentered" analysis of the data at hand. Although the acquisition of abstract logical processes must await the stage of formal operations, children between seven and eleven years of age are able to focus simultaneously on several dimensions of a situation, recognize the sequence of actions involved in apparent perceptual transformations, and reverse the direction of thinking to justify their logical conclusions (Ginsburg & Opper, 1969). The shift from primitive egocentric thinking to more concretely logical judgments around the age of six or seven years marks a fundamental developmental change. It is not merely coincidental that as these alterations in the structure of the child's thought occur, formal education is initiated, belief in Santa Claus and his imaginal colleagues comes to an end (Prentice, Schmechel, & Manosevitz, 1979), and spontaneous symbolic play is replaced by rule-guided games with peers.

Intrapsychic Development

Freud (cf. 1953) traced five stages of psychosexual development between birth and maturity: the oral (birth to one-and-one-half years), anal (one-and-one-half to three years), phallic (three to about five-and-one-half years), latency (five-and-one-half to twelve years), and genital (from puberty onward). The constructs advanced by Freud not only reflect the primary focus of bodily energy and gratification, but also draw attention to key aspects of child development and parent–child interaction during each phase. Thus, while toilet training is a principal task for the toddler in the anal stage, the broader issue is the emergence of autonomy manifest in the child's active strivings for independence and the resultant clash with authority as social restraits are imposed on the child's willful actions (Breger, 1974).

The phallic and latency stages are central to the period explored in the present chapter. According to Freud, the phallic stage heralds the conflict between intrafamilial sexual desires—the love of a boy for his mother and a girl for her father—and the universal incest taboos which pressure for the renunciation of this "family romance." As fears of retribution or abandonment lead the child to relinquish and repress these aspirations, the child identifies more strongly with the parent of the same sex, thereby developing a sense of guilt, the internalized representation of parental punishment and disapproval (Lidz, 1976). Harsh demands of conscience are often inferred from children's increased fearfulness, nightmares, and anxieties during this period (Jersild & Holmes, 1935). Yet as conscience becomes established and the intrafamilial turbulence subsides, the child becomes more independent and dependable, a resolution which expedites childhood entry into latency, a phase during which the autonomous acquisition of culturally prized skills, values, and roles is paramount.

In a more general sense, the child in the Oedipal transition must relinquish feelings of being the mother's primary source of affection and interest and accept a more delimited position in the family unit (Lidz, 1976). While the fate of the Oedipal situation depends on a variety of factors, a firm coalition between parents who maintain boundaries between the two generations denies a child the opportunity to fill an empty space in the adult generation. Rather, the youngster enters the "latency period" properly established as a boy or girl in relation to the adult parents.

During latency, gender identification with the same-sex parent is strengthened by peer play which heightens competence and social skills. Psychoanalytic thought (cf. Freud) offers relatively little regarding this period, which is viewed primarily as a moratorium between the psychosexual demands of the Oedipal period and the pubertal launching of the genital stage of development. However, Erickson's account of sociocultural aspects of childhood development reveals this period to be far from latent.

Psychosocial Development

Erickson (1950) mapped the sociocultural crises in each of "eight ages of man" which influence the development of personality and identity. Thus, according to Erickson, the opportunity to establish an enduring pattern of basic trust over mistrust is created by caregiving which combines the sensitive appreciation of the baby's needs with a strong personal reliability. Also completed by four or five years of age is the establishment of autonomy over shame and doubt, a crisis which parallels the regulation of toileting behavior advanced by psychoanalytic theorists. Erickson's third stage concludes as children resolve the Oedipal transition and, having tamed their exuberant imaginations and learned necessary self-restraint, find their interest in and capacities for relationships shifting to persons outside the family. The basic crisis for these preschoolers is between initiative, which enables them to undertake, plan, and carry out their activities, and guilt (resulting from both the Oedipal conflict and the rigidity of the developing superego) over what they wish to do.

With the development of trust, autonomy, and initiative during the preschool years, children separate themselves from the objects of their first attachment, their parents, and confront the crisis (crucial for the present chapter) of industry versus inferiority. Entry into school symbolizes the issues of this period. Children now begin to function in the world beyond their homes, establish positions in a peer group, and win recognition by their own efforts. In so doing, their self-concept, value systems, and cognitive capacities change. Unless children acquire a sense of industry during this time, they develop pervasive feelings of inferiority and inadequacy (Erickson, 1950). Assurance of belonging gained from being accepted as an integral part of the peer group becomes evident (Lidz, 1976). A sense of responsibility, the willingness and capacity to live up to expectations, evolves as children "prove" that they can be relied on for their skills. Self-concepts which emerge during this period are highly dependent on peer group standards—rules framed within the context of the classroom or playground setting. As elaborated by Sullivan (1953), children's valuation of belonging and being an active, loyal, reliable, and responsible member of the group (as well as having a special friend or "chum") reflects movement toward intimacy beyond the family. It is against this backdrop of ever-widening social and intellectual competence, concurrent lessening of intrapsychic anxiety and fearfulness, and preoccupation with growing and learning *outside* the family, that childhood illness may have its greatest impact.

Chronic Illness from a Child's Perspective

How does a child experience the diagnosis and treatment of chronic illness? What variables define, for the schoolchild, the significance of handicapping conditions? Obviously, pediatric health care professionals can neither sanction a respite from the normal demands of childhood nor endow the child with advantageous emotional, cognitive, and social maturity. It is with existing strengths and weaknesses that ill children face the kaleidoscopic series of events which can precipitate psychological distress, modify life-style, erode self-concept, and impair social relationships (Heisler & Friedman, 1981).

Consider the cognitive dilemmas and discrepancies introduced to a child with epilepsy by symptom onset, diagnostic medical procedures, treatment regimens, and even hospitalization (cf. Steward & Steward, 1981; Whitt, 1982; Whitt, Dykstra, & Taylor, 1979). The initial seizure is often associated with intense alarm and excitement (Bridge, 1947). Preceded only by vague feelings of apprehension or an unfamiliar sensory aura, alterations of consciousness may cloud the child's awareness of the seizure. Awakening to find his or her family near panic and the physician prescribing daily medication, the child may comprehend little of what has happened. Descriptions of the seizure episode may be colored by the observer's anxiety—not infrequently voiced as, "it was like the devil was in you." The task of defining the parameters and consequences of the illness and pediatric care phenomena lies ahead for the child. Clearly, however, whatever transpired must have been serious!

Neurological examination, electroencephalography, and computerized axial tomography contribute little more to a child's understanding. Indeed, the diagnostic emphasis on the brain and its "waves" may especially bewilder the youngster, who perceives the body as "a bag of bones and blood" (Perrin & Gerrity, 1981). Even for the schoolchild, probing into the adequacy of the organ system which "makes you think smart," raises significant apprehensions (Whitt, 1982). Physicians, who arrive at diagnostic conclusions by linking together the physical symptomatology, clinical history, and laboratory data like interlocking pieces of a puzzle, may fail to recognize the child's perplexity and neglect to explain the illness and medical procedures. Alternately, health care professionals may offer explanations mismatched to the child's cognitive level. Anecdotal illustrations of the resultant "quaint" character of children's perceptions of illness (e.g., "a demon [edema] in my belly"; the withdrawn diabetic child's fear that she would "die of Beetes") are common to most medical centers (Bibace & Walsh, 1979; Perrin & Gerrity, 1981; Whitt, 1982).

In the absence of medical clarity, interactions with other significant persons may further validate the child's illness distortions. Hospitalization for observation and/or continuous EEG monitoring may precipitate feelings of helplessness, isolation, and abandonment if the child is separated from supportive caregivers. "Doctor shopping" in search of a more palatable diagnosis may confirm distress as well as entail repetition of confusing physical exams. Parental anxiety, fears, and guilt often prompt untoward alterations of attitudes and behavior toward the "sick" child. Fortunately, parents generally become overprotective and indulgent, rather than rejecting their now "defective" offspring, blaming the child for financial inconvenience, or neglecting necessary medical care. Any amendment to time-honored patterns of parent–child interaction, discipline, and family routine, however, puzzles the child, giving rise to questions of causality which, like the illness itself, require explanation. Many children with chronic illness conclude, "I know I'm very sick (or dying) because everyone treats me differently. Before I became ill, my parents never let me get away with bad behavior. Now, I can even hit my little sister without being punished" (Whitt et al., 1979; Whitt, 1982). Unexplained "kindness" by previously rivalrous siblings (who may later resent deprivation of parental attention) or surges of sympathetic gift-giving by relatives and friends may similarly attest to the serious nature of an illness for the young child, particularly when followed by estrangement as these persons no longer "know what to say."

Peer, classmate, and teacher reactions may also be disconcerting to the child struggling to define the parameters of his or her illness. Classmates seeking to establish boundaries which reassure them that they will not fall victim to these frightening seizures may exclude the "crippled," "retarded," or "crazy" child from group games because "epilepsy is contagious." Having a chronically ill child in the classroom often evokes affective responses from the teacher which mirror those seen in parents. Teachers may shower the child with favored classroom tasks, allow voluntary participation in academic activities, and/or tolerate inappropriate behavior. A lack of information about epilepsy, inadequate preparation for dealing with seizure episodes, concerns about managing added classroom stress, or related educational frustrations may lead other teachers to detach emotionally from the student (Deasy-Spinetta, 1981; Isaacs & McElroy, 1980). The consequences of these reactions—solicitude, anxiety, or withdrawal—create an unsettled academic climate and stress the teachers upon whose stability classroom performance depends. "Resolution" is sometimes achieved through rationalized separation of the child into special programs or isolation in the care of a homebound teacher.

Once the mismatch is identified between the child's inner experience of illness onset and the maturational constraints on his or her abilities to master these dilemmas, the potentially devastating impact of chronic illness and handicapping conditions on childhood development follows rather easily. Faced with disruption of the family system, adults who become increasingly solicitous regarding minor life events, limitations on previously enjoyed activities, and distinctive treatment from classmates and siblings, the chronically ill child's apprehension may spiral about what it is that has provoked such change and chaos (Whitt et al., 1979). Unwilling to merely accept the gaps in their knowledge created by developmental limitations and voids in adult communication, children often complete their "understanding" of illness with idiosyncratic interpretations, embrace their "differences" from other children, and modify their self-concepts to include a "defective" body and the "sick role" life-style. In contrast to the determined spirit which characterizes much of childhood development, this more vulnerable self-image often sets in motion an enduring cycle of loss of control, increasing dependency, and helplessness. The child, in a sense, becomes a prisoner of the illness, guarded by well-intentioned parents who shield him from the demands and expectations necessary to activate underlying potential and gain access to the social world (Kearsley, 1979). The resultant absence of mastery, competence, and initiative may further isolate the child, particularly during the school years when industry and peer group participation are paramount. Finally, feelings of vulnerability and inadequacy may become self-fulfilling if, paradoxically, the child withdraws from developmental contention and sustains (or even provokes) interpersonal rejection in order to maintain the now internalized identity as a vulnerable, crippled, socially abandoned person who must depend on close family members for needed care.

Impact of Chronic Illness on the Child

Pediatric professionals attempting to investigate the impact of chronic pediatric illness or design preventive programs of comprehensive health care confront a thorny network of factors which influence the child's cognitive appraisal, emotional reactions, coping strategies, therapeutic compliance, and ultimate adaptation to a handicapping condition. Early psychodynamic studies tended to cast mastery of environmental stress in terms of intrapsychic defense mechanisms which allow individuals to maintain psychological equilibrium (Mechanic, 1974). Noting individual patterns of adaptation which exceeded the apparent limits of predisposing personality characteristics, other investigators have explored both the general phenomenon of adjustment to life change (cf. Holmes & Rahe, 1967; Coddington, 1972) and the more specific issues of individual vulnerability, coping strategies, and adaptation to severe illness or injury (e.g., Weisman, 1978). These clinicians (e.g. Caplan, 1981; Kaplan, 1981, Lipowski, 1969; White, 1974) have outlined sequential phases of individual efforts exerted to cope with life changes including loss of significant relationships, separations, unexpected successes or failures, and milestones of family life—birth, school entry, graduation, and so on. As a result, clinicians and empiricists alike increasingly recognize the complex of biopsychosocial determinants which affect children's mastery of acute stress and chronic disease.

Consider the clinical and empirical questions raised by the variability in illness, child background, disease course, family structure, and social support network which characterize this population. For example, what relative importance is the child's age, sex, intelligence, or premorbid personality style in coping with the onset of a handicapping condition (Geist, 1979)? To what extent does initial coping prophesy a child's adaptation throughout the disease course? What is the primary stress to adjustment—illness onset and diagnosis, prolonged treatment, fear of relapse, chronic ambiguity, alteration of normal routines, or concerns about future competence? How do illnesses vary in their interference with development? Does suddenness of disease onset, absence of concretely experienced disease symptoms, existence of threat to life, presence of painful, restrictive, or intrusive treatment procedures, or discontinuity of physician–child relationships directly impede childhood adjustment? Or is adaptation to illness and health care variables modulated by the family's appraisal of significant threat? How do disease characteristics (i.e., organ system complexity, symptom perceptual cues, functional deficits) interact developmentally with the child's capacity for logical thought to first limit, then allow, illness comprehension? Can family coping with illness onset maintain the child's developmental status quo against the pulls of increased dependency, yet effectively place advances toward future childhood initiative, industry, and competence "on hold" until the completion of medical treatment (van Eys, 1981)? Is "reentry" into the community a universal and problematic stage of the adaptation process, or do these difficulties exist only for children who disengage, taking an extended hiatus from social development?

While broad in scope and difficult to answer empirically, these questions translate rather easily into the day-to-day experiences of the chronically ill child. Practical issues, as illustrated by a child's response to blood drawing or intravenous chemotherapy, provide the context for attitudinal transactions which shape the child's understanding, self-concept, and sense of control. Is protest to painful procedures viewed as a healthy or pathognomonic sign? Do pediatric caregivers accept passive compliance as a symbol of adjustment, or might they consider the possibility of inhibition in a child reconciled to poorly understood but punitive retribution? The answers to these questions, as well as the many unasked, are frequently prefaced, "it depends on several variables," a qualification which acknowledges the multifactorial, transactional, and developmental nature of children's adaptation.

A Conceptual Framework of Child Adaptation to Chronic Illness

Exploration of the impact of chronic childhood illness requires a conceptual framework which encompasses multiple developmental factors, illness variables, and social transactions (Cohen & Lazarus, 1979; Drotar, 1981; Mechanic, 1974). Childhood adaptation to chronic illness is a continuing process; onset is not the only illness stress. The feelings and attitudes toward chronic illness, self-concept patterns, and illness roles which evolve over time necessitate a model which reflects, at any point of inspection, the current balance among influences from both inside and outside the nuclear family and health care system.

The framework (modified from Pless & Pinkerton, 1975) presented in Figure 4.1 illustrates the complex of transactional systems—some interlocking, some overlapping, some encased one within another—which interact with and affect the child's appraisal of threat or security, coping strategies, self-concept, and adjustment to chronic illness (Zigler, in press). Successive cycles of adjustment (or maladjustment) evolve developmentally, spurred by symptomatic improvement (or deterioration); maturational gains (or losses) in the child's cognitive or affective capacity for coping; efficacious (or detrimental) communication with health care professionals; stability (or alterations) in the routines of family, school, and community interaction; and enhanced social relationships (or rejection and isolation).

Despite a voluminous clinical literature on childhood chronic illness and handicapping conditions, few empirical studies adequately assess or control the variables included in the framework in Figure 4.1. This is not surprising; the patient population of most medical centers is insufficient to allow valid group comparisons of children even minimally categorized for type of illness; child age, intelligence, premorbid personality, and coping style; family pattern of adjustment; and socioeconomic status. As a result, most studies have focused on intellectual functioning or isolated personality traits, often combining illness types and/or studying camp children who, while more accessible, may also be more autonomous, come from higher functioning families, or have better controlled illness symptomatology. Pless and Pinkerton (1975) provide an excellent review of the hypotheses and trends found in this literature, as do earlier reviews by Chapman, Loeb, and Gibbons (1956) and Vernon and associates (1965). In

Figure 4.1. Conceptual Framework of Child Adaptation to Chronic Illness. (Modified from Pless & Pinkerton, 1975).

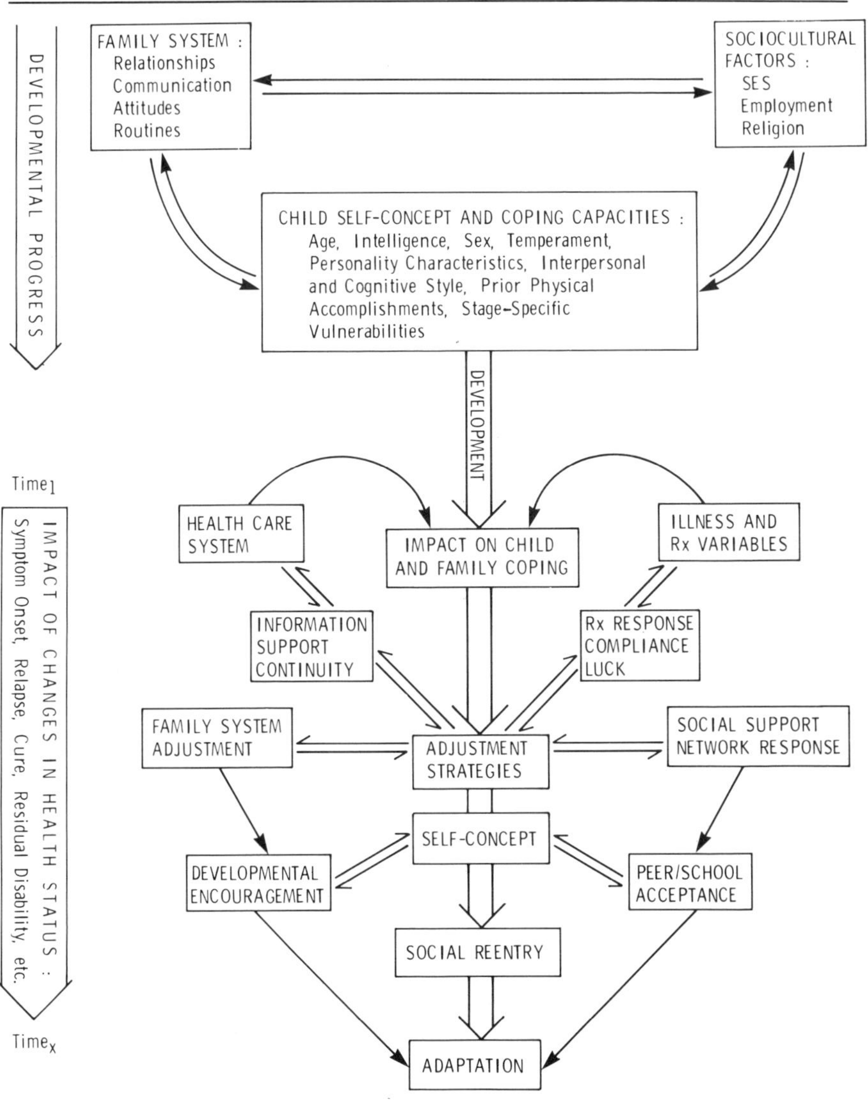

general, the available research supports the application of a multifactorial developmental framework, which may be clarified by inspecting selected findings from four areas: (1) children's reactions to illness and treatment demands; (2) children's comprehension of illness and medical procedures; (3) the impact of changing patterns of family routine and interactional style; and (4) long-term childhood adjustment to chronic illness.

Children's Reactions to Illness and Treatment Demands

A primary threat to childhood development of competence and security is the chronic illness or handicapping condition itself (Magrab & Calcagno, 1978). One has only to contrast children's enjoyment of a school drama or a playground game of softball with the rigors of regular renal dialysis to recognize the new priorities chronic illness may introduce. Excellent accounts of children's reactions to illness and treatment demands are found in Magrab (1978), Mattsson (1972), Nagera (1978), Prugh and Eckhardt (1980), and Vernon et al. (1965).

In general, children's behavioral responses include eating problems; sleep disturbances; enuresis or encopresis; tics; regression to more immature levels of behavioral and social functioning; depression, restlessness, and anxiety; fears of death; hypochondriacal concerns or delusions regarding bodily functions; phobic reactions to hospitals, medical staff, injections, and the like; frightened withdrawal from interpersonal contact; and hysterical symptomatology (Chapman et al., 1956). Prugh and Eckhardt (1980) organized children's responses to illness into the sequential phases of impact, recoil, and restitution. *Impact* encompasses the behavioral regression, bodily preoccupations, needs for nurturance, and massive denial of future outcome which accompany fears of death or "annihilation of the self." Lessening of the child's denial and regressive self-preoccupation, "mourning for the loss of self," and attempts to reestablish control over his or her environment mark the *recoil* phase. Finally, *restitution* brings increasing acceptance of the illness outcome, altered self-image, and the implications for an uncertain future.

Mattsson (1972), in addition to enumerating patterns which emerge in the child's and family's coping responses, summarizes the general interactions between illness and stage-specific developmental vulnerabilities. For example, restrictions on mobility due to orthopedic casting, bed rest, or isolation procedures run counter to very young children's reliance on motor activity to discharge tension, express dissatisfaction and aggression, and master environmental changes (Levy, 1944; Mattson, 1972; McDermott & Akina, 1972). Similarly, the observation that injections, infusions, and surgery often arouse more anxiety in the young child than the discomfort appears to warrant is linked to the universal childhood fears of bodily mutilation prevalent during the Oedipal stage (Mattsson, 1972;

Prugh et al., 1953). Although strides in cognitive and affective development better enable the school-age child to relinquish this earlier propensity (of children under seven) to view illness as punishment for real or imagined misdeeds, illness has implications for him as well. Particularly significant are situations of lengthy hospital care which foster renewed parent–child "closeness" at a time when normal relationship patterns are widening toward a more exclusive peer focus.

Certain health care phenomena also present specific interferences to the child's growth. Illnesses differ along dimensions including type, age at and suddenness of onset, course of disease, severity (life-threat), visibility of symptomatology, mental manifestations, need for hospitalization, and type (motor, sensory, cosmetic), duration, and severity of physical disability (Magrab & Calcagno, 1978; Pless & Douglas, 1971; Pless & Graham, 1970; Pless & Roghmann, 1971). It is generally assumed that the more severe a child's disability and the more visible the physical manifestations are to others, the more likely and extensive will be the child's emotional reactions. While most investigations find that children with chronic illness demonstrate psychological disturbance more frequently than healthy children of similar backgrounds (e.g., Pless & Roghmann, 1971; Rutter, Tizard, & Whitmore, 1970), some studies (Bruhn, Hampton, & Chandler, 1971; McAnarney, Pless, Satterwhite, & Friedman, 1974) report that children with diseases which produce little significant disability (e.g., epilepsy) may have more psychosocial problems than their physically disabled peers. Barker, Wright, and Gonick's (1953) concept of "marginality" acknowledged the heightened ambiguity experienced by children with minimal disabilities. These youngsters neither enjoy the benefit of being "normal" nor evoke the environmental support and allowances accorded more clearly handicapped children (Heisler & Friedman, 1981). Furthermore, although the nondisabled chronically ill child is unlikely to be regarded by others as "sick," hospital appointments and prescribed treatment serve as repeated reminders of his or her imperfect health (McAnarney et al., 1974).

Illness treatment requirements also vary considerably. Aggressive childhood cancer protocols are undoubtedly more stressful than the short-term symptomatic treatments prescribed for many other illnesses (Spinetta & Maloney, 1975; Spinetta, Rigler, & Karon, 1973). The emotional valence of illness changes when clinic visits take precedence over school attendance, when reverse isolation precludes peer interaction, and when apprehension about death supplants worry about getting braces. Moreover, a child's assessment of the effectiveness of these medical demands may be hindered if physical signs of improvement are indeterminate or when expectations for cure, symptom relief, or palliation vary over the course of the illness. For example, briefly consider the impact of three illnesses: epilepsy, end-stage renal disease, and leukemia.

Epilepsy. When anticonvulsant medication adequately controls their seizures, children with epilepsy may have little clear treatment-related interference. Poor seizure control, associated attentional deficits and behavioral side effects from near-toxic doses of drugs may be the only physical obstacles to daily functioning. However, issues of autonomy, self-concept, and peer relationships are frequently affected to some degree in the life of the child with epilepsy (Heisler & Friedman, 1981). Anxious anticipation of another seizure; rejection or taunting by peers frightened by seizure episodes; cultural mythology which equates epilepsy with mental illness, retardation, and behavioral aberrations (Bagley, 1972); and educational policies or societal regulations which delay major adolescent rites of passage—graduation and obtaining a driver's license—are but a few of the problems which may prolong dependency and reinforce a "crippled" self-concept.

End-stage Renal Disease. The majority of children with nephrotic syndrome respond to treatment and do not progress to end-stage kidney failure (Magrab & Papadopoulou, 1978). Individuals who do lose renal functioning choose between death and prolonged dependence on dialysis procedures (i.e., hemodialysis, peritoneal dialysis, CAPD) or transplantation. The problems imposed by dialysis are many, including the time commitment of several hours, three or more days per week, which may prevent normal participation in school and social activities (Abram, 1970). Security is difficult to achieve when perpetuation of life requires attachment to a machine. In addition to stimulating fantasies of bleeding to death (hemodialysis) or bursting as the abdominal cavity is repeatedly filled with fluid (peritoneal dialysis/CAPD), the immobility and dependency associated with extended time on the "artificial kidney" limit the child's growth of competence, mastery, and control. Moreover, since kidney machines are often located at distant medical centers, travel requirements may further diminish school attendance, limit peer interaction, and foster symbiotic ties to parental (usually maternal) caregivers—factors which run counter to the normal process of childhood development.

While kidney transplantation is an often desired outcome, it, too, is fraught with difficulties (Magrab & Papadopoulou, 1978). The idea of having a foreign body inside oneself can be extremely disturbing to a child recipient (Malekzadeh, Pennisi, Uittenbogaart, Korsch, Fine, & Main, 1976). What each child expects from transplantation is a life free from physical pain, restrictions of activity, and dietary constraints. Yet the early post-transplant period is characterized by anxiety, fear of rejection crises, surgical complications, infections, and daily variations of the blood, urea, nitrogen, and creatinine which constantly torment the child, family, and medical staff (Korsch, Negrete, Gardner, Weinstock, Mercer, Grushkin, & Fine, 1973; Magrab & Papadopoulou, 1978). Side effects secondary to the immunosuppressive drugs, the obesity and "moon faced" appearance secondary to steroid therapy, or failure to resume normal rates of growth may further threaten the child's psychological adjustment. If the kidney transplant fails, further crises emerge. Return to dialysis and physical pain is difficult for many children to tolerate; some children react with depressive symptoms, prolonged physical discomfort, or severe withdrawal (Bouras, Silvestre, Broyer, & Raimbault, 1976).

Leukemia. Children with leukemia face a different constellation of symptom and treatment interferences (e.g., Brunnquell & Hall, 1982). The word *cancer* evokes fears born during an era predating existing successes in long-term survivorship. Treatment is frequently painful. Bone marrow extraction, intrathecal spinal injections, and intravenous chemotherapy continue at close regular intervals over several years during which the child may experience hair loss, develop conditioned anticipatory nausea, and undergo a significant loss or gain in body weight. Despite these effects, the child in remission feels well, a paradox confusing when a drop in white blood count necessitates reverse isolation.

In summary, children's reactions to illness and handicapping conditions derive from many sources. Ambiguity regarding the illness etiology, uncertain expectations for symptomatic improvement or cure, and threat to life may interrupt future-oriented goals. Rigorous treatment procedures over which the child lacks control, increased symbiosis with parents and caregivers, loss of privacy, patterns of recurring clinic visits and hospitalization, fears of relapse or transplant rejection, and the avoidance of threat implicit in isolation precautions weaken previous childhood accomplishments. Although many clinicians hope that children will "get used to" illness stresses, empirical findings do not support this conclusion (Katz, Kellerman, & Seigel, 1980; Patenaude, Szymanski, & Rappeport, 1979; Powazek, Goff, Schyving, & Paulson, 1978). The risk is clear. In the absence of effective informational and emotional support (cf. McCollum, 1981; Reddihough, Landau, Jones, & Rickards, 1977; Visintainer & Wolfer, 1975), children may abandon active attempts to master the situation in favor of a more passive acquiescence to their illness.

Children's Understanding of Illness

Communication of disease concepts and medical treatment procedures to children is a difficult task for the pediatric health care system (Korsch, 1973; MacCarthy, 1974). Although the efficacy of pediatric care may depend at times upon the child's comprehension of illness and active participation in ongoing treatment, pediatric professionals are often uncertain as to what is "concrete" information for each child (Whitt et al., 1979; Whitt & Dykstra, 1981). Like comprehension of birth (Bernstein & Cowan, 1975), death (Childers & Wimmer, 1971; Koocher, 1973), religion (Elkind, 1962), and humor (McGhee, 1974; Shultz, 1974; Whitt & Prentice, 1977), children's views of bodily functions, illness, and hospitalization not only differ qualitatively from adult perspectives but also vary substantially according to the child's stage of development (Whitt et al., 1979).

Recent investigators (Bibace & Walsh, 1979, 1980; Carandang, Folkins, Hines, & Steward, 1979; Myers-Vando, Steward, Folkins, & Hines, 1979; Newhauser, Amsterdam, Hines, & Steward, 1978; Perrin & Gerrity, 1981; Simeonsson, Buckley, & Monson, 1979; Steward & Steward, 1981; Whitt et al., 1979) have postulated a maturational progression of children's understanding of illness causality, health care, and medical treatment procedures which parallels the theory of intellectual development advanced by Piaget (cf. 1963/1947). Further research is required to disentangle the confounded effects of age, Piagetian stage of cognitive development, stress of treatment procedures and/or hospitalization, and personality characteristics on children's illness conceptions; to clarify the perceptual salience of illness symptom cues (Whitt et al., 1979); and to assess the quality of physician explanations (Whitt & Dykstra, 1981). (For further discussion see methodological critique by Whitt, 1982). This conceptual framework, however, may guide professionals in providing illness explanations which are both accurate and within the child's cognitive capacity for understanding.

The available data (Bibace & Walsh, 1979, 1980; Perrin & Gerrity, 1981; Simeonsson et al., 1979) suggest a developmental taxonomy of children's comprehension which progresses in discrete stages from magical, egocentric causality toward a more abstract, comprehensive understanding of health and illness phenomena. In general terms, the research cited suggests that given the cognition characteristic of children less than four years of age, explanations and reason may be secondary to the protective presence of emotionally supportive caregivers (Blos, 1978). Even older preoperational stage children, despite their rapid cognitive and linguistic maturation, are unlikely to fully understand internal organ systems, link together illness symptoms, or assimilate the mechanisms of therapeutic change. Explanations for these children must be perceptually based, with an ear tuned to the reverberations of the inevitable distortions (for illustrations, see Whitt et al., 1979; Whitt, 1982). With the onset of concrete operational thinking around seven years, the child begins to comprehend the relationship between one observable occurrence (e.g., ingesting a "germ") and a perceptual cue from the illness (e.g., chicken pox sores). Disease now may be attributed to germs, albeit with little recognition of the interaction between these etiologic agents and the susceptibility of internal organ systems. Only with the onset of formal operational thinking around eleven or twelve years does the child have the capacity to comprehend illness in the abstract terms of unseen physiological systems whose disfunction is manifest by external symptom cues. This capacity for abstract thought and the ability to understand the contributory interactions between illness agents and bodily susceptibility marks a fresh opportunity for preadolescent participation in preventive health care.

Changing Relationships among Social Systems and Children with Chronic Illness

Children's responses to stress are heavily influenced by changes in the attitudes, interpersonal relationships, communication patterns, and structured routines of their social support networks (Caplan, 1978; Heisler & Friedman, 1981; Mattsson, 1972; Whitt, Brantley, & Wise, 1982). Chronic childhood illness precipitates novel family challenges which thwart habitual problem-solving mechanisms, resulting in disequilibrium accompanied by feelings of anxiety, fear, anger, and guilt which may further contribute to the disorganization (Moos & Tsu, 1977). The effects on families (see, e.g., summaries by Kaplan, 1981; Kessler, 1977; Magrab & Calcagno, 1978; Mattsson, 1972; Moos & Tsu, 1977; Pond, 1979; Spinetta, 1978, 1981; Talbot & Howell, 1971; and Chapter 5 herein by Drotar, Crawford, & Bush) may include (1) parental mourning—denial, anger, acceptance—in response to relinquishing expectations for a healthy offspring; (2) parental disappointment, shame, or guilt over the child's unmet needs, parenting practices, or genetic heritage; (3) parental anxiety leading to overprotective, restrictive, or overindulgent caregiving; (4) concentration on the sick child to the extent that the needs of other famiy members may be neglected; (5) parental resentment or anger over the financial burden and temporal demands of medical treatment; (6) parental disinterest, neglect, or rejection of the "abnormal" child; (7) distortion and impoverishment of family life, parental fatigue, or depression; (8) sibling resentment of the patient's favored status; (9) sibling vulnerability to overprotective parental attitudes and caregiving practices; and (10) family grief and depression in premature anticipation of the sick child's death.

The adequacy of family functioning in spite of these effects affirms the child's coping. Indeed, in a rare empirical attempt to evaluate this contextual variable, Pless, Roghmann, and Haggerty (1972) found that families who obtained low indices of functioning were nearly twice as likely to have poorly adjusted sick children as families that functioned well. Likewise, Spinetta and his colleagues (e.g., Spinetta, 1981; Spinetta, McLaren, Deasy-Spinetta, Kung, Schwartz, and Hartman, 1981) reported the efficacy of family coping strategies and support mechanisms which encourage children with cancer to maintain a normal life, while participating as fully and successfully as possible in family, community, and regular school activities.

Children seem to recognize shifts in parental attitudes through changing interpersonal patterns of cognitive, affective, and behavioral transactions. Children may either protest these changes or accommodate to them. As previously noted, for example, the child with leukemia often requires reverse isolation during periods when white cell counts drop below the level necessary to fight off infection. When these counts return to normal, parents often are wary of discontinuing this secure arrangement, preferring to avoid risking any exposure to infection. Some children "buy into" this parental anxiety and sick role implications for imposed dependency, activity restrictions, and isolation from peers. One child was sullen and unresponsive even within the safety of her isolation room until an outside visit behind a protective mask gave her permission to risk greater activity and emotional mastery of her situation. Other children actively protest change, behaviorally demanding greater choice (e.g., of physician providing or arm receiving an injection) and control, as if to prove to themselves their continued competence. More stoic, or even counterphobic, protest may include denial of the illness to the extent that it may interfere with medical treatment compliance (Mattsson, 1972).

The ultimate return to family, peer, school, and community group interactions may not be unobtrusive for children with cosmetic disability (e.g., hair loss), surgical scars, or other physical anomalies. Yet, particularly for the child undergoing rigorous outpatient treatment, school participation offers a rare opportunity, devoid of medical focus, for chronically ill children to exercise control, gain competence, and prepare for the future like their peers (Deasy-Spinetta, 1981).

The relationship between family functioning and child adaptation to chronic illness and handicapping conditions requires further investigation. It is unclear which family system characteristics most influence childhood adaptation (or maladjustment). Chapter 5 by Drotar and his colleagues develops these issues more comprehensively. It should be apparent, however, that the distinction between child and family adaptation to illness is a false dichotomy, as is the categorization of "good" or "bad" coping when divorced from understanding the mode, function, and outcome of these strategies (Drotar, 1981). While "negative" changes in parent–child interactions are powerful determinants of children's attitudes, self-concept, and adjustment strategies, other family strategies (i.e., adaptive denial) for coping with the shock of illness diagnosis or treatment demands may herald renewed normal striving within the constraints of the child's impairment.

Long-term Adaptation to Chronic Childhood Illness

Thus far, this chapter has pursued the chronically ill child's potential for emotional and behavioral disturbance. In general, one might conclude (cf. Pless & Pinkerton, 1975) that: (1) *as a group*, children with chronic physical disorders have a greater frequency of maladjustment than their healthy peers of comparable backgrounds; (2) disease characteristics including age at onset, manner of progression, severity, prognosis, duration, and associated disability influence child and family adaptation; (3) pre-illness intelligence, coping style, personality, and other assets (attractiveness, charm, special skills, etc.) may prejudice childhood responses to disease; and (4) family functioning—the strength, warmth, and resilience of relationships within the system—and parental attitudes about the illness, its effects on their lives, and the day-to-day burdens it imposes, significantly influence the child's capacity for coping.

Clearly, children with chronic disease are "at risk" for emotional disorders (Green, 1965). But to what extent are these children destined to become deviant from their healthy peers? Estimates of the preponderance and severity of childhood maladjustment are disparate, a problem traceable to a prevalence of inadequate conceptual design and measurement techniques (Johnson, 1980). Comparison of research reports is complicated by variability in the target illnesses studies (e.g., controlled diabetes vs. leukemia in relapse), population sampled (e.g., psychiatric referrals vs. children attending diabetes camp), comprehensiveness of study period (e.g., longitudinal observations following diagnosis vs. single cross-sectional assessment), and relevance of measures (e.g., multifactorial assessment of the child and family system vs. testing of isolated personality traits). Furthermore, relatively few investigations have assessed social competence (cf. Anderson & Messick, 1974), as contrasted to the absence of psychopathology, or attempted to understand the strengths and tactics of children and families who cope well with chronic illness. Therefore, statements regarding the impact of childhood illness on personality functioning must be limited to available comparisons of group (e.g., ill vs. healthy children) data. Generalizations implying long-term maladjustment as it either applies *a priori* to an *individual* child or continues independent of illness and family system variables need to be expressed cautiously. A few studies may illustrate the more optimistic perspective of childhood adaptation to chronic illness.

Korsch and colleagues (1973) reported that after one year the personality and family functioning of thirty-five children transplanted successfully for end-stage renal disease had returned to pre-illness equilibrium comparable to control groups of other chronically ill or well children. The stress-maintaining role of illness and treatment was also emphasized by Poznanski, Miller, Salguero, and Kelsh (1978), who found a "striking correlation" between the areas of adjustment measured (school, social relationships, self-perception, and depressive feelings) and the status of the kidney transplant. They concluded that a thriving graft is mirrored by a more successful psychosocial adjustment, while the reverse is equally true. In another sample (Tavormina, Kastner, Slater, & Watt, 1976), 144 children with mild disability obtained scores on measures of personality dimensions and self-concept which matched the distribution patterns of "normal" children. Paradoxically, children's self-report of "normalcy" may indicate the adaptive denial of anxieties and impaired self-image, a mechanism now understood to foster adaptation to chronic disability (Heisler & Friedman, 1981; Kagen-Goodheart, 1977; Koocher & O'Malley, 1981; Lazarus, 1981; O'Malley, Koocher, Foster, & Slavin, 1979; Spinetta, 1981). On the basis of the individual differences and strengths demonstrated by their sample, however, the authors argue that a focus on "deviance" obscures the successful adaptation of most children with physical handicaps.

Awareness of the multiple factors influencing the emotional outcome of childhood chronic illness does not necessitate a pessimistic view for a specific child. Rather, this knowledge may bolster efforts to clarify individual differences and strategies for competent adaptation (cf. Lazarus, 1974; Weisman, 1978). Furthermore, aspects of social readjustment often not apparent to the medical care team may be more significant than previously appreciated. Bedell, Giordani, Amour, Tavormina, and Boll (1977) found that chronically ill children who experienced higher demands for social readjustment had poorer self-concepts than children with a lower, more normal amount of life stress. Although the camp population sampled limits generalization to independently functioning children, these results indicate the need to monitor life change events, not just illness stresses, as the child returns to normal activities.

Future efforts to redress the empirical neglect of successful adaptation may find "reentry" to be a key construct (cf. Hoffman & Futterman, 1971; Kagen-Goodheart, 1977; Koocher & O'Malley, 1981; Whitt et al., 1982). Renewed social competence and the sustained reinvolvement in transactions with family, peer, school, and community networks may be clearer indications of long-term adaptation than is the absence of psychopathology demonstrated on isolated measures of personality functioning.

Conclusions and Implications for the Pediatric Health Care System

Hopefully, awareness of characteristics associated with poor adjustment including (1) moderate to severe disability; (2) illnesses beginning before six years of age or during adolescence; (3) "marginal" sensory or cosmetic disorders; (4) families where low functioning—dissatisfaction with aspects of the marriage, difficulties with communication, or a lack of cohesiveness and mutual support—interferes with stability under stress; and (5) the absence of child and parent knowledge of the illness (Pless & Satterwhite, 1975), will lead to more effective and comprehensive care of children with chronic illness and their families. Central to the described conceptual framework are implications for the identification of family systems "at risk" for adaptational problems, preventive care programs, models of interdisciplinary team functioning, and directions for further research.

Identification of "At-risk" Children and Families

Chronic illness and handicapping conditions require that pediatric clinicians know the psychosocial characteristics of the children and families under their care. Pless and Satterwhite (1973) doubt that many pediatricians fully acquire or use information about families. This is particularly true at teaching hospitals and treatment centers where rotation of interns and residents necessarily leads to service changes and breaks in continuity of care. Efforts to minimize patterns of multiple caregivers and establish a "coordinating pediatrician" who takes responsibility for evaluating special needs, seeking solutions, and interpreting treatment plans may improve communication with families and help to establish a supportive, trusting relationship (Battle, 1972; Kanthor, Pless, Satterwhite, & Myers, 1974; Koocher & O'Malley, 1981). In this context, regular "emotional checkups" may target children and families for whom allocation of greater support efforts or alteration of normal patient care practices may be necessary. Family and child advocates (Satterwhite, 1978) and/or clinical protocols assessing parent–child conflict (Boll, Dimino, & Mattsson, 1978), parenting stress (Burke & Abidin, 1980), family functioning (Moos, 1974; Pless & Satterwhite, 1973; Spinetta, 1981; Stein & Riessman, 1980), or flexibility of family routines (Jensen, James, Boyce, & Hartnett, 1982; Whitt et al., 1982) prove to be useful adjuncts to the primary doctor–family relationship.

Programs of Comprehensive Preventive Care

As the tasks inherent to the challenge of chronic illness—coping with pain and incapacitation; dealing with the hospital environment and treatment procedures; developing adequate relationships with professional staff; preserving reasonable emotional balance, satisfactory self-image, and stable family and peer relationships; and preparing for an uncertain future—are identified (cf. Moos & Tsu, 1977), effective coping strategies may be *strengthened* by a comprehensive program of preventive pediatric care (Brantley, Stable, & Whitt, 1981; Spinetta, 1981). A number of activities are helpful.

First, in addition to the identification of a "coordinating pediatrician," it is invaluable to provide continuity of routine medical, nursing, and psychosocial professionals who, by recognizing the central role of families, accepting coping strategies as necessary tools for maintaining homeostasis, and by welcoming parents as competent co-managers of their child's care, create an emotionally supportive and cognitively honest context for health care. Pediatric clinicians who accept parental shock and disbelief as adaptive reactions to the discovery of their child's life-threatening illness will provide ample time and repetition necessary for families to fully "hear" the information and formulate questions. These physicians also recognize the appropriateness of depression and the adaptive nature of denial when exercised in the service of quality of life (Koocher & O'Malley, 1981; O'Malley et al., 1979; Spinetta, 1981; Vance, Fazan, Satterwhite, & Pless, 1980).

Special programs also may lessen the stress and uncertainty for the child patient. The importance of preparation for hospital admission (e.g., Melamed, Meyer, Gee, & Soule, 1976; Oremland & Oremland, 1972; Siegel, 1976), medical and surgical procedures (e.g., Melamed & Siegel, 1975; Petrillo & Sanger, 1980; Visintainer & Wolfer, 1975; Wolfer & Visintainer, 1979), and repeated discussion of illness phenomena and treatment regimes (e.g., Kellerman, Rigler, Siegel, & Katz, 1977; Spinetta & Deasy-Spinetta, 1981; Whitt et al., 1979) cannot be overemphasized. Hospital recreation provides children both an oasis of normal activity in the midst of unfamiliar routines and the chance to master surgical procedures, casting, injections, and other traumas by actively playing out the doctor–patient experience (Association for the Care of Children in Hospitals, 1979). Application of behavioral therapies (e.g., Magrab, 1975) relaxation and hypnosis (e.g., Gardner & Olness, 1981; Hartman, 1981; Moore, 1981; Zeltzer, Dash, & Holland, 1979), guided fantasy (e.g., Johnson, Martin, Whitt, & Weisz, 1980), and biofeedback (e.g., Davis, Saunders, Creer, & Chai, 1973; Knudson-Cooper, 1981), as well as more traditional psychotherapies (cf., Johnson, 1979), may both aid pain management and foster the sense of control necessary to engage optimistically in the activities of daily living (Nannis, Susman, Strope, Woodruff, Hersh, Levine, & Pizzo, 1982). Finally, opportunities for supportive interactions with other children having similar physical conditions (e.g., Magrab, 1975; Sheridan, 1975), outreach to the often neglected siblings and fathers of these patients (Lavigne & Ryan, 1979; Spinetta, 1981), and liaison efforts with teachers and others who may be pivotal in the child's "reentry" into community and school participation (e.g., Brantley et al., 1981; Deasy-Spinetta, 1981; Gliebe, 1979; Koocher & O'Malley, 1981; Spinetta & Deasy-Spinetta, 1981) have a place in the comprehensive care of chronically ill children.

Interdisciplinary Team Functioning

Physicians, however well-intentioned, vary considerably in their psychosocial care of chronically ill children and their families. Techniques for pain control, guided fantasy, hypnosis, and relaxation therapy are not often found in the repertoire of the pediatric clinician. Even if residency or fellowship training programs emphasized these skills, the demands of psychosocial care for chronically ill children outstrip the time and energy of the physician alone (Anthony, 1973). While expert problem-centered consultation is available at many medical centers (Naylor & Mattsson, 1973), organized team efforts to anticipate common patterns of family adaptational difficulty may provide more comprehensive support for the child and family than do reactions on an ad hoc basis (Brantley et al., 1981; Strauss & Glaser, 1975). Interdisciplinary teams of health care professionals representing medicine, nursing, mental health, education, physical therapy, nutrition, and recreation among others, not only provide varied competence, but also offer mutual support against the frustration, feelings of impotence, and ultimate "burnout" faced in the task of caring for chronically ill children over long periods of time (Heisler & Friedman, 1981; Koenig, 1981; Whitt, Hunter, Dykstra, Lauria, Stabler, & Taylor, 1981).

Need for Further Research

Finally, as our conceptual framework increasingly encompasses the complexities of the problem, clinical investigators can apply available methodology and multivariate measurement technology to broaden our understanding of the child characteristics; the illness- and treatment-related phenomena; and the features of the physical, family, health care, and sociocultural environments which facilitate children's adaptation to chronic illness and handicapping conditions. If, indeed, many families succeed in coping by using psychological mechanisms such as adaptive denial, a major task of clinical investigators is to identify other characteristics which auger well for mastery of illness demands. Kucia, Drotar, Doershuk, Stern, Boat, and Matthews (1979), for example, discovered more creative problem-solving patterns in families of well-adjusted children with cystic fibrosis, a characteristic which may be invaluable in reconciling the demands of daily physical treatment with the routines of family life.

In summary, the strength, courage, and determination of children who live fully challenge us to address the problems of chronic childhood illness with optimism, not despair. Hopefully, advances in medicine, psychosocial care strategies, and clinical research will offer increasingly effective support for children and families struggling to live, adapt well, and maintain their quality of life.

References

Abram, H. S. Survival by machine: The psychological stress of chronic hemodialysis. *Psychiatry in Medicine*, 1970, *1*, 37–51.

Anderson, S., & Messick, S. Social competency in young children. *Developmental Psychology*, 1974, *10*, 282–293.

Anthony, E. J. *The child in his family: The impact of disease and death*. New York: Wiley, 1973.

Association for the Care of Children in Hospitals. Child Life Activity Study Section Position Paper. Washington, D.C.: ACCH, 1979.

Bagley, C. Social prejudice and the adjustment of people with epilepsy. *Epilepsia*, 1972, *13*, 33–45.

Barker, R. G., Wright, B. A., & Gonick, M. A. *Adjustment to physical handicap and illness: A survey of the social psychology of physique and disability*. New York: Social Science Research Council, 1953.

Battle, C. U. The role of the pediatrician as ombudsman in the health care of the young handicapped child. *Pediatrics*, 1972, *50*, 916–922.

Bedell, J. R., Giordani, B., Amour, J. L., Tavormina, J., & Boll, T. Life stress and the psychological and medical adjustment of chronically ill children. *Journal of Psychosomatic Research*, 1977, *21*, 237–242.

Bernstein, A. C., & Cowan, P. A. Children's concepts of how people get babies. *Child Development*, 1975, *46*, 77–91.

Bibace, R., & Walsh, M. E. Developmental stages in children's conceptions of illness. G. C. Stone, F. Cohen, & N. E. Adler (Eds.), *Health psychology*. San Francisco: Jossey-Bass, 1979.

Bibace, R., & Walsh, M. E. Development of children's concepts of illness. *Pediatrics*, 1980, *66*, 912–917.

Blos, P. Children think about illness: Their concepts and beliefs. E. Gellert, (Ed.), *Psychosocial aspects of pediatric care*. New York: Grune & Stratton, 1978.

Boll, T. J., Dimino, E., & Mattsson, A. E. Parenting attitudes: The role of personality style and childhood long-term illness. *Journal of Psychosomatic Research*, 1978, *22*, 209–213.

Bouras, M., Silvestre, D., Broyer, M., & Raimbault, G. Renal transplantation in children: A psychological survey. *Clinical Nephrology*, 1976, *6*, 478–482.

Brantley, H. T., Stabler, B., & Whitt, J. K. Program considerations in comprehensive care of chronically ill children. *Journal of Pediatric Psychology*, 1981, *6*, 229–237.

Breger, L. *From instinct to identity: The development of personality*. Englewood Cliffs, N.J.: Prentice-Hall, 1974.

Bridge, E. M. Emotional disturbances in epileptic children. *Nervous Children*, 1947, *6*, 11–21.

Bruhn, J. G., Hampton, J. W., & Chandler, B. C. Clinical marginality and psychological adjustment in hemophilia. *Journal of Psychosomatic Research*, 1971, *15*, 207–213.

Brunnquell, D., & Hall, M. D. Issues in the psychological care of pediatric oncology patients. *American Journal of Orthopsychiatry*, 1982, *52*, 32–44.

Burke, W. T., & Abidin, R. R. Parenting stress index: A family system assessment approach. In R. R. Abidin (Ed.), *Parent education and intervention handbook*. Springfield, Ill.: Charles C. Thomas, 1980.

Caplan, G. Family support systems in a changing world. In E. J. Anthony & C. Chiland (Eds.), *The child and his family: Children and their parents in a changing world*. New York: Wiley, 1978.

Caplan, G. Mastery of stress: Psychosocial aspects. *American Journal of Psychiatry*, 1981, *138*, 413–420.

Carandang, M. L. A., Folkins, C. H., Hines, P. A., & Steward, M. S. The role of cognitive level and sibling illness in children's conceptualization of illness. *American Journal of Orthopsychiatry*, 1979, *49*, 474–481.

Chapman, A. H., Loeb, D. G., & Gibbons, M. J. Psychiatric aspects of hospitalizing children. *Archives of Pediatrics*, 1956, *73*, 77–88.

Childers, P., & Wimmer, M. The concept of death in early childhood. *Child Development*, 1971, *42*, 1299–1301.

Coddington, R. D. The significance of life events as etiologic factors in the diseases of children. *Journal of Psychosomatic Research*, 1972, *16*, 7–18.

Cohen, F., & Lazarus, R. Coping with the stress of illness. In G. C. Stone, F. Cohen, & N. E. Adler (Eds.), *Health psychology*. San Francisco: Jossey-Bass, 1979.

Davis, M. H., Saunders, D. R., Creer, T. L., & Chai, H. Relaxation training facilitated by biofeedback apparatus as a supplemental treatment in bronchial asthma. *Journal of Psychosomatic Research*, 1973, *17*, 121–128.

Deasy-Spinetta, P. The school and the child with cancer. In J. J. Spinetta & P. Deasy-Spinetta (Eds.), *Living with childhood cancer*. St. Louis: Mosby, 1981.

Drotar, D. Psychological perspectives in chronic childhood illness. *Journal of Pediatric Psychology*, 1981, *6*, 211–228.

Elkind, D. The child's conception of his religious denomination. *Journal of Genetic Psychology*, 1962, *101*, 185–193.

Engel, G. L. *Psychological development in health and disease*. Philadelphia: Saunders, 1962.

Erikson, E. H. *Childhood and society*. New York: Norton, 1950.

Freud, S. Three essays on the theory of sexuality. In *The standard edition of the complete psychological works of Sigmund Freud* (Vol. VII). London: Hogarth Press, 1953.)

Gardner, G. G., & Olness, K. *Hypnosis and hypnotherapy with children*. New York: Grune & Stratton, 1981.

Geist, R. A. Onset of chronic illness in children and adolescents: Psychotherapeutic and consultative intervention. *American Journal of Orthopsychiatry*. 1979, *49*, 4–23.

Ginsburg, H., & Opper, S. *Piaget's theory of intellectual development*. Englewood Cliffs, N.J.: Prentice-Hall, 1969.

Gliebe, W. A. Involuntary deviance: Schooling and epileptic children. *Journal of School Health*, 1979, *49*, 88–92.

Green, M. The management of long-term nonlife-threatening illnesses. In M. Green & R. J. Haggerty (Eds.), *Ambulatory pediatrics*. Philadelphia: Saunders, 1965.

Haggerty, R., Roghmann, K. J., & Pless, I. B. *Child health and the community*. New York: Wiley, 1975.

Hartman, G. A. Hypnosis as an adjunct in the treatment of childhood cancer. In J. J. Spinetta & P. Deasy-Spinetta (Eds.), *Living with childhood cancer*. St. Louis: Mosby, 1981.

Heisler, A. B., & Friedman, S. B. Social and psychological considerations in chronic disease: With particular reference to the management of seizure disorders. *Journal of Pediatric Psychology*, 1981, *6*, 239–250.

Hoffman, I., & Futterman, E. H. Coping with waiting. *Comprehensive Psychiatry*, 1971, *12*, 67–81.

Holmes, T. H., & Rahe, R. H. The social readjustment rating scale. *Journal of Psychosomatic Research*, 1967, *11*, 213–218.

Isaacs, J., & McElroy, M. R. Psychosocial aspects of chronic illness in children. *Journal of School Health*, 1980, *50*, 318–321.

Jensen, E. W., James, S. A., Boyce, W. T., & Hartnett, S. A. The family routines inventory: Development and validation. Unpublished manuscript, University of North Carolina, 1982.

Jersild, A. T., & Holmes, F. B. Children's fears. *Child Development Monographs*, 1935.

Johnson, M. R. Mental health interventions with medically ill children: A review of the literature 1970–1977. *Journal of Pediatric Psychology*, 1979, *4*, 147–163.

Johnson, M. R., Martin, B., Whitt, J. K., & Weisz, J. Anxiety reduction through fantasy in chronically ill and normal children. Paper presented at the meeting of the American Psychological Association, Montreal, September 1980.

Johnson, S. B. Psychosocial factors in juvenile diabetes: A review. *Journal of Behavioral Medicine*, 1980, *3*, 95–115.

Kagen-Goodheart, L. Re-entry: Living with childhood cancer. *American Journal of Orthopsychiatry*, 1977, *47*, 651–658.

Kanthor, H., Pless, B., Satterwhite, B., & Myers, G. Areas of responsibility in the health care of multiply handicapped children. *Pediatrics*, 1974, *54*, 779–785.

Kaplan, D. M. Interventions for acute stress experiences. In J. J. Spinetta & P. Deasy-Spinetta (Eds.), *Living with childhood cancer*. St. Louis: Mosby, 1981.

Katz, E. R., Kellerman, J., & Siegel, S. E. Behavioral distress in children with cancer undergoing medical procedures: Developmental considerations. *Journal of Consulting and Clinical Psychology*, 1980, *48*, 356–365.

Kearsley, R. B. Iatrogenic retardation: A syndrome of learned incompetence. In R. B. Kearsley & I. E. Sigel (Eds.), *Infants at risk*. Hillsdale, N.J.: Lawrence Erlbaum, 1979.

Kellerman, J., Rigler, D., Siegel, S., & Katz, E. R. Disease-related communication and depression in pediatric cancer patients. *Journal of Pediatric Psychology*, 1977, *2*, 52–53.

Kessler, J. W. Parenting the handicapped child. *Pediatric Annals*, 1977, *6*, 654–661.

Knudson-Cooper, M. S. Relaxation and biofeedback training in the treatment of severely burned children. *Journal of Burn Care and Rehabilitation*, 1981, *2*, 102–110.

Koenig, H. M. Reflections of a pediatric cancer specialist. In J. J. Spinetta & P. Deasy-Spinetta (Eds.), *Living with childhood cancer*. St. Louis: Mosby, 1981.

Koocher, C. P. Childhood, death, and cognitive development. *Developmental Psychology*, 1973, *9*, 369–375.

Koocher, C. P., & O'Malley, J. E. (Eds.). *The Damocles syndrome: Psychosocial consequences of surviving childhood cancer*. New York: McGraw-Hill, 1981.

Korsch, B. M. The pediatrician's approach to his patient. *American Journal of Diseases of Children*, 1973, *126*, 146–148.

Korsch, B. M., Negrete, V. F., Gardner, J. E., Weinstock, C., Mercer, A. S., Grushkin, C. M., & Fine, R. N. Kidney transplantation in children: Psychological follow-up study on child and family. *Journal of Pediatrics*, 1973, *83*, 399–408.

Kucia, C., Drotar, D., Doershuk, C., Stern, R. C., Boat, T. F., & Matthews, L. Home observation of family interaction and childhood adjustment to cystic fibrosis. *Journal of Pediatric Psychology*, 1979, *4*, 189–196.

Lavigne, J. V., & Ryan, M. Psychologic adjustment of siblings of children with chronic illness. *Pediatrics*, 1979, *63*, 616–627.

Lazarus, R. S. Psychological stress and coping in adaptation and illness. *International Journal of Psychiatry in Medicine*, 1974, *5*, 321–333.

Lazarus, R. S. The costs and benefits of denial. In J. J. Spinetta & P. Deasy-Spinetta (Eds.), *Living with childhood cancer*. St. Louis: Mosby, 1981.

Levy, D. M. On the problem of movement restraint. *American Journal of Orthopsychiatry*, 1944, *14*, 644–671.

Lidz, T. *The person, his and her development throughout the life cycle*. New York: Basic Books, 1976.

Lipowski, Z. J. Psychosocial aspects of disease. *Annals of Internal Medicine*, 1969, *71*, 1197–1206.

Lipowski, Z. J. Physical illness, the individual and the coping process. *Psychiatry in Medicine*, 1970, *1*, 91–102.

MacCarthy, D. Communication between children and doctors. *Developmental Medicine and Child Neurology*, 1974, *16*, 279–285.

Magrab, P. Psychological management and renal dialysis. *Journal of Clinical Psychology,* 1975, *4,* 38–41.

Magrab, P. (Ed.). *Psychological management of pediatric problems* (Vol. 1). *Early life conditions and chronic diseases*. Baltimore: University Park Press, 1978.

Magrab, P. R., & Calcagno, P. L. Psychological impact of chronic pediatric conditions. In P. R. Magrab (Eds.), *Psychological management of pediatric problems*. Baltimore: University Park Press, 1978.

Magrab, P. R., & Papadopoulou, Z. L. Renal disease. In P. R. Magrab (Ed.), *Psychological management of pediatric problems*. Baltimore: University Park Press, 1978.

Malekzadeh, M. H., Pennisi, A. J., Uittenbogaart, C. H., Korsch, B. M., Fine, R. N., & Main, M. E. Current issues in pediatric renal transplantation. *Pediatric Clinics of North America,* 1976, *23,* 857–872.

Mattsson, A. Long-term physical illness in childhood: A challenge to psychosocial adaptation. *Pediatrics,* 1972, *50,* 801–811.

McAnarney, E. R., Pless, I. B., Satterwhite, B., & Friedman, S. B. Psychological problems of children with chronic juvenile arthritis. *Pediatrics,* 1974, *53,* 523–528.

McCollum, A. T. *The chronically ill child*. New Haven: Yale University Press, 1981.

McDermott, J. F., & Akina, E. Understanding and improving the personality development of children with physical handicaps. *Clinical Pediatrics,* 1972, *11,* 130–134.

McGhee, P. E. Cognitive mastery and children's humor. *Psychological Bulletin,* 1974, *81,* 721–730.

Mechanic, D. Social structure and personal adaptation: Some neglected dimensions. In G. V. Coelho, D. A. Hamburg, & J. T. Adams (Eds.), *Coping and adaptation*. New York: Basic Books, 1974.

Melamed, B. G., & Siegel, L. J. Reduction of anxiety in children facing hospitalization and surgery by use of filmed modeling. *Journal of Consulting and Clinical Psychology,* 1975, *43,* 511–521.

Melamed, B. G., Meyer, R., Gee, C., & Soule, L. The influence of time and type of preparation on children's adjustment to hospitalization. *Journal of Pediatric Psychology,* 1976, *1,* 31–37.

Moore, C. L. Hypnosis: An adjunct to pediatric consultation. *American Journal of Clinical Hypnosis,* 1981, *23,* 211–216.

Moos, R. H. *The family environment scale preliminary manual*. Palo Alto, Calif.: Consulting Psychologist Press, 1974.

Moos, R. H., & Tsu, V. D. The crisis of physical illness: An overview. In R. H. Moos (Ed.), *Coping with physical illness*. New York: Plenum, 1977.

Myers-Vando, R., Steward, M. S., Folkins, C. H., & Hines, P. The effects of congenital heart disease on cognitive development, illness causality concepts, and vulnerability. *American Journal of Orthopsychiatry,* 1979, *49,* 617–625.

Nagera, H. Children's reactions to hospitalization and illness. *Child Psychiatry and Human Development,* 1978, *9,* 3–19.

Nannis, E. D., Susman, E. J., Strope, B. E., Woodruff, P. J., Hersh, S. P.,

Levine, A. S., & Pizzo, P. A. Correlates of control in pediatric cancer patients and their families. *Journal of Pediatric Psychology*, 1982, *7*, 75–84.

Naylor, K. A., & Mattsson, A. "For the sake of the children": Trials and tribulations of child psychiatry-liaison service. *Psychiatry in Medicine*, 1973, *4*, 389–402.

Newhauser, C., Amsterdam, B., Hines, P., & Steward, M. Children's concepts of healing: Cognitive development and locus of control factors. *American Journal of Orthopsychiatry*, 1978, *48*, 335–341.

O'Malley, T. E., Koocher, G., Foster, D., & Slavin, L. Psychiatric sequelae of surviving childhood cancer. *American Journal of Orthopsychiatry*, 1979, *49*, 608–616.

Oremland, E. K., & Oremland, J. D. (Eds.). *The effects of hospitalization on children; models for their care*. Springfield, Ill.: Charles C. Thomas, 1972.

Papalia, D. E., & Olds, S. W. *A child's world: Infancy through adolescence*. New York: McGraw-Hill, 1975.

Patenaude, A. F., Szymanski, L., & Rappeport, J. Psychological costs of bone marrow transplantation in children. *American Journal of Orthopsychiatry*, 1979, *49*, 409–422.

Perrin, E. C., & Gerrity, P. S. There's a demon in your belly: Children's understanding of illness. *Pediatrics*, 1981, *67*, 841–849.

Petrillo, M., & Sanger, S. *Emotional care of hospitalized children: An environmental approach*. Philadelphia: Lippincott, 1980.

Piaget, J. [The origins of intelligence in children] (M. Cook, Trans.). New York: International Universities Press, 1952. (Originally published 1936.)

Piaget, J. [The psychology of intelligence] (C. K. Ogden, Ed.). Patterson, N.J.: Littlefield, Adams, 1963. (Originally published, 1947.)

Pless, I. B., & Douglas, I. W. B. Chronic illness in childhood: Part I. Epidemiological and clinical characteristics. *Pediatrics*, 1971, *47*, 405–414.

Pless, I. B., & Graham, P. Epidemiology of physical disorder. In M. Rutter, J. Tizard, & K. Whitmore (Eds.), *Education, health, and behavior*. London: Longmans, Green, 1970.

Pless, I. B., & Pinkerton, P. *Chronic childhood disorders: Promoting patterns of adjustment*. Chicago: Year Book Medical Publishers, 1975.

Pless, I. B., & Roghmann, K. J. Chronic illness and its consequences: Observations based on three epidemiological surveys. *Journal of Pediatrics*, 1971, *79*, 351–359.

Pless, I. B., Roghmann, K., & Haggerty, R. F. Chronic illness, family functioning, and psychological adjustment: A model for the allocation of preventive mental health services. *International Journal of Epidemiology*, 1972, *1*, 271–277.

Pless, I. B., & Satterwhite, B. B. A measure of family functioning and its application. *Social Science and Medicine*, 1973, *7*, 613–621.

Pless, I. B., & Satterwhite, B. B. Chronic illness. In R. J. Haggerty, K. Roghmann, & I. B. Pless (Eds.), *Child health and the community*. New York: Wiley, 1975.

Pond, H. Parental attitudes toward children with a chronic medical disorder: Special reference to diabetes mellitus. *Diabetes Care*, 1979, *2*, 425–431.

Powazek, M., Goff, J. R., Schyving, J., & Paulson, M. A. Emotional reactions of children to isolation in a cancer hospital. *Journal of Pediatrics*, 1978, *92*, 834–837.

Poznanski, E. O., Miller, E., Salguero, C., & Kelsh, R. C. Quality of life for long-term survivors of end-stage renal disease. *Journal of the American Medical Association*, 1978, *239*, 2343–2347.

Prentice, N. M., Schmechel, L. K., & Manosevitz, M. Children's belief in Santa Claus: A developmental study of fantasy and causality. *Journal of Child Psychiatry*, 1979, *18*, 658–667.

Prugh, D. G., & Eckhardt, L. O. Children's reactions to illness, hospitalization, and surgery. In A. Freedman & H. Kaplan (Eds.), *Comprehensive textbook of psychiatry*. Baltimore: Williams & Wilkins, 1974.

Prugh, D. G., & Eckhardt, L. O. Stages and phases in the response of children and adolescents to illness or injury. In B. W. Camp (Ed.), *Advances in behavioral pediatrics* (Vol. 1). Greenwich, Conn.: Jai Press, 1980.

Prugh, D. G., Staub, E. M., Sands, H. H., Kirschbaum, R. M., & Lenihan, B. S. A study of the emotional reactions of children and families to hospitalization and illness. *American Journal of Orthopsychiatry*, 1953, *23*, 70–106.

Reddihough, D. S., Landau, L., Jones, H. J., & Rickards, W. S. Family anxieties in childhood asthma. *Australian Paediatric Journal*, 1977, *13*, 295–298.

Rutter, M. Invulnerability, or why some children are not damaged by stress. In S. J. Shamsie (Ed.), *New directions in children's mental health*. New York: Spectrum, 1979.

Rutter, M., Tizard, J., & Whitmore, K. *Education, health, and behavior*. London: Longmans, Green, 1970.

Satterwhite, B. B. Impact of chronic illness on child and family: An overview based on five surveys with implications for management. *International Journal of Rehabilitation Research*, 1978, *1*, 7–17.

Sheridan, M. S. Talk time for hospitalized children. *Social Work*, 1975, *20*, 40–44.

Shultz, T. R. Development of the appreciation of riddles. *Child Development*, 1974, *45*, 100–105.

Siegel, L. J. Preparation of children for hospitalization: A selected review of the research literature. *Journal of Pediatric Psychology*, 1976, *1*, 26–30.

Simeonsson, R. J., Buckley, L., & Monson, L. Conceptions of illness causality in hospitalized children. *Journal of Pediatric Psychology*, 1979, *4*, 77–84.

Spinetta, J. J. Communication patterns in families dealing with life-threatening illness. In O. J. Z. Sahler (Ed.), *The child and death*. St. Louis: Mosby, 1978.

Spinetta, J. J. Adjustment and adaptation in children with cancer: A 3-year study. In J. J. Spinetta & P. Deasy-Spinetta (Eds.), *Living with childhood cancer*. St. Louis: Mosby, 1981.

Spinetta, J. J., & Deasy-Spinetta, P. Talking with children who have a life-threatening illness. In J. J. Spinetta & P. Deasy-Spinetta (Eds.), *Living with childhood cancer*. St. Louis: Mosby, 1981.

Spinetta, J. J., & Maloney, L. J. Death anxiety in the out-patient leukemic child. *Pediatrics*, 1975, *56*, 1034–1037.

Spinetta, J. J., McLaren, H. H., Deasy-Spinetta, P. M., Kung, F. H., Schwartz, D. B., & Hartman, G. A. *Adjustment and adaptation in parents of children with cancer*. Unpublished manuscript, San Diego State University, 1981.

Spinetta, J. J., Rigler, D., & Karon, M. Anxiety in the dying child. *Pediatrics*, 1973, *52*, 841–845.

Stein, R. E. K., & Riessman, C. K. The development of an impact-on-family scale: Preliminary findings. *Medical Care*, 1980, *18*, 465–472.

Steward, M. S., & Steward, D. S. Children's concepts of medical procedures. In R. Bibace & M. Walsh (Eds.), *The development of children's conceptions of health and related phenomena*. New York: Jossey-Bass, 1981.

Strauss, A. L., & Glaser, B. G. *Chronic illness and the quality of life*. St. Louis: Mosby, 1975.

Sullivan, H. S. *The interpersonal theory of psychiatry*. New York: Norton, 1953.

Talbot, N. B., & Howell, M. C. Social and behavioral causes and consequences of disease among children. In N. B. Talbot, J. Kagan, & L. Eisenberg (Eds.), *Behavioral science in pediatric medicine*. Philadelphia: Saunders, 1971.

Tavormina, J. B., Kastner, L. S., Slater, P. M., & Watt, S. L. Chronically ill children: A psychologically and emotionally deviant population? *Journal of Abnormal Child Psychology*, 1976, *4*, 99–110.

Vance, J. C., Fazan, L. E., Satterwhite, B., & Pless, I. B. Effects of nephrotic syndrome on the family: A controlled study. *Pediatrics*, 1980, *65*, 948–955.

van Eys, J. The truly cured child: The realistic and necessary goal in pediatric oncology. In J. J. Spinetta & P. Deasy-Spinetta (Eds.), *Living with childhood cancer*. St. Louis: Mosby, 1981.

Vernon, D. T. A., Foley, J. M., Sipowicz, R. R., & Schulman, J. L. *The psychological responses of children to hospitalization and illness*. Springfield, Ill.: Charles C. Thomas, 1965.

Visintainer, M. A., & Wolfer, J. A. Psychological preparation for surgical pediatric patients: The effect on children's and parents' stress responses and adjustment. *Pediatrics*, 1975, *56*, 187–202.

Weisman, A. D. Coping with illness. In T. P. Hackett & N. H. Cassem (Eds.), *Massachusetts General Hospital handbook of general hospital psychiatry*. St. Louis: Mosby, 1978.

White, R. W. Motivation reconsidered: The concept of competence. *Psychological Review*, 1959, *66*, 297–333.

White, R. W. Strategies of adaptation: An attempt at systematic description. In G. B. Coelho, D. A. Hamburg, & J. E. Adams (Eds.), *Coping and adaptation*. New York: Basic Books, 1974.

Whitt, J. K. Children's understanding of illness: Developmental considerations and pediatric intervention. In M. Wolraich & D. K. Routh (Eds.), *Advances in behavioral pediatrics* (Vol. 3). Greenwich, Conn.: Jai Press, 1982.

Whitt, J. K., Brantley, H. T., & Wise, E. Family, child, and school factors in the academic "re-entry" of children with chronic illness. Unpublished research report to The Spencer Foundation, University of North Carolina at Chapel Hill, 1982.

Whitt, J. K., & Dykstra, W. Patterns and content of physicians' communication with physically ill children. Unpublished manuscript, University of North Carolina at Chapel Hill, 1981.

Whitt, J. K., Dykstra, W., & Taylor, C. A. Children's conceptions of illness and cognitive development: Implications for pediatric practitioners. *Clinical Pediatrics*, 1979, *18*, 327–339.

Whitt, J. K., Hunter, R. S., Dykstra, W., Lauria, M. M., Stabler, B., & Taylor, C. A. Pediatric liaison psychiatry: A forum for separation and loss. *International Journal of Psychiatry in Medicine*, 1981, *11*, 59–68.

Whitt, J. K., & Prentice, N. M. Cognitive processes in the development of children's enjoyment and comprehension of joking riddles. *Developmental Psychology*, 1977, *13*, 129–136.

Wolfer, J. A., & Visintainer, M. A. Prehospital psychological preparation for tonsillectomy patients: Effects on children's and parents' adjustments. *Pediatrics*, 1979, *64*, 646–655.

Zeltzer, L., Dash, J., & Holland, J. P. Hypnotically induced pain control in sickle cell anemia. *Pediatrics*, 1979, *64*, 533–535.

Zigler, E. Handicapped children and their families. In Schopler, E., & Mesibov, G. B. (Eds.), *The effects of autism on the family*. New York: Plenum, in press.

5 The Family Context of Childhood Chronic Illness: Implications for Psychosocial Intervention

Dennis Drotar, Peggy Crawford, and Marcy Bush

Although it has long been recognized that the presence of a chronic illness has a profound effect on family life (Anthony, 1970; Parsons & Fox, 1952), methods of research and mental health intervention concerning childhood chronic illness have been dominated by a focus on the individual child (Becker, 1972; Bergmann, 1965; Freud, 1952). Moreover, in traditional medical models of comprehensive care, primary emphasis is placed on the professional caregiver's management of a given chronic disease and its symptoms rather than on relations with family members. Although the focus on individual adjustment has certainly advanced our understanding of children's coping (Mattson, 1972), the neglect of family-centered perspectives in the psychosocial management of childhood chronic illess has had a number of undesirable consequences. For example, child-centered comprehensive care does not recognize the family's position as a powerful context of socialization and support for the chronically ill child (Caplan & Killea, 1976; Power & Dell Orto, 1980). Since chronically ill children learn strategies of coping and adaptation to treatment regimens from their transactions with family members, the quality of intrafamilial coping is a critical component of the child's ability to negotiate the stressful demands of disease-related regimens, socialize with physically healthy peers, and function effectively in school and at work. Moreover, a transactional, family-oriented framework (Bell & Harper, 1977; Belsky, 1981; Sameroff, 1975) can consider the emotional impact of illness-related stress on parents, siblings, and extended family members, and on the family as a system and the need for psychosocial intervention with family units. A family systems' perspective is critical in planning mental health interventions for chronically ill children who are initially identified as having individual adjustment problems that are more properly construed as related to family dysfunction. A family-oriented perspective also has a number of important implications for comprehensive pediatric care. The physical care of a chronic illness takes place in a highly constrained interpersonal arena from which family and physician cannot easily exit; involvement of family members as respected participants in medical care and decision making lessens this constraint (Drotar, Ganofsky, Makker, & DeMaio, 1981c). Finally, a family-oriented approach to comprehensive care recognizes the potential of preventive interventions for enhancement of family life, coping, and stress management throughout the course of the child's illness. This state-of-the-art description of the family context of childhood chronic illness considers the unique applications of a family perspective to comprehensive medical care, mental health intervention, and research concerning childhood chronic illness.

The Family and Childhood Chronic Illness

Family development includes identifiable stages in the life cycle (Carter & McGoldrick, 1980) as well as complex pathways of direct and indirect influence (Parke, 1979). Although childhood chronic illness can disrupt family development, interpersonal relations, and allocation of resources, wide individual variations in family adjustment prior to illness onset and disease course makes one-to-one generalizations between illness-related stress and outcome impossible.

Individual chronic illnesses differ widely with respect to the organ system that is affected, the course of disease, the nature, visibility, and degree of physical symptoms, the demands of treatment regimens, age of onset and etiology, physical impairment, and threat to life (Mattson, 1972; Steinhauer, Muskin, & Rae Grant, 1974). Consequently, the specific nature of a family's task in integrating treatment regimens into their life differs greatly from illness to illness and even within a given illness. Yet irrespective of differences in illness, each and every family must cope with such general problems as (1) allocation of emotional resources to ill versus well members, (2) sharing of parental versus child responsibilities concerning the treatment regimen, (3) managing transactions with physicians and health care personnel, and (4) coping with hospitalizations and anxieties concerning the child's present and future physical vulnerability. Day-to-day treatment regimes require parents to negotiate parental roles and responsibilities, time, energy, and finances and to reconcile career versus family demands (Meyerowitz & Kaplan, 1967; Pless & Satterwhite, 1975; Turk, 1967; Vance, Fazan, Satterwhite & Pless, 1980). Beyond these concrete demands, the experience of a chronic illness forces family members to confront such personally troubling questions pertaining to the meaning of the illness, as "Why did this illness happen?" "Why is it occurring in our family?" The demands of illness-related stresses may also change the balance and structure of interpersonal relations within the family in ways that may affect the mental health of members. For example, assumption of sole responsibility for treatment regimen and physician visits by the mother may aggravate preexisting communication problems between the parents. In addition, the inevitable prospect of parental involvement in childrens' physical treatments may contribute to a maladaptive violation of customary psychological boundaries between parent and child. The fact that the child's care inevitably takes time and attention away from well siblings may also change childrearing patterns, thus potentiating dysfunctional family coalitions. The presence of a physically sick child can provide a ready vehicle for scapegoating of the child as a means of deflecting attention from other family problems, especially marital conflicts (Minuchin, 1974).

The presence of a child with a chronic illness also forces parents to consider the psychological meaning of the child's damage in their relationship and cope with feelings about the illness which can affect the quality of the relationship (Drotar, Baskiewicz, Irvin, Kennell, & Klaus, 1975). A chronic illness also poses a unique childrearing burden to parents who must master their own anxieties to the extent that they can help their child cope adaptively with the arduous demands of a treatment regimen. Helping the child cope with significant illness-related demands yet behave as a physically healthy child in other life contexts is an understandably difficult task that taxes even the most competent of parents (McCollum & Gibson, 1970).

The stresses of a chronic illness intersect with family and individual developmental issues in important ways. For example, having a child with a chronic illness may present a special burden on the newly married couple who is in process of stabilizing a family identity. The presence of a chronically ill child may threaten extended family members by intensifying concerns about death and/or dependency between parents and grandparents. Moreover, developmental transitions in the child's life can be very much affected by a chronic illness. For example, in the case of life-threatening illness, anxieties about the future may disrupt the child's ability to individuate from the family in line with societal expectations (Drotar, 1975). For this reason, it is no accident that the psychological problems of chronically ill children often present at critical times in development, such as the beginning of school or onset of adolescence, which require increased demands for independence (Drotar, 1978).

Empirical Studies of the Family Context of Childhood Chronic Illness

Family Functioning and Children's Mental Health

Although empirical investigations of family factors and childhood chronic illness are still relatively rare as compared to studies of individual adjustment, available studies have underscored the central importance of the family context as an influence on chronically ill children's mental health. For example, Pless, Roghmann, and Haggerty (1972) compared a sample of chronically ill children and a matched group of physically healthy children on a comprehensive battery of measures including responses from the child, parents, and teachers and an index of family functioning. Chronically ill children with the greatest risk for psychological impairment as judged by a composite index were from families with lower family functioning scores. Hence, family functioning was shown to be an important mediator of adjustment and one which operated in concert with other variables to affect individual adjustment.

Others have considered the relationship of family environment to the individual adjustment of chronically ill children. For example, Moise (1980) studied the adjustment of thirty-three school-aged children and adolescents with sickle cell anemia using a comprehensive objective assessment of psychological adjustment as perceived by the patients themselves, parents, and teachers. Family cohesion, as assessed by the Moos Family Environment Scale (Moos & Moos, 1976) was positively correlated with a composite measure of psychosocial adjustment. The better adjusted children among a highly stressed, impoverished sample came from more cohesive families.

Kucia, Drotar, Doershuk, Stern, Boat, and Matthews' (1979) observations of family problem solving indicated that families of well-adjusted children (as judged by physicians and parental ratings) demonstrated more creative solutions to structured problem-solving tasks than those of maladjusted children. The association of family creativity with positive adjustment is consistent with studies (e.g., Odom, Seeman, Newbrough, 1971) which indicate that families of well-adjusted children are more able to consider alternatives than those of poorly adjusted children. In addition, fathers of the well-adjusted children displayed more creativity and positive support than those of maladjusted children. This pattern, which occurred in families of male children but not of females, suggests that paternal flexibility and support may have been particularly important to the adjustment of boys. Finally, this study was noteworthy for the absence of differences in positive support or communication between families of well- versus poorly adjusted children and the fact that the families of maladjusted children had higher success scores than those with adjusted children. This study demonstrated that there is no simple relationship between children's maladjustment and family transaction.

A similar theme characterized Bush's (1981) study of the family concept and childhood adjustment of juvenile diabetics, emotionally disturbed children, and physically healthy children. Bush found a strong relationship between individual adjustment and perceptions of family across the entire sample. Moreover, the fact that maternal, paternal, and siblings' ratings for family satisfaction were significantly related to their own individual adjustment indicated that an individual's subjective experience of family may be a salient but heretofore neglected factor in adjustment. Bush's (1981) findings also contrast with clinical descriptions of families of chronically ill children as conflict ridden or ineffective and indicate that chronic childhood illness does not inevitably disrupt individual adjustment or family effectiveness.

Parental Mental Health

Since parents of chronically ill children must cope with extraordinarily difficult life circumstances including compromised finances, restriction of career mobility, and the demands of treatment regimens (Meyerowitz & Kaplan, 1967; Turk, 1967), it is not surprising that they find the experience stressful. Subjective feelings of depression and worry are common features of parental response to chronic illness (Koocher & O'Malley, 1981; Lawler, Nakielny, & Wright, 1966; Pless & Satterwhite, 1975). Although the subjective stresses of a chronic illness on parents have been well described, the specific effects on parental mental health are less well understood. For example, Lawler et al. (1966) found that most parents experienced considerable emotional upset, with eight of the thirty-eight mothers judged as clinically depressed. Tropauer, Franz, and Dilgard (1970) also noted maternal depression and guilt, but found that most mothers were able to perform effectively despite the stresses with which they were faced. Gayton, Friedman, Tavormina, and Tucker's (1977) controlled investigation found that the fathers of children with cystic fibrosis scored significantly higher on the MMPI Lie, Hypochondriasis, Hysteria, and Psychopathic Deviate scales then did fathers of healthy children. Mothers scored significantly higher on the Depression and Masculinity-Femininity scales. Although such studies point to a potential association of childhood chronic illness and parental maladjustment, the implications for childrens' mental health are not known. For example, among physically healthy children, the presence of severe parental psychopathology does not inevitably lead to childhood behavior disorder (Anthony, 1969). The way the child is involved in the parental disturbance appears to be more critical than the nature of parental disturbance per se. However, there is precious little empirical information concerning how chronically ill children perceive the impact of their own disease on their parents' emotional life and family life in general.

Marital Relationship

The demands of a chronic illness stress the parents' relationship and may disrupt their childrearing capacities, ability to support one another, and hence, the mental health of the chronically ill child. For example, Crain, Sussman, and Weil (1966) found that parents of diabetics demonstrated less agreement on child management and more marital conflict than parents of normal children. In addition, parents of children with cancer experience increased marital strain (Lansky, Cairns, Hassanein, Wehr, & Lowman, 1978), particularly around the time of diagnosis, as do the parents of children who had undergone kidney transplant (Korsch, Negrete, Gardner, Weinstock, Mercer, Grushkin, & Fine, 1973). Although childhood chronic illness presents an undeniable strain to parental relationships, it does not appear to be a causal agent in marital separation and/or divorce. Although clinical lore has it that chronic illness inevitably results in a high rate of family breakdown or divorce (Bruhn, 1977), more systematic studies have indicated that the marriages of parents of children with chronic illness, including life-threatening conditions, are no more unstable than those of healthy children (Koocher & O'Malley, 1981).

On the other hand, the consequences of heightened marital strain for the development of the chronically ill child are not well defined. What may be even more damaging than marital strain per se are changes in family alignments, including parents' difficulties in maintaining appropriate boundaries concerning their children's privacy or the development of maladaptive coalitions with one parent to the exclusion of the other (Minuchin, 1974). Furthermore, one of the most potentially intriguing but ill-understood phenomena is the possibility that a chronic illness may strengthen family unity and adaptation. For example, Pless and Satterwhite (1975) noted that parents felt that chronic illness had been a unifying force in the family, which had increased family members' sensitivity to each other. In addition, eight of sixteen parent couples of hemophiliac children felt the illness had enhanced family closeness (Markova, MacDonald, & Forbes, 1979) and parents of leukemic children in long-term remission felt the experience had altered their values and priorities in life and generated personal growth (Obetz, Swerson, McCarthy, Gilchrist, & Burgat, 1980). These findings suggest that a family's capacity to perceive meaning in the chronic illness experience may well be an important mediator of children's mental health (Venter, 1980).

Sibling Mental Health

Physically healthy siblings must cope with the anxieties imposed by their sib's chronic illness, the special parental attention and nurturance given to the ill child, and stresses faced by parents. Clinical observations have suggested that siblings experience adjustment problems (Binger, Ablin, Feurstein, Kushner, Rogers, & Mikkelson, 1969), some of which have been documented in controlled studies. For example, Lavigne and Ryan's (1979) study of the adjustment of siblings of cardiology, hematology, and plastic surgery patients indicated that siblings of patients were more withdrawn and irritable than healthy controls. Siblings of children with visible handicaps were most severely affected. Similar findings were reported by Tew and Lawrence (1973), who found that siblings of spina bifida patients were four times more likely to evidence maladjustment then were siblings of controls, and by Vance et al. (1980), who noted that the physical and emotional health of siblings of children with nephrotic syndrome were more impaired than that of siblings of healthy controls.

On the other hand, the results of other recent well-designed studies indicate that the general mental health of siblings of chronically ill children is not necessarily impaired but that their social adaptation may be vulnerable. Cairns, Clark, Smith, and Lansky (1979) found siblings of children with cancer to have "normal" self-concepts but higher perceived social isolation. Breslau, Weitzman, and Messenger's (1981) well-designed, comprehensive study of families of pediatric patients with cystic fibrosis, cerebral palsy, myelodysplasia, and multiple handicaps indicated that siblings of disabled children did not manifest higher rates of severe psychologic impairment or greater overall symptomatology when compared to control subjects. Siblings did score significantly higher, however, on two scales measuring interpersonal aggression with peers and within the school. Level of disability or nature of illness did not relate to sibling adjustment. Finally, in other recent controlled studies the adjustment of siblings of cystic fibrosis patients (Gayton et al., 1977; Drotar, Doershuk, Boat, Stern, Matthews, & Boyer 1981b) and juvenile diabetics (Bush, 1981) was not found to be impaired relative to comparison groups. Discrepancies in these findings may relate to differences in measures, patient populations, and/or the nature of comprehensive care afforded to families in various centers. The way in which a chronic illness affects the long-term relationship among siblings, which is a salient developmental influence (Bank & Kahn, 1976), remains an intriguing but unanswered question.

General Family Influences

Since research and clinical observation of family adjustment have generally concentrated on the mental health of individual members, little is known about the generalized effects of chronic illness on the family as a system. One area that may be affected by a chronic illness, however, is intrafamilial role patterns. In an interesting example of family-oriented research, Ritchie (1981) found that in contrast to families with a physically healthy child, families with an epileptic child had an autocratic, matriarchial structure which was more efficient in problem solving. Crain et al. (1966) found significantly lower goal consensus and increased role tension of family members of juvenile diabetics in comparison to healthy controls. Moreover, the capacity of family members to perform their usual roles was reduced.

Clinical observations suggest that family members' abilities to discuss the child's disease with one another, which may be a clinically relevant aspect of their adjustment, can be compromised. For example, Turk (1967) found that parents of cystic fibrosis children were able to discuss the child's management with each other, but did not discuss the illness with their other children, family, or friends. Sixty percent never discussed the diagnosis with the child. Parents of children in long-term leukemia remission (more than four years) also reported difficulty talking with each other about the illness or discussing it with the child (Obetz et al., 1980). It is quite possible that such patterns of communication may isolate parents from each other, from their children, and from social support networks, with negative consequences on children's mental health (Tropauer et al., 1970). For example, the consistent finding of a positive association between openness of family and parental communication about disease-related issues and childhood adaptation to childhood cancer (Lascari & Stehbens 1973; O'Malley & Koocher, 1981; Spinetta & Maloney 1978; Spinetta, Sarner, & Sheposh, 1981) underscores the potential importance of openness of disease-related communication for childhood adjustment.

One of the most neglected areas of research concerns the family's ability to transact adaptively with persons in other contexts, such as the school and the medical system. As yet, the factors which distinguish families who manage to encourage their chronically ill children to transact competently with others outside the family from those who cannot are largely unknown.

Family-centered Comprehensive Care of Chronically Ill Children

Although family-related research concerning childhood chronic illness is still very much in preliminary stages, the tenor of findings certainly supports the rationale for family-centered comprehensive care. Family-centered comprehensive care may be defined as the systematic inclusion of family members and subgroups in the child's physical care in ways that create a consistent family context for the discussion and long-term management of disease-related stress. Although many large centers for the treatment of chronic illness have established comprehensive care programs which purport to involve family members in the child's care, the mere designation of a given program as "family centered" or as "comprehensive" does not necessarily mean that medical or psychological care is consistently structured in line with a family-centered approach. In practice, the *content* and *structure* of care varies widely across different centers with respect (1) to nature and continuity of contact between physicians, health care professionals, and family; (2) the focus of care, for example, disease related versus family centered; (3) the structure of leadership and decision making; (4) the nature of interdisciplinary communication and planning; and (5) the quality of interpersonal support provided by caregivers. In some settings, physicians and nurses provide the sole ongoing contact with family members while mental health professionals work only with those children judged as having severe adjustment problems. Other programs feature shared professional contact with children and families over the entire course of the illness. Disease-related issues such as the child's physical status or compliance with regimens are the sole focus of some comprehensive-care programs. In others, the impact of disease on family, academic, and social adjustment are considered in close conjunction with physical care (Brantley, Stabler, & Whitt 1981; Drotar et al., 1981c; Heisler & Friedman, 1981; Koocher, Sourkes, & Keane, 1979). In practice, there are extraordinary obstacles to the implementation of family-centered care of chronically ill children.

For example, it is important to recognize that most pediatricians have had much more experience with the hospital-based management of chronically ill children's acute physical problems than with the continuous care of the chronically ill in home or community settings. As a consequence, they may not have had sufficient training to play a major role in counseling, advising, or coordinating services for the families of chronically ill children (Kanthor, Pless, Satterwhite, Myers, 1974; Pless, Satterwhite, & Van Vechten, 1976). Moreover, most chronically ill children receive their care in highly specialized centers, located in large pediatric training hospitals (Kanthor et al., 1974), where structural and organizational problems (Mechanic, 1972; Tefft & Simeonsson, 1979) can impede communication among professionals as well as between physician and family members. For example, in the highly subspecialized hospital culture, it is not uncommon for a single professional discipline to have access to only a small part of the total information concerning a chronically ill child and family (Mechanic, 1972). Moreover, the time pressures, the emphasis on action, and the absence of privacy that are prevalent in pediatric hospitals can severely constrain the quality of caregivers' transactions with families

(Drotar, Benjamin, Chwast, Litt, & Vajner, 1981a). Relating to chronically ill children and their families may also frustrate physicians (Artiss & Levine, 1973; Ford, Liske, & Ort, 1963) because this work requires the kind of communication skills which are not usually emphasized in pediatric training (Haggerty, Roghmann, & Pless, 1975). Moreover, physical treatments for chronic life-threatening conditions such as cancer and renal failure can dramatically affect the quality of life, as well as raise profound ethical questions and uncertainties for caregivers and families alike (Fox & Swazey 1978; Illich, 1976; Katz & Capron, 1975), which severely disrupt the quality of communication between physician and family members.

Although the nature of physician–family transactions which occur in the context of physical treatment have not been systematically documented, preliminary evidence indicates that they are less than optimal. For example, social-emotional issues appear to be neglected in communicating with parents about well-child care (Korsch & Morris, 1968) and evaded in the care of adolescents with certain chronic conditions (Raimbault, Cachin, Limal, Elincheff, & Rappaport, 1975). Other potentially maladaptive features of physician–family transaction include emphasis on technical versus emotional issues (Osherson, & Anarasingham, 1981) and withholding information, particularly from patients with serious conditions (McIntosh, 1974). Limiting disclosure of information to chronically ill children and families may be particularly problematic in view of the fact that both open and early communication about serious disease appears to be positively related to psychological adjustment (Koocher & O'Malley, 1981).

Despite the very real difficulties of implementing a family-centered approach to chronically ill children, a number of clinicians have recognized the potential importance of family-centered care and have recommended consistent involvement of family members at point of initial diagnosis (Ablin, Binger, Stein, Kushner, Rogers, & Mikkelson, 1971), during periods of crisis (Drotar & Ganofsky, 1976), and as part of long-term management (Power & Dell Orto, 1980). Unfortunately, with the exception of outcome studies concerning family-centered treatment of psychosomatic illnesses (Minuchin, Rosman, & Baker, 1978), systematic studies of the efficacy of family-centered versus alternative treatment modalities for comprehensive care and mental health interventions concerning chronically ill children have not been conducted (Friedrich, 1977; Johnson, 1979). Nevertheless, extensive clinical experiences with various chronic illness groups over an extended period of time (Drotar & Ganofsky, 1976; Drotar et al., 1981b; Ganofsky, Drotar, & Makker, in press; Koocher et al., 1979; Sourkes, 1977) indicate many potential advantages to integrating family-centered mental health services within the context of the child's comprehensive care. For example, preliminary evidence indicates that family-centered comprehensive care programming may enhance patient compliance in potentially problematic areas (Ganofsky, Drotar & Makker, in press), allow a surprising number of severe mental health problems to be managed within the pediatric setting (Drotar & Ganofsky, 1976), and facilitate family acceptance of psychological interventions, when they are needed.

One of the key principles in a family-centered framework is consistent attention to the impact of childhood chronic illness on *all* family members, not only on the affected child. Family-centered approaches also differ dramatically from traditional chronic illness management in the consistent involvement of family members in discussions of the child's physical treatment, treatment regimens, and decision making concerning the illness. For this reason, a family-centered approach is best implemented from the outset of the disease rather than subsequently in response to disease-related crises. Although it may appear deceptively easy to involve family members in the child's care, in practice it is very difficult to determine who to involve, at what point in the child's care, and for what purpose. As a consequence, professional caregivers who work with families are sorely in need of a conceptual framework to guide their interventions. Our experience indicates that a structural family-systems perspective which was developed out of psychotherapy with families of children with chronic, psychosomatic illness (Minuchin, 1974; Minuchin et al., 1978) has many potential advantages as a guiding framework for the family-centered care of chronically ill children. The structural approach focuses on the observable patterns through which family members relate to one another to carry out important functions, particularly stress management and integration of the illness in family life. Other salient concepts include the attention to subsystems—that is, parents, siblings—within the family, each of which is very important to the quality of total family coping. Since the parents' relationship is considered to be especially critical for the quality of the child's coping, parents are often the focal point of the professional's contact with the family. Through direct observation of family transactions, the clinician can determine how family subsystems operate with respect to one another, particularly how various family members are included or not included in family tasks. The concept of boundary, which refers to the transactional rules that define which family members participate in various activities and how, is particularly relevant to work with chronically ill children and their families. Successful management of a chronic illness requires a delicate balance between parental support and overinvolvement in the child's treatment regimen as well as between concern and preoccupation with the child's physical vulnerability. On the other hand, one of the hallmark characteristics of dysfunctional family units is the consistent violation of boundaries by inappropriate intrusion of family members into functions that are the domain of other members (Minuchin et al., 1978). The alignment of family relationships, including coalitions, which involve joint action of two members against another are also important, particularly because the visibility of a chronic illness provides a ready vehicle for "detouring" of other intrafamilial conflicts onto the chronically ill child.

The structural approach also suggests specific interventions which are quite compatible with the action-oriented pediatric setting. For example, it is often useful to support individual autonomy by stopping family members from talking for one another and by highlighting the chronically ill child's right to individual action and decision making. Other "natural" structural interventions involve supporting the parents' relationship, involving fathers and siblings in the child's care, and reinforcing the family's ability to communicate together and make decisions.

Illustrations of Family-centered Interventions with Chronically Ill Children and Their Families

The potential applicability of a family-centered approach to the comprehensive care of the chronically ill child is illustrated in the following case examples taken from the authors' experiences with families of children with a range of chronic illnesses, particularly diabetes, renal failure, and life-threatening illnesses such as cystic fibrosis. The context of the present work is a large university-based medical center, where the authors have collaborated with physicians and other caregivers in providing care for chronically ill children. The following situations were chosen to reflect a range of clinical situations which are commonly found in chronic illness work. The present approaches to intervention were developed over fifteen years of cumulative experience in pediatric comprehensive care and mental health interventions with chronically ill children.

A Family Approach to the Diagnosis of Chronic Illness

The professional's contact with the family of a chronically ill child begins at the point of diagnosis. At the outset of treatment, the professional who wishes to adopt a family perspective is at a marked disadvantage owing to a lack of knowledge of the family. For this reason initial contacts with the family are best structured to involve family groups and subgroups rather than only mother and child (Ablin et al., 1971). The way these initial contacts are structured may have critical import for the family's subsequent transactions with professional caregivers. For example, if only the mother is involved in contacts with professionals, then the family may receive the message that it is important for her (rather than anyone else) to be involved in subsequent contacts with staff. The disadvantages of a mother-centered approach to comprehensive care is that it places an unreasonable responsibility on an already highly stressed caregiver, may disrupt the parents' capacities to support one another, and may isolate the father from the child's care. A more adaptive model of family-centered comprehensive care involves as many salient family members as possible at point of initial diagnosis, but places primary focus on the parents' relationship. An example of a family-centered approach to the initial discussion of the diagnosis of a chronic disease is shown in the following situation:

Dawn is a seven-year-old child who was diagnosed as having diabetes following a mild onset of symptoms. The parents were shocked to be told that Dawn had a chronic illness requiring lifelong treatment with insulin.

At the beginning of the hospitalization, Dawn's father asked many questions about the diagnosis and treatment of diabetes, in an attempt to confirm in his own mind the reality of his daughter's condition. During the brief four or five day hospitalization, family members learned new information and many skills including insulin injections, urine testing, diet, and recognition and treatment of symptoms.

In Dawn's case, we included her two older sisters in educational sessions as well. Allowing siblings to share in this process helped take some of the mystery out of the hospitalization and the disease. Dawn's parents were very supportive of their daughters' involvement and decided that Dawn's sisters could share responsibility with her for the after-school urine testing and recording.

Inclusion of as many family members as possible in educational sessions not only allows family members to act as supports to each other but may bring out family strengths that were not otherwise obvious. Moreover, family discussions can also stimulate much-needed group feedback. For example, one family member may ask a novel question which exposes the whole family group to new and important information. This process also encourages family members to share concerns and worries. It is important to recognize that the diagnosis of a chronic illness requires family members to assimilate a great deal of new information and skills very quickly and at a time when they are highly stressed. For this reason, the behaviors learned in the initial hospitalization are best construed as survival skills. Understandably, many parents of chronically ill children express concern about taking their newly diagnosed child home where they must carry out unfamiliar responsibilities outside of the protective hospital environment. Consequently, following initial diagnosis, we find it particularly helpful to have regular phone contact with families to review symptoms and treatment regimens. Each of these phone contacts serves as support, education, and an opportunity to provide positive reinforcement to the family.

It is important to recognize that just as the course of the family's contacts with professionals concerning the initial diagnosis of a chronic illness should be structured with the family in mind, so should all subsequent contacts. Professional energies are often concentrated on the crisis period of initial diagnosis, which, while important, is but one point in the family's ongoing experience of a chronic illness. Ongoing monitoring of the family's adjustment, help with participation in care, and involvement in decision making may provide more critical support than intervention which is restricted to the period of initial diagnosis.

Including Siblings in the Chronically Ill Child's Care

Siblings often have a great many worries about what is happening to their chronically ill brother or sister. Moreover, they may feel "left out" and deprived of parental attention. Our experience indicates that siblings also can be significant sources of support for the chronically ill child over the entire course of the illness, but *only* if they are informed and involved. Informing siblings about the illness makes their experience more understandable and less frightening and can facilitate their development. Productive structuring of sibling involvement was shown in the following case of a seven-year-old diabetic child, Abbie, and her eight-year-old brother, Jamie:

From the beginning Abbie's parents were sensitive to Jamie's feelings about Abbie's illness and hospitalization. The parents planned for one of them to be home each night with Jamie to maintain some level of usual family activity for him and themselves. Some of this time was spent talking with him about Abbie's diabetes. Thus, Jamie was able to share his concern that he was in some way responsible for Abbie's getting diabetes. His parents reassured him that this just was not true and described for him how well Abbie was again feeling.

These parents encouraged the children to keep in daily phone contact with each other. When we suggested that Jamie visit Abbie, they readily agreed. Jamie was included in family educational sessions, which provided him an opportunity to observe urine testing and injections and to ask questions. He seemed reassured to know that Abbie could still play sports and eat with him at McDonald's.

After discharge the family was encouraged to attend clinic visits together, which they often did.

Enhancing Family Decision Making

One of the most important principles of family-centered comprehensive care is the involvement of family members in decision making concerning the child's physical care. It is important to recognize that the presence of a chronic illness inevitably poses extraordinary constraints because staff and family are locked into a treatment course in which neither can exit but where neither is completely comfortable. For this reason, clashes of expectations between physician and family members are not uncommon. For example, families may expect the physician to cure the child's problem and may express chronic disappointment and frustration when this does not occur. In turn, physicians may be similarly frustrated by the chronic nature of the child's condition. Family and staff must participate in encounters in which neither has complete control of the situation but where each needs the others. One potential approach to this inherent dilemma involves consistent sharing of information about the disease, decision making, and responsibility. This kind of collaboration, which is not easily sanctioned in the authoritarian hospital culture (Friedson, 1970), has a number of important advantages. First, attention to family members' concerns lessens the sense of helplessness that is ordinarily part and parcel of coping with a chronic illness. As families experience their feelings as being heard and their wishes as being respected, they may be more likely to integrate arduous treatment regimens into family life, which become truly "theirs" rather than the alien orders of a fearsome authority. The experience of sharing decision making and responsibility for regimens also allows for more honest transaction between staff and family. Professional caregivers do not have to pretend that they know all the answers. Family members can admit more of their anxieties and misgivings. Over the course of time, as the family begins to appreciate the partnership that is generated, a family-oriented perspective may result in enhanced compliance with regimens. Finally, a family-centered framework provides a strategy for working with difficult and troubling decisions that often arise in the course of a chronic illness. For example, compelling family decisions are raised by chronic illnesses such as renal failure which involve decisions concerning choice of treatment, for example, dialysis versus organ transplantation.

Special Problems: Engaging the Absent Father

The adaptive integration of a chronic illness into family life is a slow process which does not always occur without setbacks. Some families with maladaptive methods of stress management appear to resolve the initial crisis of a chronic illness only to "break down" at a subsequent time. One of the most common dysfunctional arrangements occurs when when one parent (usually the mother) assumes the entire responsibility for the management of the disease. This pattern of adjustment may be successful for a short while, but as the stresses mount, dysfunction may be expressed in the child's noncompliance and/or disruptions in the medical regimen. In such instances, it may be critical to reorient the family to the illness by including formerly absent family members in the process. Since family members have often reached a stable pattern of adaptation which is very difficult to counter, however, it may be very difficult to accomplish a reorientation without a concerted effort from the professional caregiver to involve family members. For example, a home visit can be used both as a method of family observation and as an intervention technique to engage absent family members, such as the father. A maladaptive focus on the mother–child dyad can be shifted to include the father through strenuous efforts on the part of the professional caregiver. Our work underscores the need for flexible methods and extreme persistence in working with families.

Helping the Family in Disease-related Crises

The course of childhood chronic illness is often marked by disease-related crises of acute illness, physical deterioration, or the threat of death. Each of these events requires family support, unity, and control, which are most difficult to achieve, especially in the culture of the acute care hospital (Drotar, 1976; Drotar et al., 1981c). In the face of the extreme anxiety and feelings of helplessness that can surround crisis situations, physicians and nursing staff may focus time and attention on the individual child's physical status rather than on the family, thus contributing to further emotional isolation. One important principle of crisis management involves the professional caregivers' support of family control by encouraging their participation in the child's care, which is illustrated in the following case example:

Gina is an eight year old with juvenile diabetes. Diagnosed at age three years, Gina had not been hospitalized since her diagnosis. Her parents have managed the usual colds and sore throats without many diabetes-related problems. Following a bout of gastroenteritis, she became dehydrated and looked very ill, reminding the parents of her initial hospitalization with diabetic ketoacidosis. Gina's parents were instructed to monitor her progress by measuring all urines and testing them for sugar and acetone, checking her weight every three to four hours, and watching for signs of dehydration and ketoacidosis. Initially, we kept in phone contact every one to two hours to evaluate Gina's condition and make suggestions about type and amount of insulin and fluids. Perhaps the most important function of this frequent contact was the support to her parents, who were dealing with a scary and new experience. During the day Gina's parents saw progress as she stopped vomiting, gained weight, and looked considerably better. Although this process required much time from both parents and professional, it was time well spent. An expensive hospitalization was prevented by keeping the family at home and intact. The event also served as a day-long educational session in which the family learned when to give extra insulin, assess dehydration, and deal with vomiting. The parents in fact successfully treated their own child—an accomplishment which enhanced the family's competency and self-confidence.

The experience of life-threatening illness is a tragic family predicament which disrupts relationships within the family and threatens every member (Drotar, 1978; McCollum & Gibson, 1970). The terminally ill child requires continual support at a time when each and every family member experiences psychological pain. Because family members are reacting in individual ways to this stress, they may be fearful of sharing their experience. Consequently, in such situations, professional caregivers often have to take the lead and assume responsibility for structuring transactions with family members so that each family member's concerns are recognized.

The structuring of contacts to bring family members together in a common forum to share their concerns is important. Despite great concern for one another, family members' anxieties can prevent them from recognizing and appreciating one another's feelings. Opening up the painful disease-related realities for discussion not only affords family members the experience of clarifying perspectives but enhances their control over the experience. A structural framework can be useful to organize the intervention in a crisis. For example, the parents' isolation can be lessened through discussions of their mutual reactions to the specific situation. Isolated by the multiple demands of their child's illness, parents may not have had sufficient time to share their feelings. Supporting the parents' relationships also helps to counter the child's tendency to divide his parents by complaining to mother about father. The identification of the parents as a unit in their own right who have worries that are independent of yet related to the child's predicament supports the child's individuation and allows him or her to clarify feelings. As a child begins to express feelings about the disease, he or she can become more able to adaptively utilize his or her parents' support without losing control of feelings.

Family-centered Mental Health Intervention

In addition to applications in comprehensive pediatric care, a family-centered perspective can also provide an invaluable means of intervening with mental health disturbances associated with chronic illness in children. Clinical observations of family problem-solving communication and disease-related coping (Power & Dell Orto, 1980) can reveal potentially maladaptive family alignments such as overly close parent–child relationships and suggest treatments that address these problems (Jaffe, 1978). Family therapy is a primary treatment modality for emotional disturbances that are rooted in longstanding dysfunctional relationships which culminate in overprotection or scapegoating of the ill child (Minuchin et al., 1978). As with physically healthy children, problems that are initially construed by parents and/or by medical caregivers as examples of individual adjustment problems may actually be highly intertwined with family influences. A family-oriented approach to mental health treatment can help address and rectify the counterproductive labeling of the ill child as the sole focus of disturbance. Moreover, family-systems-based therapeutic intervention provides a method to address the role of the family in a way that cannot ordinarily be achieved through individual treatment alone, as shown in the following treatment of an adolescent adjustment problem:

Jay, a sixteen-year-old boy with cystic fibrosis, was referred by his physician because of his parents' concerns that he was not doing well in school and did not have sufficient friends. The eldest and firstborn son, Jay was a high school junior who was in good physical condition for someone with his disease. Although he did relatively well in school, his parents considered him an underachiever. He did not date or socialize with peers very much but carved out swimming as an arena to demonstrate his competence. In an individual interview, Jay was defensive, felt blamed by his parents, and was quite critical of their expectations of him. The parents had very high expectations of Jay and themselves and often criticized him in small but important ways, which was very much apparent in a family interview. Family interaction was characterized by a series of unresolved tugs-of-war. Jay resisted passively as his parents relentlessly continued their criticism.

Parental messages about Jay's socialization and independence were contradictory. Although the parents expected Jay to venture out more on his own, they harbored a great many fears about his future, and subtly undercut his efforts toward independence. For example, his mother, who was a teacher, often had occasion to observe Jay at school and commented on his failure to socialize with friends in the cafeteria. Jay's father expressed concern that Jay would become sick when he left home for college and admitted his disappointment in him. The parents also did not expect nearly so much of Jay's healthy sister as they did of him. They eventually noted that because Jay was so sick, "We tried very hard to force him to be as competent as possible, but maybe we overdid it." The parents could not easily see that they derogated Jay and perceived him as damaged.

With support, Jay eventually confronted his parents with "You act like there has always been something wrong with me, you expect things to happen." As the themes of criticism and failure were linked to Jay's illness, it became possible for the parents to give up some of their overprotectiveness to allow Jay to make some of his own mistakes. Jay and his father were encouraged to discuss their differences, with marked lessening of the tension and isolation between them. At the same time, Jay's mother was confronted with her protection of Jay and asked to begin the difficult task of allowing his independence. Finally, Jay's sister was brought into the discussion as the parents began to explore their differing perceptions of her and Jay.

Although Jay's situation initially presented solely in terms of his individual problems, they were better understood in relation to family problems including: (1) denial of illness-related anxieties which were expressed as concerns about Jay and his emotional state; (2) a maladaptive family coalition of mother and son with the father isolated; and (3) undue focus on parental anxieties and expectations on Jay to the neglect of his physically healthy sibling. Short-term, focused, family-centered intervention was guided by structural principles in which potentially dysfunctional parent–child alignments (in this instance, the overly invested mother–son relationship) were countered and alternate relationship pathways (father–son) encouraged. In addition, the parental anxieties about Jay as a "vulnerable child" (Green & Solnit, 1964), which had very much colored their perceptions, were addressed, thus encouraging the parents to frame their view of him as a more normal child. Finally, Jay's sibling was brought into the family arena so that he was not the sole focus of parental attention. In this instance, Jay's special sensitivity to his parents' vigilance and labeling of him as "disturbed" would have most likely precluded successful intervention if approached solely from an individual perspective. Furthermore, it would have been next to impossible to recognize the pervasive nature of maladaptive family influences from individual interventions with Jay and his parents alone. On the other hand, with the special perspective afforded by family interviews, it became clear that Jay's upset with his parents' criticisms corresponded to the reality of their labeling rather than an internalized distortion. As a consequence of this recognition, familial contributions to his difficulties became easier to address in treatment.

Discrepant Family Cultures and Life-styles

Parents and family members must enter an alien hospital culture, depend on unfamiliar professionals, and entrust the care of their child to a myriad of settings and persons. Successful comprehensive care involves a healthy respect for family values, culture, and participation in decision making. The need to appreciate family culture is especially important in large medical centers which draw patients from disparate ethnic and socioeconomic backgrounds. Understanding of family culture is complicated, however, by the fact that professional staff are generally from relatively homogeneous middle-class backgrounds and may not have sufficient experience with complex variations of American family life, particularly among poor families from varying racial and ethnic backgrounds (Stack, 1974). Without appreciation of the particular cultural meaning of a given behavior, the staff may label patterns of family life as deviant that are more properly considered as understandable reflections of family culture. In such instances, the staff's "diagnosis" of a family can actually reflect misunderstanding of family members' behavior which relates more to the staff's own stress than it does to the family's psychopathology. In turn, family members may sense this misunderstanding and become increasingly disturbed. The difficulties of working with complex variations in family structure are compounded by the fact that the staff must transact with family members who are also under great stress. Given this circumstance, it is especially important to avoid premature judgments concerning the family "pathology" and to involve as many family members as possible so that their stories can be heard. With additional information about family life, seemingly deviant and contradictory family behavior can be clarified, often with beneficial effects on family–staff relations.

Ethnic or Cultural Minority Families

The following case illustrates how understanding of the family culture allowed the staff to provide more sensitive and effective support to a critically ill child:

John, an eleven-year-old boy with acute leukemia diagnosed during his current admission, experienced massive internal bleeding and difficulty breathing; he was critically ill. The nurses were quite concerned about John's family. They felt that the family denied the seriousness of John's condition and had their own ideas concerning his care. For example, his aunt's idea that John's condition could be cured with herbs disturbed the staff greatly. As we met to formulate a therapeutic approach to this family, a more coherent picture of their constellation and culture emerged. John was the eldest son of parents who had been separated during most of his life. He had long been cared for by his mother, maternal grandmother, and aunt, who were of the Black Muslim faith. His grandmother had long been the dominant force in the family, which was quite close knit and included a large number of relatives who wished to visit John because of his precarious physical condition. The family was quite devoted to John, and his illness was a severe blow to everyone. Although the family had been made aware of the critical nature of John's condition, they could not easily express their grief in words. However, their constant attendance, their demands to participate in his care, and their annoyance with the staff were testimony to their great concern about the boy.

As family members' reactions became more understandable, the staff could express admiration for the family's courage in the face of tragedy. We tried to enhance their comfort in our setting by allowing greater participation and affirmed the family's culture by offering John a special hospital tray, in keeping with their religious and cultural preferences. In addition, the staff eventually accommodated to the presence of John's extended family and provided a great deal of support for him.

Divorced and Reconstituted Families

One of the more challenging situations for the clinician who works with chronically ill children involves work with families who have complex living arrangements owing to divorce, separation, and/or remarriage. Disparate living arrangements and/or continuing conflicts between the parents can often obscure responsibilities and procedures for decision making concerning illness regimens. In such situations, the professional caregiver can be put in an untenable, confusing situation created by separate dealings with individual parents, who are fighting with one another via the child's care. Successful intervention with such families often requires a shift in perspective toward the total "family," by emphasizing negotiations with both parents and clarification of their responsibilities.

The Highly Fragmented Family

Unfortunately, not all chronically ill children live in the kinds of families that can provide the emotional and physical support necessary for optimal management of chronic illness. Some chronically ill children live in highly fragmented, chaotic family situations which do not provide a coherent nurturing network and thus do not easily lend themselves to a family-intervention approach owing to their disorganization. In such instances, an understanding of the complexity of the family arrangement can help structure basic principles of management, including (1) expectation of at least minimal standards of care from the parents and (2) maintenance of a close relationship with the child, who is helped to understand and deal with the impact of family stresses on his care.

Implications

The integration of a family-centered perspective in the comprehensive care of chronically ill children faces a number of formidable obstacles, including lack of family-related perspectives in the training of professional caregivers, the prevalence of disease or deficit models of physical and psychosocial care (Mohr, 1977), organizational pressures which fragment care, and the authoritarian culture of the hospital (Friedson, 1970). As a consequence of such compelling forces, very few comprehensive-care programs are initially planned in accord with a family-centered approach, particularly one with a preventive perspective. In many comprehensive-care programs, mental health interventions are directed toward disease or mental health crises, which are usually treated as individual problems construed as a problem of individual anxiety, anger, or "hatefulness" (Groves, 1978). Yet over the course of their experience, many seasoned clinicians have come to recognize the wisdom of seeing the child's problems as embedded in a larger context and have begun to involve family members consistently in the child's care. Experience with family-centered approaches has many potential benefits for professional development, particularly in facilitating diagnostic and theraputic expertise. For example, when one has had experiences with large numbers of families, patterns that were formerly seen as quite deviant can be understood more on their own terms and with increasing respect for family individuality. Moreover, with experience, the prospect of talking with siblings and fathers becomes more natural and comfortable. Finally, a family-centered model of comprehensive care can also enhance the humanization of patient care and facilitate long-range planning for family mental health needs.

There is a critical need for systematic outcome studies in which family-centered methods are compared to different models of intervention and for documentation of the structure of family-centered care (e.g., which family members are involved, at what point in time, for what purpose) in various centers. The families' experience of family-centered comprehensive care is yet another ill-studied but very important question for future research. Are families who have been seen from a family perspective more satisfied with care than those seen from an individual vantage point? Does family-centered care result in enhanced compliance? The prospective study of families coping with the stress of a chronic illness at various points of post-illness contact also provides a unique opportunity to study stress-related change and transition in families that are for the most part emotionally healthy. The process by which developmental transitions in individual development (e.g., onset of adolescence) or disease-related stress (e.g., physical deterioration) interact with family development is a critical target area for future study.

Finally, it should also be recognized that a family-centered framework is not a panacea for the awesome stress and human tragedy that can accompany chronic illness. By including the total family, the clinician is privy to more of the family's world and hence to more of their pain.

Professionals who work closely with chronically ill children and their families cannot help but be touched and, at times, severely stressed by these poignant encounters. The need to remain open and available to multiple family members while somehow not unduly stressing oneself is an inherent dilemma for the professional. On the other hand, the potential for understanding is much greater when the family context is recognized and appreciated on its own terms. The families of the chronically ill have much to teach us about human resilience in the face of severe and chronic stress. Let us hope that we can become sufficiently sensitive to family communication and culture to learn this lesson.

References

Ablin, A. R., Binger, C. M., Stein, R. C., Kushner, T. H., Roger, S., & Mikkelsen, C. A. A conference with the family of a leukemic child. *American Journal of Diseases of Children*, 1971, *122*, 362–366.

Anthony, E. J. A clinical evaluation of children with psychotic parents. *American Journal of Psychiatry*, 1969, *126*, 2–10.

Anthony, E. F. The impact of mental and physical illness on family life. *American Journal of Psychiatry*, 1970, *127*, 138–145.

Artiss, K. L., & Levine, A. S. Doctor–patient relation in severe illness. *New England Journal of Medicine*, 1973, *283*, 1210–1214.

Bank, S., & Kahn, M. Sisterhood–brotherhood is powerful: Sibling systems and family therapy. *Annual Progress in Child Psychiatry and Child Development*, 1976, 493–519.

Becker, R. D. Therapeutic approaches to psychopathological reactions to hospitalization. *International Journal of Child Psychotherapy*, 1972, *1*, 65–96.

Bell, R. Q., & Harper, L. V. *Child effects on adults*. Hillsdale, N.J.: Lawrence Erlbaum Associates, 1977.

Belsky, J. Early human experience: A family perspective. *Developmental Psychology*, 1981, *17* (1), 3–23.

Bergmann, T. *Children in the hospital*. New York: International Universities Press, 1965.

Binger, C. M., Ablin, A. R., Feuerstein, R. C., Kushner, J. H., Rogers, S., & Mikkelson, C. Childhood leukemia: Emotional impact on patient and family. *New England Journal of Medicine*, 1969, *280*, 414–421.

Brantley, H. T., Stabler, B., & Whitt, J. K. Program considerations in comprehensive care of chronically ill children. *Journal of Pediatric Psychology*, 1981, *6*, 229–238.

Breslau, N., Weitzman, M., & Messenger, K. Psychologic functioning of siblings of disabled children. *Pediatrics*, 1981, *67*, 344–353.

Bruhn, J. G. Effects of chronic illness on the family. *Journal of Family Practice*, 1977, *4* 1057–1060.

Bush, M. Family concept and adjustment of siblings and parents of children with chronic illness and emotional disorder. Unpublished Master's thesis. Case Western Reserve University, 1981.

Cairns, N. V., Clark, G. M., Smith, S. P., & Lansky, S. B. Adaptation of siblings to childhood malignancy. *Journal of Pediatrics,* 1979, *95,* 484–487.

Caplan, G., & Killea, M. *Support systems and mutual help: Multidisciplinary explorations*. New York: Grune & Stratton, 1976.

Carter, E. A., & McGoldrick, M. *The family life cycle: A framework for family therapy*. New York: Gardner Press, 1980.

Crain, A. R., Sussman, M. B., & Weil, W. B. Effects of a diabetic child on marital integration and related measures of family functioning. *Journal of Health and Human Behavior,* 1966, *13,* 122–127.

Drotar, D. The treatment of a severe anxiety reaction in an adolescent boy following renal transplantation. *Journal of the American Academy of Child Psychiatry,* 1975, *14,* 451–462.

Drotar, D. Psychological consultation in the pediatric hospital. *Professional Psychology,* 1976, *7,* 72–80.

Drotar, D. Adaptational problems of children and adolescents with cystic fibrosis. *Journal of Pediatric Psychology,* 1978, *3,* 45–50.

Drotar, D., Baskiewicz, A., Irvin, N., Kennell, J., & Klaus, M. The adaptation of parents to the birth of an infant with a congenital malformation: A hypothethical model. *Pediatrics,* 1975, *56,* 710–717.

Drotar, D., Benjamin, P., Chwast, R., Litt, C., & Vajner, P. The role of the psychologist in pediatric outpatient and inpatient settings. In J. Tuma (Ed.), *The practice of pediatric psychology*. New York: Wiley, 1981. (a)

Drotar, D., Doershuk, C. F., Boat, T. F., Stern, R. C., Matthews, L., & Boyer, W. Psychosocial functioning of children with cystic fibrosis. *Pediatrics,* 1981, *67,* 338–343. (b)

Drotar, D., & Ganofsky, M. A. Mental health intervention with children and adolescents with end-stage renal failure. *International Journal of Psychiatry in Medicine,* 1976, *7,* 181–194.

Drotar, D., Ganofsky, M. A., Makker, S. P., & DeMaio, D. A family-oriented supportive approach to renal transplantation in children. In N. Levy, (Ed.), *Psychological factors in hemodialysis and transplantation*. New York: Plenum, 1981. (c)

Ford, A. B., Liske, R. E., & Ort, R. S. Reactions of physicians and medical students to chronic illness. *Journal of Chronic Disease,* 1963, *15,* 785–794.

Fox, R. C., & Swazey, J. P. *The courage to fail: A social view of organ transplantation and dialysis*. Chicago: University of Chicago Press, 1978.

Friedrich, W. N. Ameliorating the psychological impact of chronic physical disease on the child and family. *Journal of Pediatric Psychology,* 1977, *2,* 26–31.

Friedson, E. *The profession of medicine*. New York, Dodd, Mead, 1970.

Freud, A. The role of bodily illness in the mental life of children. *Psychoanalytic Study of the Child,* 1952, *7,* 69–81.

Ganofsky, M. A., Drotar, D., & Makker, S. Growing-up with renal failure—problems and perspectives. In N. Levy (Ed.), *Psychonephrology. II. Psychological factors in hemodialysis and transplantation*. New York: Plenum Press, in press.

Gayton, W. F., Friedman, S. B., Tavorimina, T. F., & Tucker, F. Children with cystic fibrosis: Psychological test findings of patients, siblings and parents. *Pediatrics*, 1977, *59*, 888–894.

Green, M., & Solnit, A. F. Reactions to the threatened loss of a child: A vulnerable child syndrome. *Pediatrics*, 1964, *34*, 58–66.

Groves, J. E. Taking care of the hateful patient. *New England Journal of Medicine*, 1978, *8*, 883–887.

Haggerty, R., Roghmann, K. J., & Pless, I. B. *Child health and the community*. New York: Wiley, 1975.

Heisler, A. B., & Friedman, S. B. Social and psychological considerations in chronic disease: with particular references to the management of seizure disorders. *Journal of Pediatric Psychology*, 1981, *6*, 239–250.

Illich, I. *Medical nemesis: The expropriation of health*. New York: Random House, 1976.

Jaffe, D. T. The role of family therapy in treating physical illness. *Hospital and Community Psychiatry*, 1978, *29*, 169–174.

Johnson, M. R. Mental health interventions with medically ill children. A review of the literature 1970–1977. *Journal of Pediatric Psychology*, 1979, *4*, 147–163.

Kanthor, H., Pless, I. B., Satterwhite, B., & Myers, G. Areas of responsibility in the health care of multiply handicapped children. *Pediatrics*, 1974, *54*, 779–786.

Katz, J., & Capron, A. M. *Catastrophic diseases: Who decides what?* New York: Russell Sage, 1975.

Koocher, G. P., & O'Malley, J. E. *The Damocles Syndrome, psychological consequences of surviving childhood cancer*. New York: McGraw-Hill, 1981.

Koocher, G. P., Sourkes, B. M., & Keane, W. M. Pediatric oncology consultation: A generalization model for medical settings. *Professional Psychology*, 1979, *10*, 467–474.

Korsch, B. M., Negrete, V. F., Gardner, J. E., Weinstock, C. L., Mercer, A. S., Grushkin, C. M., & Fine, R. N. Kidney transplantation in children: Psychosocial follow up study on child and family. *Journal of Pediatrics*, 1973, *83*, 339–408.

Korsch, B. M., & Morris, M. Gaps in doctor–patient communication. Patients' response to medical advice. *New England Journal of Medicine*, 1968, *280*, 535–540.

Kucia, C., Drotar, D., Doershuk, C., Stern, R. C., Boat, T. F., & Mathews, L. Home observations of family interaction and childhood adjustment to cystic fibrosis. *Journal of Pediatric Psychology*, 1979, *4*, 479–489.

Lansky, S. B., Cairns, N. U., Haasanein, R., Wehr, J., & Lowman, J. T. Childhood cancer: Parental discord and divorce. *Pediatrics*, 1978, *65*, 184–190.

Lascari, A., & Stehbens, J. The reactions of families to childhood leukemia: An evaluation of a program of emotional management. *Clinical Pediatrics*, 1973, *12*, 210–214.

Lavigne, J. V., & Ryan, M. Psychological adjustment of siblings of children with chronic illness. *Pediatrics*, 1979, *63* (4), 616–627.

Lawler, R. N., Nakielny, W., & Wright, N. Pychological implications of cystic fibrosis. *Canadian Medical Association Journal*, 1966, *94*, 1043–1046.

Markova, I., MacDonald, K., & Forbes, C. Impact of hemophilia on childrearing practices and parental cooperation. *Journal of Child Psychology/Psychiatry*, 1979, *21*, 153–161.

Mattson, A. Long-term physical illness in childhood: A challenge to psychosocial adaptation. *Pediatrics*, 1972, *50*, 801–811.

McCollum, A. T., & Gibson, L. Family adaptation to the child with cystic fibrosis. *Journal of Pediatrics*, 1970, *77*, 574–578.

McIntosh, J. Processes of communication, information seeking, and control associated with cancer. *Social Science and Medicine*, 1974, *8*, 157–187.

Mechanic, D. *Public expectations and health care*. New York: Wiley, 1972.

Meyerowitz, J. H., & Kaplan, H. B. Familial responses to stress: The case of cystic fibrosis. *Social Science and Medicine*, 1967, *1*, 249–262.

Minuchin, S. *Families and family therapy*. Cambridge, Mass.: Harvard University Press, 1974.

Minuchin, S., Rosman, B., & Baker, L. *Psychosomatic families*. Cambridge, Mass.: Harvard University Press. 1978.

Mohr, R. Paradigms in the clinical psychology of a chronic illness. Paper presented at a meeting of the American Psychological Association, Washington, D.C., September 1977.

Moise, J. R. Psychosocial adjustment of children and adolescents with sickle cell anemia. Unpublished master's thesis. Case Western Reserve University, 1980.

Moos, R., & Moos, B. A typology of family social environments. *Family Process*, 1976, *15*, 357–371.

Obetz, W. S., Swerson, W. M., McCarty, C. A., Gilchrist, G. S., & Burgat, E. O. Children who survive malignant disease: Emotional adaptation of the children and families. In J. L. Schulman & M. J. Kupst (Eds.), *The child with cancer*. Springfield, Ill.: Charles C. Thomas, 1980.

Odom, L., Seeman, J., & Newbrough, J. R. A study of family communication patterns and personality intergration in children. *Child Psychiatry and Human Development*, 1971, *1*, 275–385.

O'Malley, J. C., & Koocher, G. *The da mocles syndrome: Psychosocial consequences of surviving childhood cancer*. New York: McGraw Hill, 1981.

Osherson, S., & Amarasingham, L. R. The machine metaphor in medicine. In E. Mischler, L. R. Amarasingham, S. D. Osherson, S. T. Hauser, N. E. Waxler, & R. Liem (Eds.), *Social contexts of health, illness and patient care*. Cambridge: Cambridge University Press, 1981.

Parke, R. Perspectives on father infant interaction: In J. E. Osofsky (Ed.), *Handbook of infant development*. New York: Wiley, 1979.

Parsons, T., & Fox, R. Illness, therapy and the modern urban American family. *Journal of Social Issues*, 1952, *8*, 31–44.

Pless, I. B., Roghmann, K., & Haggerty, R. F. Chronic illness, family functioning, and psychological adjustment: A model for the allocation of preventive mental health services. *International Journal of Epidemiology*, 1972, *1*, 271–277.

Pless, I. B., & Satterwhite, B. B. Chronic illness. In R. Haggerty & I. Pless (Eds.), *Child health and community*. New York: Wiley, 1975.

Pless, I. B., Satterwhite, B., & Van Vechten, D. Chronic illness in childhood: A regional survey of care. *Pediatrics*, 1976, *58*, 37–46.

Power, P. W., & Dell Orto, A. E. (Eds.). *Role of the family in the rehabilitation of the physically disabled*. Baltimore: University Park Press, 1980.

Raimbault, G., Cachin, O., Limal, J. M., Elincheff, C., & Rappaport, L. Aspects of communication between patients and doctors: An analysis of the discourse in medical interviews. *Pediatrics*, 1975, *55*, 401–405.

Ritchie, K. Research note: Interaction in the families of epileptic children. *Journal of Child Psychology and Psychiatry*, 1981, *22*, 65–71.

Sameroff, A. Transactional models in early social relations. *Human Development*, 1975, *18*, 65–79.

Sourkes, B. Facilitating family coping with childhood cancer. *Journal of Pediatric Psychology*, 1977, *2*, 65–68.

Spinetta, J. J., & Maloney, L. J. The child with cancer: Patterns of communication and denial. *Journal of Consulting and Clinical Psychology*, 1978, *46*, 540–541.

Spinetta, J. J., Sheposh, J. P., & Swarner, J. A. Effective parental coping following the death of a child from cancer. *Journal of Pediatric Psychology*, 1981, *6*, 251–264.

Stack, C. B. *All our kin: Strategies for survival in a black community*. New York: Harper & Row, 1974.

Steinhauer, P. D., Muskin, D. N., & Rae Grant, Q. Psychological aspects of chronic illness. *Pediatric Clinics of North America*, 1974, *21*, 825–840.

Tefft, B. M., & Simeonsson, R. J. Psychology and the creation of health care settings. *Professional Psychology*, 1979, *10*, 558–570.

Tew, B. J., & Lawrence, K. M. Mothers, brothers and sisters of patients with spina bifida. *Developmental Medicine and Child Neurology*, 1973, *15*, Suppl. 29, 69–76.

Turk, J. Impact of cystic fibrosis on family functioning. *Pediatrics*, 1967, *34*, 67–71.

Tropauer, A., Franz, M. N., & Dilgard, V. W. Aspects of the care of children with cystic fibrosis. *American Journal of Diseases of Children*, 1970, *119*, 424–432.

Vance, J. C., Fazan, L. E., Satterwhite, B., & Pless, I. B. Effects of nephrotic syndrome on the family: A controlled study. *Pediatrics*, 1980, *65*, 948–955.

Venter, M. Chronic childhood illness/disability and familial coping. Unpublished doctoral dissertation. University of Minnesota, 1980.

III

Adolescence

6 Adolescence: A Time of Transition

Barbara D. Blumberg, M. Jane Lewis, and Elizabeth J. Susman

Literature Review

Adolescence is a key transitional period in an individual's growth, a relatively short period in which a number of developmental tasks must be accomplished at the same time that rapid physical changes occur. The necessity of accomplishing these tasks is no less important for an individual with a chronic illness than for one who is healthy. Indeed, an adolescent's development may be seen as proceeding along a given course, and although an adolescent with a chronic illness confronts emotionally and physically stressful problems that potentiate an atypical course of development, normal development processes do occur (Susman, Hollenbeck, Nannis, & Strope, 1980).

Various theorists have defined the developmental tasks of adolescence. For Erik Erikson (1963) this is a period typified by the search for identity, one in which individuals are concerned with how others see them as compared to how they see themselves. Others (Havighurst, 1951; Leventhal & Boeck, 1978; Weiner, 1976) point out that this search for identity involves the need to establish independence from parents and other adults, adjust to sexual maturation, enter into mature relationships with peers of both sexes, and begin to prepare for the future. If developmental tasks are successfully completed, the adolescent will emerge from this period with adequate self-esteem, a comfortable body image, an established identity, emotional independence, economic independence or the ability to achieve it when the completion of school or training makes it appropriate, a sexual identity, and a realistic, goal-oriented view of the future.

In their pursuit of these developmental tasks, adolescents typically exhibit certain behaviors—strong peer identification and unwillingness to appear different, assertions of independence as they test their autonomy, the need for control, an acute sense of their bodies (especially any imperfections)—that are so striking it is easy to forget the basic tasks from which they spring. This is particularly true when one is dealing with an adolescent with a chronic illness, where the illness, rather than the person, may become the focal point for attention.

When considering the pervasive nature of the tasks adolescents must undertake—development of an identity, a positive body image and self-image, a realistic orientation to the future, emotional independence—one can see the enormity of the task that lies before each person entering adolescence. For an adolescent with a chronic illness, the difficulties of achieving these tasks can be easily compounded by the manifestations of the illness and its treatment.

The particular nature of the additional stress associated with an illness will differ with each chronic condition. One recent study (Kellerman, Zeltzer, Ellenberg, Dash, & Rigler, 1980) examined adolescents with five different chronic illnesses to assess the psychological effects of illness in adolescence. One hundred sixty-eight adolescents with chronic or serious disease were compared with 394 healthy adolescents on standardized measures of trait anxiety (generalized, long-term), self-esteem, and perception of self-control over health and illness (health locus of control). Members of the adolescent patient group included patients with cancer, cardiologic disorders, diabetes mellitus, cystic fibrosis, renal disorders, and rheumatologic disorders. The findings, as reported by Kellerman and his colleagues, showed no significant differences in trait anxiety or in self-esteem between healthy and ill groups or among the various disease groups. A difference between healthy and certain ill groups did emerge when measuring health locus of control, with only the diabetes and cystic fibrosis groups showing scores similar to those of the healthy sample. Scores for the other chronically ill adolescents indicated that they saw their health as being controlled more by outside (external) factors rather than by themselves.

These findings support the hypothesis that the diagnosis of certain types of disease and all that follows this diagnosis may reduce adolescents' sense of control over their health. Adolescents with diabetes and cystic fibrosis, whose scores were similar to those of the healthy adolescents, have the potential to exert some control over their illness and its symptoms through complying with diet regimens and self-administered medication schedules. Patients with cancer, renal dysfunction, cardiac disorders, and rheumatologic disease, however, do not have such control. Instead, control over their disease and symptoms comes from medical sources [e.g., from physicians and nurses, from treatments and medications administered in medical settings] (Kellerman et al., 1980). Given that control of disease comes from external sources, the study's authors point out, attitudes indicating external locus of control on the part of these patients are not a psychologic deviance, but rather an accurate self-perception.

When anxiety levels were compared with physician prognosis, patients whose physicians rated their prognosis as "stable" were found to be less anxious than those whose physicians predicted change—even if change was for the better. This suggests that the perception of future stability is important to chronically ill adolescents. Kellerman and his co-investigators (1980) determined that additional change due to disease may be particularly anxiety provoking for adolescents, who are already experiencing multiple and rapid changes.

Despite the finding of increased anxiety when confronted with a changing prognosis, adolescents with chronic illness in general seem to have a higher tolerance for stress than do their healthy peers. In reviewing the fact that no difference in trait anxiety levels was found between ill and healthy groups, these authors point to results of a previous study (Bedell, Giordan, Amour, Tavormina, & Boll, 1977) where life stress was found to be related to anxiety in healthy children but not in patients with chronic illness. The Bedell study suggested that, for healthy children, life stress is seen as disruption, and changes are anxiety producing. For chronically ill children, varying degrees of constant or frequent life disruption are common, and they therefore develop heightened stress tolerance, learning to live with their disability and developing effective coping mechanisms. The Kellerman study (1980) of adolescents with chronic illness found support for this by noting that there was a negative correlation between anxiety and time since diagnosis, indicating that, with time, increased coping skills are developed. The adolescents appear to have learned to live with disability and to have developed mechanisms for coping with anxiety.

The overall findings of the Kellerman study point to a marked similarity in ill and healthy adolescents. Where there were differences, such as lower levels of feeling control over their health by adolescents with certain chronic illnesses, these were based on reality and did not appear to demonstrate a lack of adjustment. A related study, reported by Zeltzer, Kellerman, Ellenberg, Dash, and Rigler (1980) concerning the impact of illness in adolescents, found chronically ill adolescents to be essentially healthy psychologically and to have generally hopeful, positive outlooks. Because both of these studies were based in large part on self-administered questionnaires, denial of problems may account in part for the findings. In general, however, they may be seen as supporting those theorists and caregivers who view adolescents with chronic illness as being well-adjusted, normal adolescents, who are confronted with a stressful situation with which they must deal while also confronting the stresses that normal adolescents face.

Studies of Adolescents with Cancer

The remainder of this chapter will focus on the problems of adolescents with chronic illness from the perspective of a particular group: adolescents with cancer. Common behaviors of these patients, how they may be viewed within the spectrum of adolescent development, and actions which may help these adolescents accomplish their developmental tasks will be discussed. Many of the problematic issues considered, including a body image, peer relations, school, independence, and relations with parents, are common to variant chronic illnesses and must be dealt with by any adolescent learning to cope with a chronic debilitating condition. Consideration of psychosocial problems associated with cancer will merely provide the vehicle by which these issues can be more closely examined.

Cancer in adolescents has only recently come to be viewed as a chronic, although life-threatening, disease. It was once considered a swift and certain killer. Today, treatment techniques capable of producing remissions (disease-free states) have increased the length of survival and, in some cases, brought about apparent cures. Treatment techniques and survival rates may vary from one type of cancer to another, and not all adolescents with cancer face identical treatment courses or prognoses.

Adolescents may be diagnosed with any of a number of types of cancer, including leukemia, Hodgkin's disease, non-Hodgkin's lymphoma, and brain tumors. Certain tumors of the bone, such as Ewing's sarcoma and osteogenic sarcoma, are particularly associated with adolescents. Ovarian and testicular cancers and other forms less common to adolescents are also possible.

For the most part, cancer in adolescents is treated with chemotherapy, radiation therapy, or surgery, and often with a combination of these treatment modalities. Amputation of the affected limb is a common treatment for osteogenic sarcoma. Treatment for adolescents with all forms of cancer is aggressive, and almost always involves anticancer drugs or radiation therapy that produces numerous side effects, such as hair loss, nausea, weight loss or gain, and lowered energy levels. These affect an adolescent's appearance and ability to participate in normal activities.

In discussing adolescents with cancer, we will follow a model that addresses human development within the context of a life-threatening illness (Susman, Hollenbeck, Strope, Hersh, Levine, & Pizzo, 1980). This model assumes that physiological, social, and cognitive development continues in spite of the illness and that adolescents' reactions to the illness, although these include symptoms of stress, are not necessarily pathological, but more likely are related to appropriate development concerns of their age. In other words, while psychological development may be altered by the diagnosis of cancer, the manifestations of the disease, its life-threatening nature, and treatment regimens, development will continue.

Most adolescents with cancer cope remarkably well. The resiliency of this developmental period gives the adolescent the tools to spring back from disappointments and function despite the adversities associated with a diagnosis of cancer. Adolescents see themselves as being immortal and view death as something possible only in the distant, unforseeable future (Zeltzer, 1980).

One study (Susman & Pizzo, 1977) of adolescents on research drugs whose cancers had failed to respond to conventional treatment found that patients displayed an inordinate degree of hope in the remission-inducing potential of chemotherapy. The majority of the adolescents thought they would survive even though the odds were against them. Similar reactions are common to adults, but they may be more pronounced in adolescents, who, by virture of their youth and previous good health, may regard their bodies as indestructible.

This view of their own indestructibility may be interpreted as denial, but it may be less a manifestation of denial in the psychoanalytic sense than it is a natural adolescent reaction (Susman, Pizzo, & Poplack, 1981). However one views it, denial as exhibited by adolescent cancer patients is more often adaptive than maladaptive. Further, caregivers often reinforce this behavior. Encouraging adolescents to continue as many prediagnosis activities as possible amounts to tacit approval of some denial as a valid way of adapting to the disease. Denial becomes a problem if it impedes the treatment process or allows a patient to participate in activities against medical advice (Moore, Holton, & Martin, 1969).

Other coping mechanisms commonly observed include overcompensation, intellectualization, and anger. Overcompensation or attempts to outdo peers, when successful, may reinforce denial and support the adolescents' belief that they are normal. Intellectualization may be used in an attempt to master anxiety by repressing the emotions involved with cancer and emphasizing the rational aspect of its existence; teenagers using this defense tend to research their illness and ask many questions. Anger about the disease may be displaced to parents, siblings, or friends, and often is directed at caregivers (Moore et al., 1969).

At least one significant gap exists in the literature. A review of the literature in medicine, nursing, and the behavioral sciences conducted by the National Cancer Institute's (NCI) Office of Cancer Communications indicated that, although the psychosocial needs of adolescents, and particularly those with a serious illness such as cancer, are great, little, if any, information has been designed for them. To fill this gap and attempt to help adolescents cope with the disease, its treatment, and the impact of these on developmental tasks, NCI undertook the development of materials (e.g., National Cancer Institute, 1982a, b) addressing specific areas of concern identified by a review of the literature and confirmed by adolescents with cancer and health professionals from whom they seek care, information, and support. These include independence/dependence; body image; relations with parents, siblings, caregivers, and friends; continuation in school; future orientation; and remission and recurrence.

Eighty-nine responses from adolescent cancer patients representing four institutions, and fifty-three responses from health professionals from seven institutions participated in evaluative research of the materials during their development. This formative evaluation was designed to validate existing content, point to any information needs that were not addressed, and provide guidance for materials format. Input from participants came from questionnaires completed by health professionals and adolescents, and from personal interviews and moderated group discussions with patients.

Responses from patient and professional audiences to the materials and the concepts they contain validated previous research and anecdotal observations about adolescents with cancer. The research confirmed that patients are willing to talk about their disease and to discuss sensitive issues. It also confirmed that they have little or no access to written or audiovisual materials about their disease. In terms of their parents, adolescents were found to vacillate between wanting parental support and wanting to be independent of their parents. The adolescents were generally concerned with returning to school and conscious of any changes in appearance resulting from the disease and its treatment; they were fearful of appearing different from others. As with all teenagers, they felt acceptance by their peers at home was important. Interaction with other adolescent cancer patients met through treatment was also valued. They expressed a desire for honest yet positive information and relations with health professionals. Finally, they were found to be concerned about their futures.

Materials produced by Adria Laboratories, Inc. (1982) in cooperation with the National Cancer Institute for this group of cancer patients reflect their specific concerns and remarks. These materials include a booklet and cassette tape for adolescents and accompanying discussion guide for health professionals.

Treatment Issues: Applications and Strategies

The Zeltzer et al. study (1980) used a special illness-impact questionnaire to assess impact of the disease and treatment in several areas among the five groups of adolescents with chronic illness. The questionnaire focused on relationships with family members; school and peer activities; independence and autonomy; perceptions of personal, social, and sexual functioning; future orientation; and effects of treatment. The findings show that, of all disease groups, cancer patients reported the most disruption to their lives from the illness and its treatment. In particular, they reported the most problems due to treatment, which was perceived as causing general problems and affecting appearance, and thus body image. Adolescents with cancer were significantly more likely than those in the other disease groups to perceive the treatments as being worse than the disease. Overall, they reported the illness and treatment as having a negative impact on freedom, body image, school, and family relations.

It is this negative impact that caregivers may attempt to combat through knowledge of the obstacles cancer and its treatment pose and of the concerns of adolescents with cancer. In some cases, accurate information to counteract fears or fantasies will meet a patient's needs. For other issues, patients may need tips on how to deal with a problem, such as explaining the manifestations of their disease or treatment side-effects to friends. In this section, we will address some specific concerns and possible ways patients may deal with them.

Body Image

[Since adolescents often are more concerned about how others feel about them than how they feel about themselves,] changes in body image resulting from the disease and its treatment, such as weight loss, hair loss, or amputation of a limb, often threaten their self-esteem. These changes may be perceived by adolescents as more problematic than is the disease itself (Susman et al., 1981). Indeed, the changes may affect both their perceptions of themselves and their peer relations.

Hair loss, one of the most common side-effects of treatment, is particularly difficult for the adolescent with cancer to accept. Upon hearing of its likelihood, many react initially by saying they would rather die than lose their hair. Hair loss is indeed a dramatic, highly visible side-effect, and one for which most newly diagnosed patients are not prepared. In addition to not wanting to lose their hair because of the role it plays in enhancing physical appearance, specifically sexual attractiveness, patients realize loss of hair will set them apart from their peers. The thought of being bald is not easily accepted. In addition, some patients fear that their hair will never grow back.

Adolescents may be helped to cope with hair loss, or to accept its possibility, by being assured that their hair will grow back and by being given tips on the options they have for appropriate head coverings, such as wigs, scarves, or hats. These options should be explored early in treatment so that patients are prepared to deal with the problem when it arises.

The adolescent may also need help in learning how to respond to questions from others about what happened to their hair. Patients in the NCI materials development project reported feeling uncomfortable when people stared at them and bothered by kidding about their baldness. They advised others to be prepared for names like "onion top or skin head." They felt that preparing friends for hair loss was important. One patient urged honest answers to others' questions: "I tell them that the medicine I'm taking to cure my disease makes my hair come out" (Office of Cancer Communications, 1980).

Weight gain (from certain treatments) or loss (from the disease itself or as a side-effect of treatment) may also be alarming. Here again, adolescents face the problem of feeling different from their peers. One adolescent described her experience this way:

> When I first came up here, I weighed 118-½ pounds. When I left you know how much I weighed? . . . 88 pounds. It makes you really self-conscious to go somewhere and see people who know you [Office of Cancer Communications, 1980].

This self-conscious feeling is also experienced by those whose treatments result in weight gain. Either way, adolescents face problems in finding clothing to fit them during peak periods of weight gain or loss. Patients may need to buy or borrow clothing. Some find it possible to wear styles that minimize the change in their appearance, such as the girl who had lost weight and bought clothes "to make you look fuller, where your ribs and hipbones stick out" (Office of Cancer Communications, 1980).

A reduced level of energy is another possible side-effect of treatment. Lowered energy may produce problems in continuing normal activities. This may be perceived as a sign of weakness and a threat to independence. Forced limitation resulting from lower levels of energy causes the adolescent to feel weaker and different from peers for whom activity and vitality are viewed as being of paramount importance (Susman et al., 1981).

With amputations, adolescents feel the natural grieving for the loss of a body part and fear a resulting loss of function. They may be concerned that they will be dependent on others as a result of the amputative surgery. With loss of a leg, adolescents may fear they will never walk again or participate in other physical activities, such as sports. With loss of an arm, particularly the dominant arm, they may fear becoming dependent through loss of the ability to perform many functions such as eating, writing, or driving.

Caregivers may assist the adolescent by pointing out ways to retain independence following amputative surgery and resume as many former activities as possible. These discussions may begin before the surgery.

Caregivers can encourage immediate use of a prosthesis and point to the many amputees who participate in former activities, such as skiing, horseback riding, or motorcycling, which they once feared would be impossible for them.

Talking with others who have undergone amputative surgery and the adjustments made necessary by that surgery may be helpful. Advice provided by adolescents in the NCI materials development project suggested that amputees "get busy and find out what there is to do about it. Get yourself a prosthesis." Specifically for those who had lost a leg, they suggested: "Start walking. Try and get back on two feet again" (Office of Cancer Communications, 1980).

Amputation, of course, has a strong effect on body image and future plans and a potential effect on peer relations. One adolescent with a leg amputation explains her fears this way:

> I know young men, especially, really pay a lot of attention to looks and physical attractiveness. I wonder—will a boy accept me just the way I am? You hear them talking about how a girl's really built, or how she looks in a bathing suit and I hope they understand that they just amputated my leg, they didn't take my heart and soul and personality. I just don't know if they'll ever accept me [Darling, 1978].

Peer Relations

Adolescents with cancer may be acutely sensitive to others' reactions to changes resulting from the cancer and its treatment. The diagnosis itself has changed them, not only in their own eyes but in the eyes of others as well. Caregivers and parents may be more protective, thus interfering with the natural adolescent drive toward independence. Peers may avoid them, out of embarrassment, fear, uncertainty of how to treat the patient, or the belief that cancer is contagious. When adolescents receive a diagnosis of cancer, an unsettling change in status within the peer group probably occurs, so that regardless of where they were in the social pecking order before, after the diagnosis they are someplace different. Feeling this change does not constitute unreasonable paranoia, but the recognition of reality (Plumb & Holland, 1977). Adolescents may find it difficult to adjust to these changed perceptions and prefer limited participation to altered status.

Regardless of the adolescent's perception or self-image, however, the disease and its treatment may limit opportunities for socialization needed to maintain peer contacts and accomplish the developmental tasks in which peers play such an important role. Long periods of hospitalization and disability alter life-style. School performance becomes a problem because of frequent absence (Susman et al., 1981). Physical limitations from amputations may prevent the adolescent from driving, participating in athletics, or dancing, all of which provide social status and feelings of competence. If physical limitations do not remove these adolescents from normal socialization, they may isolate themselves through a distorted self-image and self-consciousness (Weiner, 1976).

Reactions from adolescents with cancer in the NCI materials development project indicate that this self-isolation does occur. One patient said she often felt like an outsider and believed people did not want to approach her because she had had cancer. Another patient echoes this response, saying:

> I felt that a lot of people thought they wouldn't want to get near me because I had this disease; they were afraid that I might be able to give it to them or something, and they weren't really sure whether or not they could talk to me about it. So I just tried to explain to them that I was okay and that you can't catch it. And I told them that I didn't know how I got it, it just happened [Office of Cancer Communications, 1980].

Many adolescent patients recommend telling friends the truth about cancer, its treatment, and side-effects. As one patient says: "If you don't tell them exactly what's going on then they won't know how to react to you, or how to talk to you like they did before" (Office of Cancer Communications, 1980). Friends may react in various ways. Some patients have good experiences with their friends, as in the following case:

> And I prepared one of my better friends. I told her I'm going to come home and probably I'm going to be bald, I'm probably going to look like I'm sicker than a dog. And she said okay, just as long as you're you [Office of Cancer Communications, 1980].

Others may lose friends who find the situation to be more than they can handle.

Friends who can handle the situation may be able to influence reluctant adolescents with cancer to come out of self-imposed isolation, as the following account illustrates:

> When I first got sick I didn't feel like getting involved and going to parties. After awhile I thought I'd gotten too far behind to be going to a party or anything like that. One day my friend told me that I should be getting out more so I went out on dates and stuff like that. I learned that I could still have a lot of fun. You shouldn't just stay in the house, cutting everyone off. You can have fun with people even if they know what's wrong with you [Office of Cancer Communications, 1980].

School

The return to school of the adolescent with cancer is particularly important. It represents a resumption of the adolescent's way of life before the disease, and the adolescent with cancer may gain a sense of mastery by the successful return to the role of student. In addition, it reduces the isolation from peers and their activities. As shown by the NCI findings, adolescents feel it is important to return to school, but are concerned about it (Office of Cancer Communications, 1980, 1981). There may be several reasons for this. In school they have little control over which of their peers will see them and notice any physical changes. Lowered energy levels may make it hard to keep up to past levels of performance, and they may have to miss school for treatment or when they are ill from treatment side-effects. They are concerned about how to respond to questions and how to handle any teasing or rejection. Overall, they are afraid of being thought of as different from their schoolmates and of being rejected by them.

Caregivers in cancer centers are increasingly aware of the importance of school for adolescents with cancer and may from the beginning of treatment make it clear to the adolescent that he or she is expected to return to school. Hospital schools are maintained so that patients can keep up with their classwork, and arrangements for homebound teachers may be made if the patient is at home and too ill to return to school for a period. But the eventual goal is always return to the classroom and peers. Caregivers may ease the return to school by contacting and encouraging continuing liaison with the school and teachers, offering any needed explanations or information (Blumberg, Flaherty, & Lewis, 1980; National Cancer Institute, 1980).

Independence

One constraint to living as nearly a normal life as possible is the dependence upon caregivers and family members which cancer imposes. For adolescents, this dependence occurs during a time when they have a need to assert their independence. In looking at this aspect of adolescent cancer, it has been noted that when medical treatment is prolonged, control may shift from the adolescent to the institution and its staff. Dependence and regression are reinforced by medically imposed periods of compliance and inactivity during which the adolescent is passive and has things done to him (Kellerman & Katz, 1977).

Forced into a dependent state, frustrated adolescents may rebel. It is not uncommon for them to refuse treatment, break hospital rules, miss outpatient appointments, or undertake activities they have been advised against. Although these reactions cannot be attributed solely to the feeling of dependency (fear and reluctance to appear different may also be present), striking out against established rule is clearly a key factor leading to rebellious behavior (Blumberg et al., 1980).

If no concessions are made to what adolescents see as an untenable situation, or if adolescents are not allowed to achieve some sort of autonomy within the role as patient, they may take control themselves. One way of maintaining control is noncompliance with medical treatment. Indeed, in an active struggle for control, patients may use the only thing they feel is totally theirs—their bodies—as a weapon in a final rebellion and refuse treatment altogether (Zeltzer, 1980).

Clearly, extreme forms of noncompliance must be avoided and adolescents given more control over their own lives. Hospital and outpatient clinics may need to adjust their schedules to allow some flexibility for adolescent patients to receive treatment on a schedule that conforms more closely with their lives as they were before diagnosis. Treatments may be given in late afternoon or early evening to minimize disruption to school attendance and outside activities. Sometimes postponing treatment for a short time may be necessary so that patients can attend a special event. While such changes may cause minor disruption to clinic or hospital schedules, they have the potential effect of greatly reducing the adolescent patients' feelings of helplessness and frustration (Blumberg et al., 1980).

To maintain compliance, caregivers should not only increase adolescent participation in their treatment, but also work to enhance adolescents' self-esteem and to return their sense of control so that treatments need not be the target of that control (Zeltzer, 1980). Other methods of enhancing a sense of control are relatively new and will be discussed later in this chapter under Future Trends.

Relations with Parents

The relationship between adolescents and their parents is complicated by a number of psychological issues unique to adolescents. Although teenagers are striving for independence, they have yet to achieve their goal. This is particularly true for younger adolescents. They may vacillate between the desire to be independent from parents and the need to be dependent, resenting what they see as overprotective behavior by their parents at one point and appreciating the support and protection of their parents at another (Moore et al., 1969). Problems may arise when parents react to their teenagers' cancer by trying to take care of them when, as parents, they should be learning to let go. They may attempt to maintain their authority by focusing on specifics of the adolescent's care that appear amenable to parental control (Kellerman & Katz, 1977).

A battle of wills on side issues can hinder the adolescent's adaptation to the disease and achievement of independence. Caregivers may intervene by expressing an understanding of parental concerns leading to overprotective or overindulgent behavior while supporting the adolescent's efforts at independence. Family sessions with a social worker or other mental health professional may be called for and welcomed, since parents often realize they are being overly protective but find it difficult to change. As one mother of an adolescent patient said:

> I wait on her hand and foot. I know I don't have to, but I just can't do enough. All of us baby her. I'll tell her 'don't clean your room, I'll do it,' but when I come back later she's done it herself. She knows the other kids have to clean their rooms and maybe that's why she cleans hers. Everybody wants to protect her more than she needs. She started going for walks to build up her strength and get outside for awhile. The neighbors worry about her walking around. One day one of them brought her home. She said, 'I didn't need help, but I let him do that because he wanted to' [Office of Cancer Communications, 1980].

Patients themselves may confront their parents with issues that are creating problems. As one patient says, "If you've got a problem with your parents, you should go to them and act like an adult and not a child" (Office of Cancer Communications, 1980). Although this may not always work at first, you should keep trying, according to another patient: "About the only thing you can do is sit down and talk to your parents. Sometimes they won't understand, but you just got to keep talking" (Office of Cancer Communications, 1980).

Caregivers and parents alike should be sensitive to the fact that patients may feel guilty about the extra burden their disease has placed on their families: One study (Leventhal & Boeck, 1978) found adolescent patients to be "concerned about the cost, the loss of parents' time from work and spoiled plans such as missed vacations." These investigators found a common goal for adolescent patients was getting a driver's license, thereby relieving the family of the responsibility for driving the patient to the hospital. And driving themselves to the hospital, perhaps accompanied by a friend, may increase their feeling of control.

Despite problems between patients and their parents, some patients feel they can rely on their parents more than on anyone else. As one adolescent patient said: "Your parents are your best friends, they'll never desert you" (Office of Cancer Communications, 1980). Another comments: "If you've got a good parent who will sit down and talk to you and really sympathize with your problem then you've got a lot" (Office of Cancer Communications, 1980).

Preparation for the Future

As part of the maturation process, adolescents normally look forward to what their lives will be like in the future. Most begin thinking about education, careers, marriage, and children. Adolescents with cancer, however, may be concerned about whether their disease will limit the possibilities open to them. School or employment may have to be interrupted for treatment, delaying future career plans. And the issue of marriage and childbearing may be especially problematic for the adolescent with cancer.

Sterility is a possible side-effect of some cancer treatments. Older adolescents may see their friends getting married and having children and wonder if they will be able to do so as well. In terms of having children, patients may be concerned about their ability to reproduce but be afraid to ask. As one patient said:

> Sometimes I wonder if I can have kids because of the treatment and it bothers me. I need to talk to the doctor about it but I haven't. I think it's because I may be afraid of what I might hear [Office of Cancer Communications, 1980].

In addition to the fears and threats to future plans and self-esteem that sterility may impose, those who are told they will probably not be sterile may worry about the effects of cancer therapy on the children they might have.

Such concerns are not easily answered because the long-term effects of cancer therapy are not fully known. Some studies in this area have been conducted (e.g., Li & Jaffe, 1974; Siris, Leventhal, & Vaitukaitis, 1976), the results of which indicate that, while cancer treatment may have an effect on fertility and future progeny, such a course is not inevitable.

In terms of plans for marriage, current treatment for cancer or a history of it does not preclude considering marriage. However, some adolescents may be concerned about the possibility of a recurrence of the disease and the burden they feel that would place on a spouse.

In spite of the uncertainty about the future, the adolescent cancer patient must be encouraged to make realistic plans. The responsibility of caregivers and parents is to provide the emotional support and information the adolescent needs to make sound decisions. Certainly, it must be emphasized that, with modern treatment techniques, young people do survive and go on to become productive, socially acceptable adults (Blumberg et al., 1980). As one young cancer patient said:

> I think about how good I'm going now. And when I can look back at last November, that was the worst part of my life. Then I look at this November. I'm having a great time. I'm in school, in college now, and I'm taking up early childhood education [Office of Cancer Communications, 1980].

Future Trends

In general, as adolescents with cancer survive longer and remain in the treatment system, attention to their developmental needs has increased. When dealing with adolescent patients, the emphasis is rightly less on rehabilitation, or returning the patient to a former level of functioning, than it is on fostering development and on assuring that their development continues as closely as possible to that of their age-mates. This emphasis on fostering development has created the atmosphere in which special attention is paid to the adolescent with cancer's educational, social, and developmental needs. Thus, special programs in treatment settings promote the return to school and ease the transition back to school. Hospitals and clinics have altered treatment times or regimens so that the patient's chances for recovery are not diminished, but chances for pursuing normal adolescent activities are increased. Continuation of these types of programs may be expected, and the principles they imply—fostering development, increasing a patient's feelings of autonomy and control—applied to other areas.

As research findings on adolescents with cancer accumulate, there is increasing evidence that behavior of adolescent cancer patients follows the normal developmental processes of their age. Except for those few patients who may have preexisting emotional problems, behavior of adolescent patients, even if it is not what caregivers would prefer, is not indicative of psychological maladjustment. Often adolescents are reacting to reality-based concerns. Where these issues are amenable to change, they may be addressed by competent members of a treatment team, people who are aware of the developmental tasks of adolescence and the roadblocks to these which cancer and its treatment impose, and are willing to look for solutions which take into account both medical realities and the patients' needs. With other problems which lie outside the power of the treatment center staff, such as loss of a friend because of the cancer, caregivers can offer support and understanding of the impact of this loss.

Some treatment centers employ methods such as hypnosis, biofeedback, relaxation, meditation, and yoga. These treatment modalities are intended to contain certain side-effects of treatment and enhance an adolescent patient's feelings of control of his or her body, and thus feelings of mastery and independence. They are noninvasive techniques, capable of decreasing unpleasant or uncomfortable symptoms, and may decrease reliance on drugs to control symptomatology. As an adolescent becomes adept at these techniques, the disease and treatment may interfere less with his or her life, thus allowing more time to undertake normal developmental activities (Zeltzer, 1980).

Recent research has centered not only on adolescents under treatment, but also on the quality of their lives as adults who were diagnosed and treated for cancer while adolescents (Koocher & O'Malley, 1981). As treatment advances are made and greater numbers of patients survive the experience, further research will be possible. As survival rates increase and more time has lapsed since the first strides in treatment were made, researchers are examining in greater depth both the physical and psychosocial long-term effects of having the disease as well as the long-term effects of the treatments that are currently used to extend these young people's lives.

References

Adria Laboratories. *Help Yourself: Tips for Teenagers with Cancer: Four Audio Plays—Users Guide*. Produced by Adria Laboratories, Inc., in cooperation with the National Cancer Institute, 1982.

Bedell, J. R., Giordan, B., Amour, J. L., Tavormina, J., & Boll. T. Life stress and the psychological and medical adjustment of chronically ill children. *Journal of Psychosomatic Research*, 1977, *21*, 237.

Blumberg, B., Flaherty, M., & Lewis, J. (Eds.). *Coping with cancer: A resource for the health professional*. Bethesda, Md.: National Cancer Institute, NIH Publication No. 80–2080, 1980.

Darling, L. Living with cancer. *The Washington Post*, June 24, 1978.

Erikson, E. *Childhood and society* (2nd ed.) New York: Norton, 1963.

Havighurst, R. J. *Developmental tasks and education*. New York: Longman's Green, 1951.

Kellerman, J., & Katz, E. B. The adolescent with cancer: Theoretical, clinical and research issues. *Journal of Pediatric Psychology*, 1977, *2*(3), 127–131.

Kellerman, J., Zeltzer, L., Ellenberg, L., Dash, J., & Rigler, D. Psychological effects of illness in adolescence. I. Anxiety, self-esteem, and perception of control. *The Journal of Pediatrics*, 1980, 97(1), 126–131.

Koocher, G. P., & O'Malley, J. E. *The Damocles Syndrome: Psychosocial consequences of surviving childhood cancer*. New York: McGraw-Hill, 1981.

Leventhal, G., & Boeck, M. M. The adolescent with cancer. *Proceedings of the American Cancer Society Second National Conference on Human Values and Cancer*. Cancer Society, 1978.

Li, F. P., & Jaffe, N. Progeny of childhood-cancer survivors. *The Lancet*, 1974, *2*(7882), 707–709.
Moore, C., Holton, C. P., & Martin, G. W. Psychologic problems in the management of adolescents with malignancy. *Clinical Pediatrics*, 1969, *8*(8), 464–473.
National Cancer Institute. *Students with cancer: A resource for the educator*. Bethesda, Md.: National Cancer Institute. NIH Publication No. 80–2086, 1980.
National Cancer Institute. *Help yourself: Tips for teenagers with cancer*. Produced by Adria Laboratories, Inc., in cooperation with the National Cancer Institute, 1982. (a)
National Cancer Institute. *Help yourself: Tips for teenagers with cancer: Four audio plays*. Washington, D.C.: National Cancer Institute, 1982. (b)
Office of Cancer Communications, National Cancer Institute. Adolescent coping project pretest report of adolescent cancer patient materials. Unpublished Report, September 1981.
Office of Cancer Communications, National Cancer Institute. Pretest report: Statements on issues of concern to adolescents with cancer. Unpublished Report, January 1980.
Plumb, M. M., & Holland, J. Cancer in adolescents: The symptom is the thing. *Nursing Digest*, 1977, *5*(2), 56–63.
Siris, E. S., Leventhal, B. G., & Vaitukaitis, J. L. Effects of childhood leukemia and chemotherapy on puberty and reproductive function in girls. *New England Journal of Medicine*, 1976, *294*(21), 1143–1146.
Susman, E. J., Hollenbeck, A. R., Nannis, E. D., & Strope, B. H. A developmental perspective on psychosocial aspects of childhood cancer. In J. L. Schulman & J. Kupst (Eds.), *The child with cancer*. Springfield, Ill.: Charles C. Thomas, 1980.
Susman, E. J., Hollenbeck, A. R., Strope, B. E., Hersh, S. P., Levins, A. S., & Pizzo, P. A. Separation-deprivation and childhood cancer: A conceptual re-evaluation. In J. Kellerman (Ed.), *Psychological aspects of cancer*. Springfield, Ill: Charles C. Thomas, 1980.
Susman, E., & Pizzo, P. A. Cognitive and affective changes in terminally ill adolescents. Presented at the symposium, Life-Span View of Death and Dying, 85th Annual Convention of the American Psychological Association, San Francisco, Calif., 1977.
Susman, E. J., Pizzo, P. A., & Poplack, D. G. Adolescent cancer: Getting through the aftermath. In P. Ahmed (Ed.), *Living and dying with childhood cancer*. New York: Elsevier, North Holland, 1981.
Weiner, I. B. The adolescent and his society. In J. Gallagher, F. P. Heald, & D. C. Garell (Eds.), *Medical care of the adolescent* (3rd ed.). New York: Appleton-Century-Crofts, 1976.
Zeltzer, L., Kellerman, J., Ellenberg, L., Dash, J., & Rigler, D. Psychologic effects of illness in adolescence. II. Impact of illness in adolescents—crucial issues and coping styles. *The Journal of Pediatrics*, 1980, 97(1), 132–138.
Zeltzer, L. K. The adolescent with cancer. In J. Kellerman (Ed.), *Psychological aspects of childhood cancer*. Springfield, Ill.: Charles C. Thomas, 1980.

7 The Family of the Adolescent: A Time of Challenge

Fran Z. Farrell and John J. Hutter, Jr.

Review of the Literature

Although this chapter addresses the problems faced by the family of the adolescent with cancer, the material presented is illustrative of the dynamics of a social unit with a chronically disabled adolescent member. The family is a complex social system consisting of intricately related positions with multiple sets of roles and norms (Hill, 1958) and having a variety of objectives. These objectives are a series of developmental tasks which must be successfully fulfilled if health maintenance and progress within the family cycle are to be achieved (Rowe, 1971). Individual family members and the family unit as a whole face different tasks at set transition points in the development of the family. The completion of these tasks leads to satisfaction and success with later tasks; failure to complete the tasks causes unhappiness in the family, difficulty with future tasks, and sometimes disapproval by society. The point at which a stressful event such as a diagnosis of a chronic illness occurs within the life cycle of the family can produce increased familial vulnerability if a transitional crisis is already occurring within the family organizational structure (Hymovich, 1973). During a stressful event, the equilibrium of the family unit is threatened; the security derived from accustomed means of dealing with conflict may disappear; and the expected responses from family interactions may not be forthcoming.

There is little doubt that when illness affects any member of the family there is an immediate assault on that family's sense of unity and well-being. Involvement of the family unit should begin at the time of diagnosis and continue throughout the illness (Kaplan, Smith, Grobstein, & Fischman, 1978). As each member of the family deals with the impact of the diagnosis, it is imperative that the professional help the family create methods for coping with the crisis. Many observations have been made of families which withdrew out of fear or reacted out of anger. As the family members develop purpose and a sense of involvement, their sense of value and worth will be enhanced.

The coping ability of a family is a function of the recognition and utilization of both internal and external resources of the family. The professional helps the family identify and mobilize its internal and external resources in order to maximize those abilities.

The diagnosis and treatment of a chronic illness of an adolescent affects the adolescent himself and integrity and function of the entire family. Changes which occur in the accustomed structure, patterns, and roles of the individual family members call for a reevaluation of old roles and establishment of new patterns. Although there are several studies investigating the effects of chronic illness on children, there are few controlled studies and studies which evaluate the frequency of disturbances among adolescents as a separate age-group.

The Parents

Discipline of the adolescent with cancer is often a problem. Frequently the family is overindulgent. Parents begin to tolerate behavior that they would not accept in a well child. Allowing the child to "get away with things," or buying whatever he asks for, can frighten the child by telling him that his disease is indeed serious: "He knows that only people who are not expected to live get this type of attention, and he may be feeling quite well" (Lansky, Lowman, Gyulay, & Brisco, 1976).

Another parental reaction is that of overprotectiveness. This is sometimes activated out of the parent's fear that the child will become ill again. Overprotectiveness impedes the child's development and makes the child angry at the people who are restricting his movement, which has been considerably reduced by the disease process itself (Rothenberg, 1967).

A survey of parents of children with cancer found that two-thirds of the respondents felt they had discipline problems (Lawrence, 1978). More than half of these parents attributed their problems to lack of information about what is "reasonable" in the way of behavior expectations for their child as related to the illness and treatments. One mother stated:

> It's no coincidence that the sign of cancer is the crab. My son is so grouchy and difficult to deal with when he takes steroids I feel sorry for him because he is so miserable. I know he can't help himself and yet I know that certain behavior [aggression toward his sister] cannot be allowed. I often feel confused about what to let him get away with and when to set limits [Lawrence, 1978].

The Siblings

While medical personnel and parents focus attention on the physical and, more recently, the psychosocial needs of the sick child, little time and energy are centered on the needs of the other well children in the family. Often the siblings are not personally known to the treatment team and may exist only as vague figures in the patient's background.

Siblings of the ill child must adjust to a situation where their parents' energies are directed toward the brother or sister with cancer. Siblings are acutely aware of the stresses which exist in their family following the diagnosis, in addition to any personal stresses they may have. A study by Lansky and Cairns (1979) showed siblings' concerns to be similar to the sick child's. Both siblings and patients experienced high levels of anxiety and viewed themselves as being vulnerable to catastrophic illness. Interestingly, the siblings displayed greater concern about isolation from others and dependency than the patients being tested. The siblings felt that the sick child was overindulged, but were reluctant to express negative feelings about other family members, perhaps out of fear of jeopardizing their precarious position in the family.

Feelings of jealousy, anger, guilt, and resentment surface causing immediate and acute pain. These feelings can contribute to long-term personality defects (Burton, 1975). A sibling may become attentive to the sick child's every want and need throughout the disease process because he may feel directly responsible for his brother's or sister's illness due to an outright confrontation or a secret wish for this sibling to go away or die at some point prior to the diagnosis.

> Margo, age 13, often quarrelled with her 15 year old sister. She wanted her sister's clothes, friends, and generally all the same privileges that Tina had. Following Tina's diagnosis with non-Hodgkins Lymphoma, Margo became withdrawn and obsessed with remaining at home to care for her sister. During a home visit, she verbalized her feelings about her motivations for this behavior: "I once wished that Tina would drop dead so I could have all her things for myself. It's coming true now. I caused it and I want to make up for what I said" [Sakata, 1980].

Several studies have documented the fact that chronic illness of a child within a family has ramifications throughout the family's system and causes a shift in family member interrelationships (Gogan, Koocher, Foster, & O'Malley, 1977; Peck, 1979). A recent study explored the perceptions of surviving siblings of the cancer experience (Burlington, 1980). Significant in this study is that the surviving siblings know that one of the major things which happened when their sibling became ill was that their "world changed." These changes included alterations in relationships with parents and the ill sibling, decreased social activity, and increased boredom. Other studies indicate a positive and direct relationship between open communication and the nature of change in family member relationships: as communication improves, the quality and nature of family member relationships also improve (Iles, 1979; Burlington, 1980).

Treatment Issues, Applications, and Strategies

Kaplan, Smith, and Grobstein (1972) cite the family as "a critical stress mediating system intimately involved in the adaptive efforts of all its members to master stress" (p. 140). Professional recognition and treatment of the entire family is therefore required in order to achieve success in protecting all family members threatened by the serious illness (Kaplan et al., 1972).

Kaplan, Smith, and Grobstein (1976) studied forty families three months after the death of a child due to illness. It was revealed that coping responses initially utilized by family members are predictive on long-term adaptability to stress. The severe impact of the child's death on family members and implications for supportive interventions are apparent in the study results. Only 12 percent of the study families emerged intact from the illness experience without some change in effective family functioning or without multiple problems among survivors. Seventy percent of the family members surveyed reported having one or more problems, and 80 percent of those problems occurred after the cancer diagnosis was made. Health problems among survivors were reported in 95 percent of the family members. Functional problems, which are difficulties in fulfilling major role responsibilities, were reported in 43 percent of the surviving siblings and 51 percent of the adults. The researchers' conclusion:

> The study findings support the view that the optimal period for intervention is during the early, acute stage of the crisis, immediately following the confirmation of the diagnosis, when the family is making those decisions associated with maladaptive coping and poor stress outcomes [Kaplan et al., 1976].

Financial strains, isolation between family members, and isolation from the community may greatly affect the supportive capacity of the family unit when chronic illness strikes (Calhoun, Selby, & Kind, 1976). Inordinate amounts of guilt in siblings and parents may be precipitated by the death of the sick child. This guilt may overwhelm family members and in this way interfere with the lending of mutual support (Calhoun et al., 1976).

In a case study of three adolescents with cancer, the family was identified as the most central support system for the adolescents (Farrell & Hutter, 1980). All three adolescents identified their mothers as the individuals closest to them. Their mothers were the persons with whom the adolescents shared their initial feelings.

Moore, Holton, and Marten (1960) cite the ambivalence between dependency and independence as one of the crucial challenges for parents in dealing with their adolescent who has cancer. These dependence and independence issues manifest themselves in a variety of ways. In an interview with five sets of parents of adolescents with cancer, all parents indicated that one of the crucial challenges at the time of diagnosis was their desire to protect their child from the knowledge of the implications of the diagnosis. All the parents were concerned about the degree of involvement of their children in discussions with health care professionals. Ultimately, they all recognized that the involvement of their child in the ongoing decision making with the treatment team provided the child with a heightened sense of control over his own life (Farrell, 1981).

This was supported by Nischke, Wunder, Sexauer, and Humphrey (1977), who involved their patients in a final stage conference to discuss treatment issues and decision making when the patient was no longer responding to conventional chemotherapy. This is in keeping with Karon (1973), who advocated an atmosphere of openness and honesty as essential for supportive psychological care of the adolescent with cancer.

The issues confronting the family members of an adolescent who is experiencing a chronic, disabling disease are indeed varied and challenging. When their child is ill from the treatment, the parents frequently find themselves in the role of nursing caretaker with an adolescent who tends to revert to a dependent childlike state. As soon as the ill effects of the treatment are resolved, the adolescent rebuffs parental affection. This dependent–independent cycle was cited by parents as very confusing. As one parent stated: "When she zigs I zag and we just can't seem to get our zigs and zags synchronized" (Farrell, 1981).

In summary, the need for honest and open communication would appear to be important for the adolescent patient. Open communication enhances interaction between the adolescent and his significant others and should be instituted and encouraged from the onset of diagnosis and treatment.

Interventions which enhance the quality of social interactions are indicated in order to maximize coping with the crisis inherent in chronic, disabling disease. All family systems are different in response to the stress and strain of chronic illness. In order that each family system be maintained as functional and intact as feasible, it is usually helpful to assess areas of both vulnerability and strength. Such assessment involves exploring the following areas:

1. External support systems, for example, school, peers, church;
2. Strength of marital and family member relationships;
3. Parent's fears and needs;
4. Siblings' fears, needs, and adjustment;
5. Philosophy regarding life and death (Farrell, 1977).

Acknowledgment of the entire family's involvement in the crises and of the feelings that they may have about it begins at the time of diagnosis. The goal is by timely intervention during the crises to be able to facilitate the family's reparative process and ward off emotionally painful complications.

Family network intervention utilizes a crisis intervention model which calls upon the assembled strengths of the family and its own network in order to mobilize and generate resources within the family in a productive manner. Lutwick (1965) summarized the clinical importance of the network as follows ("family" refers to the family kinship group):

> There are several classes of situations where the trained expert is of little use: in situations which are not uniform and where the minimal standards set by society are not involved—the question arises as to whether the family as a primary group might not be superior to the formal organization in these areas—the family is able to deal more easily with the idiosyncratic event because the family has more continuous contact over many different areas of life . . . the family has speedier channels for transmitting messages with no prior definition of legitimacy . . . it is less likely to have explicit rules of what is and what is not legitimate, it is more likely to consider events which have had no definition . . ." [p. 179].

Thus, family networking is particularly effective with "hard to reach families" with whom professionals have difficulty relating as they are subsequently supported by their own system. It also offers a unique opportunity to educate the entire family and other significant people in an adolescent's life about the illness and its treatment while they are assembled as a group, thereby decreasing the likelihood of misunderstanding and misconceptions. Thus the goals in a family network meeting are to increase all of the participants' understanding of the illness, its treatment, and side-effects, and also to reduce their anxieties and fears associated with the illness.

Process of Intervention

At the time of establishing the diagnosis, the physician and the social worker meet with the parents to inform them of the diagnosis, its treatment, and potential side-effects. The parents are subsequently encouraged to be present along with the adolescent and his siblings when the diagnosis and proposed treatment are given to the patient. In order to illustrate and facilitate understanding of the disease, pictures are drawn and notes taken highlighting the discussion. At this time, the patient, the siblings, and the parents will be assured that none of them did anything to bring about the illness by either their wishes or their actions. Although questions will be encouraged and answered, a special effort is made to avoid overwhelming the family with too much information. An initial assessment focuses and elicits discussion on: (1) the individual's fear and needs, (2) past experiences with any type of catastrophic illness (e.g., who was affected and what were some of the related unresolved questions and concerns), and (3) social supports and resources. The following day the social worker makes contact with the parents as well as the patient and seeks to identify questions and concerns which may have surfaced since the previous meeting. A list of immediate concerns related to such activities as childcare, household assistance, job, transportation, and other problems related to activities of daily living is then developed. The parents are invited to make a list of extended family members, friends, neighbors, schoolteachers, church associates, and other significant individuals in the adolescent's life. The adolescent is also invited to contribute to this list. The concept of family networking is introduced to the parents and patient as a means whereby everyone will have an opportunity to air their questions and concerns associated with the illness. The family meeting is subsequently scheduled within the first couple of weeks of the diagnosis. Present are the physician and the social worker, who open the meeting by introducing themselves and invite the individuals present to introduce themselves and state their relationship to the adolescent. The purpose of the meeting is to discuss the diagnosis, proposed treatment, and potential side-effects of the illness openly. The opportunity for each person to discuss his or her own concerns openly as related to the patient is invited. More specifically, the physician and social worker encourage questions in order to clarify understanding of what will be done, why, when, where, and by whom. There is a focus on the emotional responses of the individuals and acknowledgment of feelings. At this time there is an opportunity to assure individuals that feelings of confusion or shock are frequent reactions to illness and other unexpected life events and to encourage the sharing and expression of feelings. Concrete needs which the parents and the adolescent have previously identified are then presented to the group and suggestions are invited from the group toward problem resolution. Information regarding hospital and community resources is also provided. At the conclusion of the meeting there is literature pertaining to the illness that is dispensed and members of the group are invited to accompany the patient to the hospital when he receives subsequent treatment. As the adolescent receives medical treatment, there is an ongoing assessment of the emotional responses of his parents and himself relative to the illness.

The following is a case illustration of a young adolescent (L.E.) diagnosed with osteogenic sarcoma (bone cancer) with a proposed amputation of her left leg. Diagnosed three years earlier, this case will illustrate the effect and benefit of ongoing meetings with the family's system. The eldest of five children, at the time of her diagnosis she resided with her parents and siblings 300 miles from the hospital. At the time of her diagnosis she was almost twelve and her youngest sibling was two. Her mother was twenty-seven and her father was thirty-four. From the outset of the diagnosis it was essential that early ongoing assessment be carried out taking into account the developmental needs of all of the nuclear family members. The original family meeting was comprised of twenty people who chose to meet at the hospital. Their main concerns focused on: (1) the likelihood of cancer in the rest of the family, (2) what and how to tell siblings and cousins who are not present, (3) effects of chemotherapy and proposed time of treatment, (4) childcare and transportation, (5) patient's activities and/or limitations. Communication and problem sharing was facilitated during the meeting. A resolution regarding childcare and transportation was reached by the family members. Initially the patient was rather frightened and developed a strong, dependent relationship with her mother and would not allow her mother out of her sight. During the initial crisis of the amputation and immediate postoperative care, it was essential to support the adolescent patient and at the same time support the rest of the nuclear family members. Gradually health care providers and other extended family members became a significant relief for the mother, which offered L.E. a transition from mother-dependence to a more independent state. It was also crucial to take into account the needs of the nuclear family and define how these were going to be met. The mother had a long history of physical illness. Part of the restorative rehabilitative goals were set for the entire family so that the mother could continue in optimal health as she integrated a new crisis into her life. The role that the patient had assumed previously as the eldest in the family had been one of surrogate mother to the younger siblings, and this role also underwent some dramatic changes. The first six months after the diagnosis presented a challenge to the family as there was a shifting and redefinition of roles and a need for ongoing communication and support. L.E. returned to school despite initial fears of being teased over the loss of a limb and loss of hair. Of interest is that the loss of hair was far more difficult psychologically to overcome than the loss of the limb relative to self-image. The family network, comprised of extended family, helped with the childcare and transportation while the parents made numerous visits to the health care facility. L.E. adapted to her prosthesis and continued with a relatively active life in school. At age thirteen-and-one-half, the progression of cancer required an amputation of her other leg. Upon hearing the physicians state that the tumor was present in her other leg, the patient refused to participate in a family meeting where treatment options were to be discussed. The patient became very quiet, sullen, withdrawn, and refused to talk about what was bothering her. She responded to an invitation to write down her feelings, at which point she wrote, "I'm afraid to die." Upon sharing this with her mother and the social worker, she said, "There, it's out, now I feel better and let's get going. . . . Before we talk about my treatment I'm hungry and I want to eat first." On the following day, her parents and two siblings were present with the patient and both authors to discuss the proposed treatment. It was concluded that a second amputation would be necessary to provide the best chance for survival. Both parents invited her opinion, to which she remarked, "I don't want to die, let's take it off." Parents acknowledged that that too was their desire. At the conclusion of the meeting, her younger brother, age eight, knelt and scurried around the room, saying, "This is what you're going to look like when you walk." The patient and her family responded with laughter, and playful bantering between the patient and her sibling ensued. This seemed to manifest not only comic relief, but a sense of acceptance from the patient as well as the rest of the family members. A few days before her fourteenth birthday she required another operation to remove metastases (spread) of cancer to the lung. On the day of her fourteenth birthday at a small birthday party in her honor, the patient was composing a list of items she wanted for Christmas, which was only a month away. As she made the list she said out loud, "Stockings," only to be followed by a loud laugh and giggle from the patient as she said, "Sometimes I forget I don't have any legs." This resulted in some modest bantering between her and her siblings and her parents. It was evident by this interchange that "not having legs" is not an obvious interference in the interaction and life-style of the family members.

Results of family network therapy, as in any other type of psychotherapy, are extremely difficult to measure; that changes occur throughout the network, that individual's tighten significant relationships and become more aware of themselves and others, we have no doubt. The primary goal of our intervention with this particular family was accomplished—involvement of the family unit from the beginning and throughout the illness process. In this particular family there was a preexisting sense of family unity before the onset of the illness. As the family members integrated this event into the continuum of their lives, the stress of the initial amputation with the subsequent stresses of ongoing medical treatment and subsequent surgery have resulted in strengthened relationships. At this particular time, the patient is actively engaged in school and school activities. She is continuing to develop ongoing independence even though she is wheelchair bound. She continues to assist her mother in the caretaking of the younger siblings by entertaining them. As a matter of fact, she has developed great expertise in the entertainment arena. She has an interest in working with puppets, singing, and in listening to music. She enjoys creating plays with her siblings, assuming different roles and incorporating singing and dancing. She also enjoys telling jokes, and her siblings assume the role of audience as she participates in her multiple endeavors in entertainment. Her relationship with her peers seems to follow a "normal course" in that she has several friends, including a boyfriend. She spends a lot of time talking with her friends on the telephone, exchanges notes, and also enjoys attending school activities with them.

Of significance to L.E.'s self-esteem and the integrated functioning of the entire family is that she has not been viewed or treated as a victim. By involving L.E. and her entire family right from the beginning, it reduced the unknown to the familiar for all family members; thus, through knowledge, each individual was able to take and maintain control of his or her own situation. L.E. and her parents acknowledge the uncertainty within which they live as they realize there could be another metastases. Their sense of meaning in life is derived from closely shared daily activities. Ultimately, this family's main support has come from within the family and the extended family system. Despite the stresses caused by chronic illness, multiple surgeries, and prolonged treatment, they have not only maintained their close ties but transcended to a higher appreciation of day-to-day life.

A frequent challenge for the professional in working with families who have an adolescent with chronic illness is taking into account their cultural belief system and helping the family integrate their unique beliefs with the conventional medical system. The followig illustrates a blend of two different belief systems in an effort to promote optimal psychosocial and physiological help for the patient and the family. D.L., thirteen years old, died at home six months after the diagnosis of liver cancer was confirmed. He had been ill approximately six months prior to this confirmation. His parents were divorced two years prior to his illness and since the divorce he had lived with his father and twin brother in another community approximately 300 miles from his mother. His mother had relinquished care of the twin boys because of her debilitating chronic asthma. The relationships between the parents remained amicable, and the boys and their mother made frequent visits to each other. The diagnosis of cancer was confirmed in a large cancer center in the same town where the mother resided. Two weeks after the diagnosis was confirmed, a family network meeting was held by the pediatric oncology staff members. All family members, concerned friends, and relatives were invited to attend. The meeting was called so significant friends and family members could be oriented to the patient's diagnosis, present condition, prognosis, and optimal treatment modes. It was also a time for all in attendance to ask questions and express their concerns. There were approximately twenty-five people present. D.L.'s father was accompanied by D.L.'s mother and twin brother. The mother was present with both of her parents as well as a large group of her close friends, who formed a small community adhering to Eastern religious philosophy and homeopathic medical treatment. Because of D.L.'s progressive illness and poor prognosis, treatment options included purely palliative care. One week after the group meeting, the decision was made by the parents that the child would be cared for at home by his mother. Treatment options sought at this time were acupuncture, meditation, and herbal remedies. Although D. L.'s father and maternal grandparents did not object to these treatments, they held little belief in their effectiveness. The large group meeting served not only as an opportunity for the sharing and exchange of different ideas and beliefs, but also as an opportunity to identify the resources and define concrete needs which mother would need in caring for D.L. at home. Having met the members of the health care team at this large meeting, family members and concerned friends were able to create an opportunity with different members of the health care team for ongoing contact and discussion of their concerns. A relationship was established which would continue throughout the course of this child's illness, death, and up to the present time, which is a year and a half after his death. Several misunderstandings between the mother and her parents arose over the next six months of care. A member of the health care team coordinated the involvement of the parents and grandparents, which was difficult because of their differing belief systems. It was important to help the mother accept the fact that grandparents also suffer a great loss in the illness and death of a grandchild and they have a need just as parents and siblings do to help as much as they possibly can. Communication between those involved in caretaking resulted in the avoidance of conflict and resulted in promoting optimal care for D.L.

The second phase of coordinating medical care with members of the family involved the actual planning of the delivery of this care. This phase consisted of two steps: (1) identification and coordination of the medical disciplines, and (2) planning and implementation of care plans. This was accomplished by identifying two significant members of the health care team who would be the primary people involved with the family. Continuity of care could best be implemented when there existed a minimum of staff interacting with the family. Frequent communication was a key factor in delivering optimal care, and this was facilitated by frequent small family meetings. Although D.L.'s father and twin brother resided 300 miles away, it became evident that they wanted to be closely involved in the care and support. A challenge was to assist these two siblings who had been extremely close since birth to begin the disengagement process. Since they could no longer jointly engage in the activities that were typical of their age-group, it became important to help the well twin to identify means and ways that he could still spend time with his brother in sharing quiet activities which were not normally part of his life-style. They ended up spending time alone with each other engaged in conversation. The well sibling experienced his brother growing less and less interested in their conversations. In addition, he experienced D.L. "thinking things" and "feeling things that I just don't understand." "We just seem to lose closeness, it was just hard to feel what he was feeling." Since D.L.'s death, there have been several conversations with his surviving sibling, who has acknowledged that knowing about the illness and the prognosis helped him to prepare for dealing with the separation and subsequent loss of his brother. He was thankful that his parents included him at the initial group meeting because he felt that his questions about the illness were answered. He subsequently felt permission to continue talking to his parents about the illness and its treatment. He said that he had learned a lot about cancer and it helped him understand what his brother was experiencing. He found difficulty in coping with boredom when he missed his brother and the games they had played together.

The following highlights the significance of family networking in a letter written to the authors by the mother:

> . . . The love and support I found at the meeting were some of the most positive and significant events . . . later as events shaped themselves each one had a role to play in making home care possible. I'm not sure that would have happened if all had not understood the situation from the beginning.
>
> Also, because we all became familiar with each other, my family felt at ease with my friends and the professionals. Problems did come up and inevitable differences. . . . Examples could go on and on. There was an ease of communication established by the meeting which made it much easier . . . in spite of our divided family situation we had an unusual degree of harmony. . . . Though my friends would have all wanted to help anyway, the meeting unified them [personal communication, 1981].

Future Trends

As advances in medical science continue, we shall no doubt experience longer term remissions and cures of adolescents with cancer. With fewer people dying of the disease, we can expect larger populations of adolescents who currently have or have had cancer. With the reduction of resources for professionals in the social sciences, the trend is for increased use of self-help measures and interventions. Family networking, which takes advantage of the family's own resources with a minimum of professional assistance, is an expanding trend.

Interventions utilizing a family systems approach which serves to enhance coping capacity of the individual patient and the family seem warranted. The overall goal is toward the maintenance of as much normality as possible with a focus on the quality of day-to-day life.

Longitudinal cross-cultural studies of a large group of adolescents with chronic illnesses is required before we can fully understand the many problems faced by those adolescents and their families. Each family is unique and has a unique set of problems. As professionals, we can help the family define these problems, mobilize its resources, and work together closely to mitigate the possibly divisive impact of the illness. As a result of our efforts, families can surmount the sorrows, grow stronger and more closely knit, and learn to cherish and better appreciate each other.

References

Burlington, K. The cancer experience: Perceptions of surviving siblings. Unpublished thesis, University of Arizona, Tucson, Ariz., 1980.

Burton, L. *The family life of sick children: A study of families coping with a chronic illness*. London: Routledge and Kegan Paul, 1975.

Calhoun, L. G., Selby, J., & Kind, H. E. *Dealing with crisis: A guide to critical life problems*. Englewood Cliffs, N.J.: Prentice-Hall, 1976.

Farrell, F. Z. Living until death: A case study of three adolescents with cancer. Unpublished thesis, Arizona State University, Tempe, Ariz., 1977.

Farrell, F. A. Interviews with five sets of parents of adolescents with cancer. Unpublished manuscript, 1981.

Farrell, F. A., & Hutter, J. J. Living until death: Adolescents with cancer. *Health and Social Work*, 1980, *5*(4), 35–38.

Gogan, J. L., Koocher, G. P., Foster, D., & O'Malley, J. Impact of childhood cancer on siblings. *Health and Social Work*, 1977, *2*, 41–58.

Hill, R. Social stresses in the family. *Social Casework*, 1958, *39*, 139–158.

Hymovich, D. The family with a young child. In D. Hymovich & M. Barnard (Eds.), *Family Health Care*. New York: McGraw-Hill, 1973.

Iles, J. P. Children with cancer: Healthy siblings' perceptions during the illness experience. *Cancer Nursing Forum*, 1979, *2*, 371–377.

Kaplan, D. M., Smith, A., & Grobstein, R. The Problems of siblings. *Proceedings of the American Cancer Society's National Conference on Human Values and Cancer*, Atlanta, Georgia, June 22–24, 1972.

Kaplan, D. M., Smith, A., & Grobstein, R. Predicting the impact of severe illness in families. *Health and Social Work*, 1976, *1*(3), 71–82.

Kaplan, D. M., Smith, A., Grobstein, R., & Fischman, S. In C. A. Garfield (Ed.), *Psychological care of the dying patient*. New York: McGraw-Hill, 1978.

Karon, M. The physician and the adolescent with cancer. *Pediatric Clinics of North America*, 1973, *20*, 965–973.

Lansky, S. B., & Cairns, N. U. The family of the child with cancer. In *Care of the Child with Cancer*. New York: American Cancer Society, 1979.

Lansky, S. B., Lowman, J. T., Gyulay, J. E., & Brisco, K. A team approach to coping with cancer. In J. W. Cullen, B. H. Fox, & R. N. Isom (Eds.), *Cancer: The behavioral dimensions*. DHEW Publication No. (NIH) 76–1074. Bethesda, Md.: National Institutes of Health, 1976.

Lawrence, S. Results: Candlelighters discipline questionnaire. Unpublished report presented to the Division of Cancer Control and Rehabilitation, Silver Spring, Md., April 12, 1978.

Lutwick, E. Extended kin relations in an industrial democratic society. In E. Shanas & C. F. Streib (Eds.), *Social Structure and the Family*, Englewood Cliffs, N.J.: Prentice-Hall, 1965.

Moore, D. C., Holton, C. P., & Marten, G. W. Psychological problems in the management of adolescents with malignancy. *Clinical Pediatrics*, 1960, *8*, 464–473.

Nitschke, R., Wunder, S., Sexauer, C., & Humphrey, G. The final stage conference: The patient's decision on research drugs in pediatric oncology. *Journal of Pediatric Psychology*, 1977, *2*(2), 58–64.

Peck, B. Effects of childhood cancer on long-term survivors and their families. *British Medical Journal*, 1979, *1*, 1327–1329.

Rowe, G. The developmental conceptual framework to the study of the family. In F. M. Nye & F. I. Berardo (Eds.), *Emerging conceptual frameworks in family analysis*. New York: Macmillian, 1971.

Rothenberg, M. B. Reactions of those who treat children with cancer. *Pediatrics*, 1967, *40* (suppl), 507–510.

Sakata, M. K. The child with cancer: A psychosocial resource manual. Unpublished thesis, University of California, Davis, Calif., 1980.

IV

Young Adults

8 Facing Physical Disability as a Young Adult: Psychological Issues and Approaches

Robert L. Glueckauf and
Alexandra L. Quittner

Introduction

Following the life-span approach (Erikson, 1959), the primary developmental goal of early adulthood (ranging from eighteen to thirty years of age) is the formation of mature interpersonal relationships. In arriving at this goal, the young adult is confronted with difficulties in developing close ties with friends, choosing a career, and integrating sexuality into a meaningful, long-term relationship.

For persons who develop a chronic medical disorder in early adulthood, the complexity of these tasks may be greatly compounded. The reactions of family, friends, and associates may vary considerably. Some persons may react with exaggerated positive or negative displays (for example, Katz & Glass, 1978), while others may exhibit overcontrolled, stereotypic behaviors (for example, Kleck, Ono, & Hastorf, 1966). Such reactions may lead the disabled individual to believe that the behavior of others is not predictable, or that their responses are not genuine. This problem can become especially severe if the person perceives that the responses of significant others, particularly family and friends, are altered as a result of the disability. Thus, newly handicapped individuals may choose to isolate themselves from social contact and from information which might help to reduce their uncertainty about the behavior of others and about their medical condition (Glueckauf & West, 1982a).

Further complications may arise as a result of the social norms against providing constructive feedback to the physically handicapped (cf. Kelley, Hastorf, Jones, Thibault, & Usdane, 1960). Employers may experience considerable conflict in evaluating the work performance of the physically disabled young adult, especially when negative feedback is called for.

Some may hold the belief that disabled persons are fragile and respond to criticism with excessive self-condemnation or defensiveness (cf. Dunn & Herman, in press). The consequence of these misconceptions may be delays or avoidance in giving handicapped young adults information about their work behaviors. In the absence of constructive feedback, ineffective work patterns are likely to be maintained, which in turn may lead to a decline in the handicapped individual's overall performance.

A similar process is likely to occur in developing and maintaining intimate relationships with nonhandicapped individuals. Disabled young adults, especially males, may be perceived by nondisabled individuals as highly desirable friends or confidants who have no ulterior sexual motives (cf. Hahn, 1981). The ambiguity of these situations is likely to be high for the disabled individual who may interpret personal disclosures as cues for sexual involvement. If the handicapped person acts on such cues, he or she may be rebuffed and suffer losses of self-esteem. Faced with the possibility of further rejection experiences, the disabled young adult may avoid potentially intimate social contacts or possibly deny the sexual aspects of their social functioning (cf. Wagner, 1974). Hence, the transition to adulthood is likely to be a period fraught with uncertainty for disabled persons, necessitating the development of considerable skill in managing a variety of difficult interpersonal situations.

In accordance with the life-span perspective, this chapter will focus on the three major developmental tasks of early adulthood. First, the social implications of physical disability will be examined, followed by a discussion of the current therapeutic techniques to facilitate the social adjustment of handicapped young adults. Second, the effects of a disabling medical condition on vocational functioning will be addressed and recent advances in the field of vocational rehabilitation will be described. Third, the sexual consequences of physical disability will be discussed and a presentation of the current approaches to enhance sexual adjustment will follow. Finally, future directions for research on rehabilitative techniques will be examined.[1]

Social Consequences of Physical Disability

Persons who develop a chronic, disabling condition as young adults are faced with substantial alterations in their social environment (cf. Safilios-Rothschild, 1970). These changes can be located in four major areas of

[1]Spinal cord injury, rheumatoid arthritis, multiple sclerosis, and head injury have a high frequency of occurrence in early adulthood and therefore will receive special attention. Note that a discussion of the differential effects of these conditions on the psychological functioning of young adults was considered beyond the scope of this chapter.

interpersonal functioning: (1) public attitudes about physical disability, (2) the differential behavior patterns of the able-bodied toward the handicapped, (3) embarrassing social situations related to specific medical disorders, and (4) the reinforcement of dependent behaviors by health care professionals.

Prior research (Albrecht, Harasymiw, & Horne, 1977; English, 1971; Wright, 1960) has indicated that able-bodied persons share a common set of misconceptions and derogatory attitudes about physically handicapped individuals. For example, Albrecht and colleagues interviewed a random sample of Chicago residents and found that 76 percent of the participants felt that one should not expect as much from the handicapped as from the nonhandicapped. In addition, 36 percent of the subjects expected paraplegics to be bitter and 43 percent felt that most disabled persons do not marry or have children. In a laboratory study (Weinberg, 1976) two groups of college students received identical, brief descriptions of either a well-liked handicapped or a physically normal individual. Substantial differences were found in the ratings of the two groups across several behavioral dimensions. The disabled person was perceived to be less socially skilled and more dependent than the nonhandicapped individual. Note that these devaluing perceptions may be shared by those who become disabled as young adults and may lead to poor self-concept (Dixon, 1977). Further, several investigations (e.g., Comer & Piliavin, 1973) have shown that such negative self-perceptions are reflected in increased anxiety and passivity in the disabled interacting with nonhandicapped individuals.

Next, several inconsistencies have been observed in the affective and behavioral reactions of the able-bodied toward the physically handicapped. Kleck and associates have performed a series of laboratory studies examining the effects of physical deviance on face-to-face interactions. In an early study (Kleck et al., 1966) university students were randomly assigned to either a disabled or a nondisabled confederate with whom they were required to interact. Subjects interacting with the disabled confederate expressed opinions less representative of their actual beliefs, showed less variation in their behavior, and terminated the interview sooner than subjects interacting with the nonhandicapped person. In a follow-up study (Kleck, 1968) subjects in the disabled-interviewer condition reported greater liking for the interviewer, exhibited more motoric inhibition, and expressed attitudes more consistent with those assumed to be held by the disabled person than subjects in the nonhandicapped condition. The authors proposed that these results supported Goffman's (1963) earlier theoretical notions on the effects of stigma. Social encounters with stigmatized individuals are likely to be avoided and, if interaction is necessary, nondisabled persons become somewhat emotionally aroused, producing overcontrolled, stereotypic behaviors. Further, nonhandicapped persons are likely to engage in self-presentational tactics (e.g., showing immediate positive regard) to please a disabled individual and to lessen personal discomfort (cf. Schlenker, 1980).

A third major change in the disabled person's social environment can be located in the public's response to specific medical conditions. For example, persons who are partially sighted or totally blind are frequently exposed to individuals who grab their arms without warning, who talk inordinately loudly, and who talk about them as though they were not present (cf. Carroll, 1961). Social situations can be complicated for multiple sclerosis persons with gait problems or loss of balance. Such symptoms are frequently mistaken for alcohol intoxication by unwitting observers (Glueckauf & West, 1982a). As a result of social norms, physically handicapped persons may experience considerable discomfort when faced with losses of bodily control. In a study of a social discomfort Dunn (1977) asked forty cord injured veterans to fill out a questionnaire consisting of twenty potentially embarrassing social situations specifically associated with spinal cord disability. Subjects rated the level of discomfort they felt in each situation. The three most anxiety-provoking situations were having an accidental bowel movement in public, discovering a leaky external catheter at a party, and falling out of the wheelchair.

Last, typical hospital rehabilitation does not teach newly disabled young adults the social skills for successful reintegration into the community (Cogswell, 1968). Rehabilitation therapies are usually delivered in highly structured, time-limited units in which the individual passively receives instruction from the professional staff. Formal therapies are likely to permit little behavioral independence and may not encourage the patient to develop problem-solving skills (cf. Harriman & Garfunkel, 1981). Further, most treatment services are delivered by hospital nursing personnel who have received little or no training in social interaction skills. In order to complete their assigned duties, they may inadvertently reward dependent responding in the patient. In several studies on the effect of the treatment environment (Vineberg & Willems, 1971; Willems, 1972) the highest rates of patient independence appeared in activities which are the accompaniments of comprehensive rehabilitation (e.g., eating and passive recreation), while those activities which are central to the rehabilitation process (e.g., ADL training and exercise) produced the lowest rates of independence. Hence, the typical hospital environment is likely to foster dependent behaviors in newly disabled young adults. The problem-solving and social skills critical to normal daily living may not be acquired.

Social Adjustment Techniques

The psychological intervention which has shown considerable promise in facilitating the social adjustment of the disabled is assertion training (cf. Trieschmann, 1980). Assertion skills programs typically use a group approach lasting approximately eight weeks. The group consists of eight to ten members who meet once a week for one-and-one-half to two hours. Some examples of topics covered in the training are: (1) attitudes and values about physical disability, (2) instruction and practice in basic communication skills, (3) distinguishing among assertive, aggressive, and passive modes of responding, (4) practice in dealing with awkward social situations (e.g., falling out of the wheelchair, having a bladder accident), (5) instruction in stress management and relaxation techniques, and (6) maintaining support systems in the community. Assertiveness training usually receives positive patient acceptance because it appears quite different from traditional group psychotherapy approaches (Dunn & Herman, in press). Further, assertion skills programs can be run by rehabilitation professionals with a variety of counseling backgrounds, since intensive training in a particular theoretical system or process-oriented approach is not required.

The overall results of recent outcome studies with a variety of disabled populations (e.g., spinal cord injured and cerebral palsied) suggest that assertion training leads to significant improvement in social interaction skills such as refusing help and making requests for new behavior (Dunn, VanHorn, & Herman, 1981). Increases in social comfort and control of health outcomes have also been noted (Glueckauf, 1982; Morgan & Leung, 1980).

Vocational Functioning

Chronically disabled young adults are likely to confront a number of difficulties in vocational functioning. These potential difficulties may be located in a restricted range of job opportunities, transportational and architectural barriers, financial disincentives, and limited vocational rehabilitation services. First, research on vocational adjustment (Bors, 1956; Brown & Chanin, 1974; Frank, 1969; Weidman & Freehafer, 1981) has shown that the range of available occupations is substantially reduced following disability. Note, however, that the extent of vocational choice may vary with the severity of physical disability (cf. Crewe, Athelstan, & Bower, 1978). For example, persons who are quadriplegic are likely to have fewer job alternatives than individuals who are paraplegic. Quadriplegic young adults who are successful in obtaining employment typically have vocational objectives in the clerical, sales, or professional areas (cf. Dvonch, Kaplan, Grynbaum, & Rusk, 1965). However, the reduction of vocational options may not be exclusively attributable to losses of physical functioning. The perceptions of employers, the expectations of family and friends, and self-evaluations of work capacity and outcome may significantly influence the occupational decisions of handicapped young adults (cf. Felton, 1964; Schlesinger & Frank, 1974).

A second limitation in finding employment lies in transportational requirements and the architectural design of the work place. Owning an automobile may be a critical factor in the occupational adjustment of the physically disabled young adult (cf. Dvonch et al., 1965). Public transportation is usually inaccessible to individuals who rely on wheelchair devices or who have substantial motor deficits. Low-income persons, in particular, may have considerable difficulties obtaining employment outside the home. The costs of operating a vehicle large enough to hold a wheelchair and the purchase of adaptive equipment (e.g., hand controls or lifts) may be prohibitive (cf. Tanaka, 1977). The architectural plan of the work place may further restrict the occupational choices of the physically disabled. Examples of common architectural barriers are inaccessible washrooms, thick carpeting, and narrow doorways and aisles (Crewe et al., 1978). Early architectural modifications may play an important role in the success of vocational rehabilitation programs. In an innovative job development program, Hunter and Zuger (1979) contracted with New York City business firms to provide summer work experiences to seventy-one disabled high school and college students. Work environment and equipment modifications (e.g., ramps, changes in desk height) were suggested prior to job placement. The authors reported that early commitment to architectural modifications led to increases in cooperation and higher perceptions of involvement by the participating companies.

Third, financial disincentives impose a substantial limitation on the employment of physically disabled young adults. Faced with the rising costs of medical care (e.g., follow-up medical visits and supplies), many young adults may choose to remain unemployed rather than lose their government benefits. Crewe and colleagues (1978) estimated that a quadriplegic would have to make $18,000 to $20,000 a year to cover basic medical expenses. The inequities of the welfare system were outlined in the *Comprehensive Service Needs Study* (1975) and legislation permitting severely disabled persons to work without significant losses in benefits has been advocated.

Last, current vocational rehabilitation services may not adequately prepare the disabled young adult for the working world of the able-bodied. Vocational rehabilitation personnel tend to rely heavily on formal college education or training in professional, clerical, or sales work to equip the disabled young adult for future employment. A more flexible approach may be required, fitting individuals for jobs which are suited to their predisability interest (cf. Trieschmann, 1980). In a recent survey Crewe and associates (1978) compiled a list of seventy-nine vocations held by a sample of one hundred spinal cord injured persons residing in Minnesota. Several clients held physically demanding jobs for which they had considerable preinjury experience (e.g., farming, plumbing, and professional fishing guide). Using assistive devices and creative problem solving, these individuals have made successful adaptations to jobs previously considered unsuitable for the handicapped.

Vocational Rehabilitation Approaches

Upon examination of the literature two vocational rehabilitation (VR) training programs merited special attention for their level of innovation and emphasis on social interaction skills: (1) Personal Achievement Skills (PAS) training (cf. Roessler & Bolton, 1978) and (2) Threlkeld's (1979) self-help approach. The PAS program is composed of basic communication skills training, values clarification exercises, goal setting, and instruction in goal-attainment scaling. In addition, each participant receives a workbook which includes didactic information and outside assignments. Enrollment in the group typically ranges from five to eight members. The duration of the training is usually five weeks with two-hour daily sessions. The results of recent outcome investigations (e.g., Roessler, Cook, & Lillard, 1977) have shown that PAS group participants score significantly higher on the dimensions of vocational maturity, vocational functioning, and interpersonal maturity than treated controls. Further, PAS subjects make substantially higher gains in achieving work objectives than controls.

Using an innovative self-help approach, Threlkeld (1979) has provided vocational planning services to high-risk physically and emotionally handicapped adults. Group participants typically display a history of multiple social or psychological problems and considerable difficulties formulating vocational plans. The group is comprised of six to ten members. To enhance vocational planning, group participants are given VR materials, counselor manuals, training aids, and case funds normally controlled by the VR counselor (approximately $8,000). In addition, outside rehabilitation consultants are used to explain the operations and procedures of the VR system. As the participant develops rehabilitation plans, they are discussed by the peer group and cost estimates are provided. Following intensive discussion, the group members individually vote on the suitability of the plan. If the group approves the plan and cost, a check (i.e., for transportation or education) is issued to the individual. Analysis of the outcomes of the self-help program have shown mixed results. In a tristate study (Threlkeld, 1979) only 10 percent of the group members were gainfully employed at the five-month follow-up. However, 70 percent were actively pursuing specific vocational goals.

In summary, both PAS and self-help methods share a common therapeutic thrust: shifting the locus of responsibility for vocational adjustment to the disabled young adult. While their employment outcomes remain equivocal, these approaches have created heightened perceptions of responsibility and goal-oriented activity in disabled clients. In the final analysis, further research is needed to assess the effectiveness of these innovative VR strategies.

Sexual Adjustment to Physical Disability

Until the early 1970s the sexual functioning of physically disabled young adults was largely ignored by rehabilitation professionals (Cole, 1975). The introduction of sexual attitude reassessment workshops (Cole, Chilgren, & Rosenberg, 1973) and several provocative reports (e.g., Hohmann, 1972) were responsible for the development of sexual counseling services in rehabilitation facilities. Despite the growing importance ascribed to sexual health, a modicum of empirical research has been conducted in the field. Moreover, little is known about the effectiveness of sexual counseling programs for the disabled. In examining sexual adaptation to physical disability, the factors associated with the adjustment process will be considered first, followed by a discussion of current psychological approaches.

Factors in Sexual Adjustment

Four major factors are likely to play an important role in shaping the disabled person's perceptions, sexual performance, and quality of intimate relationships: (1) physiologic changes in sexual functioning, (2) the side-effects of drug therapy, (3) changes in body image, and (4) alterations in the social environment, particularly the misconceptions about the sexuality of disabled individuals and the reduction of available partners.

First, the disabled young adult's sexual response patterns may be disrupted by permanent physiologic changes and transitory symptoms. Losses of genital sensation, difficulties in getting or maintaining penile erection, and absence of orgasm are common sequelae of disabilities involving the central nervous system (e.g., low back injuries, multiple sclerosis, and spinal cord dysfunctions). During the initial phase of adjustment, these bodily disturbances may lead to increases in negative affect (e.g., anxiety and tension) and losses of self-esteem (Lovitt, 1970; Richards, 1980; Romano, 1973). In particular, young males who place a high value on sexual performance and traditional sex roles may be especially susceptible to lowered self-concept (cf. Rainwater, 1968; Trieschmann, 1980).

Transitory symptoms such as leg spasms, pain, urinary incontinence, and fatigue may also interfere with sexual functioning (cf. Barrett, 1977; Halstead, Halstead, Salhoot, Stock, & Sparks, 1978). If these symptoms are correlated with sexual activities, the disabled individual or partner may fear that regular sexual contact may exacerbate the disabled person's condition (cf. Infante, 1981). Other implications may arise if such symptoms are associated with rejection or marked increases in anxiety. Disabled individuals may avoid intimate relations and thus limit the possibility of future successful sexual experiences (cf. Hahn, 1981).

Second, drug therapy may have negative side-effects. Anti-inflamatory medications have been shown to reduce libido and alter facial appearance (Ehrlich, 1973; Richards, 1980). Other drugs including the antispasmodics (diazepam) and tricyclic antidepressants (commonly prescribed for low back pain patients) may reduce sexual interest and retard ejaculation (Couper-Smartt, 1973; Infante, 1981). Thus, the extent to which persons experience side-effects may be correlated with sexual adjustment, particularly the frequency of sexual activity and difficulties in sexual performance (cf. Weiss & Diamond, 1966). Further ambiguities may arise if handicapped individuals are not informed about the side-effects of medications. They may erroneously attribute alterations in sexual performance to internal, psychological states (e.g., anxiety or fear of rejection).

A third factor which may influence the sexual adaptation of handicapped young adults is altered body image. Following the onset of disability, the person's conception of his or her body is likely to be disrupted. The adverse effects of disability on body image have been observed particularly in early onset arthritis, which produces facial disfigurements or deformity of trunk and limbs (Hamilton, 1982). Persons with spinal-cord injuries have also reported substantial losses of perceived attractiveness. With increases in sexual experience, however, their perceptions of attractiveness have also increased (Bregman & Hadley, 1976). Further, the extent to which individuals are able to integrate the physical changes into their body image may be associated with assertiveness in sexual situations (cf. Dunn, Lloyd, & Phelps, 1979).

Last, changes in the social environment, particularly the negative expectations of nondisabled others and a decrease of available partners, may play an important role in the sexual adjustment of handicapped young adults. Nondisabled individuals typically overestimate the disabilities of handicapped persons. Able-bodied observers may formulate negative expectancies which spread beyond the actual physical disability to other areas including sexual and social functioning (cf. Heider, 1958; Wright, 1960). Thus, disabled persons, especially those who display overt physical symptoms (e.g., impaired gait, spasticity, or wheelchair use) are likely to be considered asexual or impotent by potential partners. These negative attitudes may lead to avoidance behavior in the nondisabled and, consequently, a reduction of available sexual partners (cf. Hahn, 1981; Hamilton, 1982). Successful management of these environmental constraints may depend upon the disabled person's social interaction skills, particularly the use of positive self-statements and preparing the nondisabled mate for irregularities in the sexual experience (e.g., bladder accidents and catheter removal).

Sexuality Enhancement Approaches

Psychological interventions to enhance the sexual functioning of disabled young adults have focused primarily on attitude changes (Trieschmann, 1980). Two group treatment strategies have produced significant increases in participants' ratings of comfort about sexual functioning and the use of alternate sexual practices: (1) sexual attitude reassessment workshops (e.g., Barrett & Barrett, 1978; Halstead et al., 1978; Held, Cole, Held, Anderson, & Chilgren, 1975) and (2) sexual counseling groups (e.g., Eisenberg & Rustad, 1976; Romano, 1973; Steger & Brockway, 1980).

Using a combination of explicit audiovisual materials, groups discussions, and didactic presentations, participants of sexuality attitude reassessment (SAR) workshops are first exposed to basic information about early sexual experiences and fantasies about sex and masturbation. As the training progresses, the group discussions help focus the participants on sexual values and the need for close communication between sexual partners. Last, the implications of physical disability on sexuality are addressed. A panel composed of physically handicapped individuals share their personal experiences in coping with the uncertainties of chronic, disabling conditions and the methods they have developed for enhancing sexuality. Taking a brief sexual history and basic interviewing skills are also discussed.

SAR researchers have relied heavily on self-report measures to evaluate the efficacy of the workshops. Using the Minnesota Sexuality Attitude Scale, Halstead and colleagues (1978) found significant increases in disabled participants' ($n = 59$) ratings of comfort about the use of fantasy for masturbation and three heterosexual behaviors, specifically masturbation, intercourse, and oral-genital sex. No data were collected from untreated controls. Most disabled persons were spinal cord injured (75 percent) and the remainder included persons with multiple sclerosis, muscular dystrophy, cerebral palsy, and visual impairments. The participants' level of sexual satisfaction was also assessed. Fifty-two percent reported substantial increases, whereas 48 percent of the subjects reported no changes in sexual satisfaction following training. Note that increases in comfort about alternate sexual practices were not correlated with the individuals' perceptions of overall sexual satisfaction.

Turning now to group counseling approaches, several studies (Evans, Halar, DeFreece, & Larsen, 1976; Romano & Lassiter, 1972; Wiig, 1973) have provided anecdotal evidence of the benefit of sexual counseling for disabled young adults. In one of the few reports on sexual adjustment training for brain-injured individuals, Wiig (1973) observed discrepancies between group participants' verbal messages and expressed emotions. In particular, the monotone, telegraphic speech of nonfluent aphasics tended to interfere with verbal expressions of emotions. The group treatment consisted primarily of therapist reflection and client feedback on the accuracy of reflected emotions. In post-treatment interviews 90 percent of the group participants reported gains in sexual adjustment.

Most sex education and counseling programs have been developed for spinal cord injured (SCI) persons. Romano (1973) discussed the advantages of group procedures in sexual counseling. Group interactions afforded numerous opportunities for feedback, modeling, and information on sexual adjustment. Further, the group approach was considered less threatening than individual counseling, since the SCI person was not the focus of attention. Next, Eisenberg and Rustad (1976) have provided an excellent description of a sexuality counseling program for male SCI veterans. The group participants were generally twenty to thirty years old and varied considerably on the dimensions of length of injury, extent of disability, and sexual experience. The program consisted of eight weekly sessions, each lasting approximately one-and-one-half hours. A similar format was employed for each session. Didactic presentations, including films and slides, were given first, followed by group discussion. A pamphlet developed by the authors was also used to provide basic information on sexuality and spinal cord injury. The course content covered a variety of topics such as: (1) anatomy and physiology of the sexual response following spinal cord disability, (2) marriage, divorce, and children, and (3) techniques for preparation, relaxation, and arousal. It should be noted that Eisenberg and Rustad did not present outcome data to substantiate the effectiveness of the training program.

Last, only two studies (Brockway, Steger, Berni, Ost, Williamson-Kirland, & Peck, 1978; Steger & Brockway, 1980) have systematically assessed the impact of sexual counseling for the physically handicapped young adult. The combined results of these investigations have shown that sexuality group participants (i.e., spinal cord patients and their partners) report significantly greater increases in acceptance of a variety of sexual behaviors and fewer sexual concerns than untreated spinal cord injured couples.

Future Research Directions

Two lines of research on treatment approaches to enhance the adjustment of handicapped young adults will be proposed. One direction is to conduct research on a critical vocational question: "Which VR training methods work best with which types of disabled clients?" Prior studies on the effects of VR training have largely ignored interactions between subject characteristics and treatment methods in determining career outcomes (Zadny & James, 1976). Psychological characteristics such as locus of control, need for achievement, and self-confidence may interact with treatment variables (e.g., group format and degree of structure) to produce results unaccounted for by main effects' approaches (cf. Fretz, 1981). For example, external locus of control (LOC) clients may do better in highly structured group interventions, such as PAS training, whereas internal LOC individuals may benefit more from nondirective therapies or career planning workshops. The practical utility of this research is likely to be high. VR counselors would be able to place clients in treatment programs which are suited to their personality styles, thus increasing the likelihood of positive training outcomes and employment potential.

A second direction for research is to evaluate the efficacy of peer counseling in facilitating the social adjustment of newly disabled young adults. Peer counseling approaches have been used successfully with several patient populations including substance abusers (cf. VanStone & Gilbert, 1972), mastectomy patients, and obese individuals (Gussow & Tracy, 1978). As noted previously, the rehabilitation professionals' behavior may inadvertently reinforce dependent responding in the physically disabled. Further, the favored cooperative patient, as judged by hospital staff, may actually be the one who is less independent and more passive (Albrecht & Higgins, 1977). Such passive modes of responding may lead to poor rehabilitation outcomes in the community. An alternative to the traditional medical model is the implementation of peer counseling programs. One advantage of this approach is increased acceptance of the peer counselor by the disabled client. The initial credibility of the counselors is likely to be high, since they have firsthand knowledge of clients' adjustment problems. Another advantage is the flexibility of peer counselors to interact with clients in a variety of community settings. They can accompany clients to recreational places, restaurants, and shopping centers, thus facilitating the transition from the protective environment of the home or hospital to the community setting. Several training modules have been developed to teach rehabilitation personnel basic counseling techniques (e.g., Farley & Rubin, 1981); these can be adapted for paraprofessional use. Further, rehabilitation professionals from a variety of backgrounds can use these training materials since formal instruction in a particular theoretical orientation is not required. Finally, two evaluation instruments, the Longitudinal Functional Assessment System (Alexander, 1978; Willems, 1976) and the Rehabilitation Indicators Project (Diller, Fordyce, Jacob, & Brown, 1978) may serve as measures of the impact of the peer counseling program on the psychosocial adjustment of the newly disabled young adult. Both focus on activity patterns, social contacts, and the level of independence of persons in the community.

References

Alexander, J. *Performance assessment system in spinal cord injury*. Unpublished doctoral dissertation, University of Houston, 1978.

Albrecht, G., Harasymiw, S. J., & Horne, M. *Social perception of disability*. Paper presented at the American Sociological Association Meeting, Chicago, 1977.

Albrecht, G., & Higgins, P. Rehabilitation success: The interrelationships of multiple criteria. *Journal of Health and Social Behavior*, 1977, *18*, 36–45.

Barrett, M. *Sexuality and multiple sclerosis*. Toronto: Multiple Sclerosis Society of Canada, 1977.

Barrett, A., & Barrett, M. *Guide to program planning on sexuality and multiple sclerosis*. Toronto: Multiple Sclerosis of Canada, 1978.

Bors, E. The challenge of quadraplegia. *Bulletin of Los Angeles Neurological Society*, 1956, *21*, 105–123.

Bregman, S., & Hadley, R. G. Sexual adjustment and feminine attractiveness among spinal cord injured women. *Archives of Physical Medicine and Rehabilitation*, 1976, *57*, 448–450.

Brockway, J. A., Steger, J. C., Berni, R., Ost, V. V., Williamson-Kirkland, T. E., & Peck, C. L. Effectiveness of a sex education and counseling program for spinal cord injured patients. *Sexuality and Disability*, 1978, *1*, 127–136.

Brown, B., & Chanin, I. *Patterns of education and employment: Rehabilitants from severe spinal cord injury, FY 1972–3*. Rehabilitation Research Reports, No. 30, Department of Rehabilitation, Sacramento, Calif., June 1, 1974.

Carroll, T. J. *Blindness: What it is, what it does, and how to live with it*. Boston: Little, Brown, 1961.

Cogswell, B. Self socialization: Readjustment of paraplegics in the community. *Journal of Rehabilitation*, 1968, *34*, 11–13, 35.

Cole, T. M. Sexuality and physical disabilities. *Archives of Sexual Behavior,* 1975, *4,* 389–403.

Cole, T. M., Chilgren, R., & Rosenberg, P. A new program of sex education and counseling for spinal cord injured adults and health care professionals. *Paraplegia,* 1973, *11,* 111–124.

Comer, R. J., & Piliavin, J. A. The effects of physical deviance upon face-to-face interaction: The other side. *Journal of Personality and Social Psychology,* 1973, *23,* 33–39.

Comprehensive service needs study. Urban Institute, Washington, D.C., June 23, 1975.

Couper-Smartt, J. D. A technique for surveying side-effects of tricyclic drugs with reference to reported sexual effect. *Journal of International Medical Research,* 1973, *1,* 473–476.

Crewe, N., Athelstan, G., & Bower, A. *Employment after spinal cord injury: A handbook for counselors.* Minneapolis: Department of Physical Medicine and Rehabilitation, University of Minnesota, 1978.

Diller, L., Fordyce, W., Jacob, D., & Brown M. *Activity pattern indicators.* Rehabilitation Indicators Project, New York University Medical Center, 1978.

Dixon, J. K. Coping with prejudice: Attitudes of handicapped persons towards the handicapped. *Journal of Chronic Diseases,* 1977, *58,* 247–260.

Dunn, M. Social discomfort in the patient with spinal cord injury. *Archives of Physical Medicine and Rehabilitation,* 1977, *58,* 257–260.

Dunn, M., & Herman, S. M. Assertiveness and social skills training in physical disability. In D. M. Doleys, R. L. Meridity, & R. Ciminero (Eds.), *Behavioral psychology in medicine: Assessment and treatment strategies.* New York: Plenum, in press.

Dunn, M., Lloyd, E., & Phelps, G. Sexual assertiveness in spinal cord injury. *Sexuality and Disability,* 1979, *2,* 293–300.

Dunn, M., VanHorn, E., & Herman, S. H. Social skills and spinal cord injury: A comparison of three training procedures. *Behavior Therapy,* 1981, *12,* 153–154.

Dvonch, P., Kaplan, L., Grynbaum, B., & Rusk, H. Vocational findings in post disability employment of patients with spinal cord dysfunction. *Archives of Physical Medicine and Rehabilitation,* 1965, *46,* 761–766.

Ehrlich, G. E. Sexual problems of the arthritic patient. In G. E. Ehrlich (Ed.), *Total management of the arthritic patient.* Philadelphia: J. B. Lippincott, 1973.

Eisenberg, M., & Rustad, L. Sex education and counseling program on a spinal cord injury service. *Archives of Physical Medicine and Rehabilitation,* 1976, *57,* 135–140.

English, R. Correlates of stigma toward physically disabled persons. *Rehabilitation Research and Practice Review,* 1971, *2,* 1–17.

Erikson, E. *Identity and the life cycle.* New York: University Press, 1959.

Evans, R., Halar, E., DeFreece, A., & Larsen, G. Multi-disciplinary approach to sex education of spinal cord injured patients. *Physical Therapy,* 1976, *56,* 541–545.

Farley, R. C., & Rubin, S. E. *Systematic interviewing skills*. Hot Springs: University of Arkansas, 1981.

Felton, J. Blocks to employment of paralytics. *Rehabilitation Record*, 1964, *5*, 35–37.

Frank, D. S. *The multi-troubled jobseeker: The case of the jobless worker with a convulsive disorder*. Three Cities Employment, Training, Counseling Program. Washington, D.C.: Epilepsy Foundation of America, 1969.

Fretz, B. R. Evaluating the effectiveness of career interventions. *Journal of Counseling Psychology*, 1981, *28*, 77–90.

Glueckauf, R. Assertion training for disabled persons in wheelchairs. Paper presented at the 43rd annual meeting of the Canadian Psychological Association, June 1982.

Glueckauf, R., & West, S. *The uncertainties of coping with the epilepsies: A social-psychological perspective*. Manuscript submitted for publication, 1982. (a)

Glueckauf, R., & West, S. *The uncertainties of coping with multiple sclerosis: A social-psychological perspective*. Manuscript submitted for publication, 1982. (b)

Goffman, Erving. *Stigma*. Englewood Cliffs, N.J.: Prentice-Hall, 1963.

Gussow, Z., & Tracy, G. The role of self-help in adaptation to chronic illness and disability. *Nursing Digest*, 1978, *6*, 23–35.

Hahn, H. The social component of sexuality and disability: Some problems and proposals. *Sexuality and Disability*, 1981, *14*, 220–233.

Halstead, L., Halstead, M., Salhoot, J., Stock, D., & Sparks, R. Sexual attitudes, behavior, and satisfaction for able bodied and disabled participants attending workshops in human sexuality. *Archives of Physical Medicine and Rehabilitation*, 1978, *59*, 497–501.

Hamilton, A. Sexual problems in arthritis and allied conditions. *International Rehabilitation Medicine*, 1982, *3*, 38–42.

Harriman, M., & Garfunkel, M. The value of self-help groups in spinal cord injury rehabilitation. *SCI Digest*, 1981, *3*, 26–33.

Heider, F. *The psychology of interpersonal relations*. New York: Wiley, 1958.

Held, J., Cole, T., Held, C., Anderson, C., & Chilgren, R. Sexual attitude reassessment workshops: Effect on spinal cord injured adults, their partners, and rehabilitation professionals. *Archives of Physical Medicine and Rehabilitation*, 1975, *56*, 14–18.

Hohmann, G. W. Considerations in management of psychosexual readjustment in the cord injured male. *Rehabilitation Psychology*, 1972, *19*, 50–58.

Hunter, P., & Zuger, R. Easing the transition from school to work for students with severe physical disabilities: A summer work experience. *Rehabilitation Literature*, 1979, *40*, 298–304.

Infante, M. C. Sexual dysfunction in the patient with chronic back pain. *Sexuality and Disability*, 1981, *4*, 173–178.

Katz, I., & Glass, D. C. An ambivalence-amplification theory of behavior toward the stigmatized. In W. Austin & S. Worchel (Eds.), *The social psychology of intergroup relations*. Monterey, Calif.: Brooks/Cole, 1978.

Kelley, H., Hastorf, A. H., Jones, E. E., Thibaut, J. W., & Usdane, W. H. Some implications of social psychological theory for research on the handicapped. In L. H. Lofquist (Ed.), *Psychological research and rehabilitation*. Washington, D.C.: APA, 1960.

Kleck, R. Physical stigma and nonverbal cues omitted in face-to-face interactions. *Human Relations*, 1968, *21*, 19–28.

Kleck, R., Ono, H., & Hastorf, A. H. The effects of physical deviance upon face-to-face interaction. *Human Relations*, 1966, *19*, 425–436.

Lovitt, R. Sexual adjustment of spinal cord injury patients. *Rehabilitation Research and Practice Review*, 1970, *1*, 25–29.

Morgan, B., & Leung, P. Effects of assertion training on acceptance of disability by physically disabled university students. *Journal of Counseling Psychology*, 1980, *27*, 209–212.

Rainwater, L. Some aspects of lower class sexual behavior. *Medical Aspects of Human Sexuality*, 1968, *2*, 15–25.

Richards, J. S. Sex and arthritis. *Sexuality and Disability*, 1980, *3*, 95–104.

Roessler, R. & Bolton, B. *Psychosocial adjustment to disability*. Baltimore: University Park Press, 1978.

Roessler, R., Cook, D., & Lillard, D. Effects of systematic group counseling on work adjustment clients. *Journal of Counseling Psychology*, 1977, *24*, 313–317.

Romano, M. Sexual counseling in groups. *Journal of Sex Research*, 1973, *9*, 69–78.

Romano, M., & Lassiter, R. Sexual counseling with the spinal cord injured. *Archives of Physical Medicine and Rehabilitation*, 1972, *53*, 568–572.

Safilios-Rothschild, C. *The sociology and social psychology of disability and rehabilitation*. New York: Random House, 1970.

Schlenker, B. R. *Impression management: The self-concept, social identity, and interpersonal relation*. Monterey, Calif.: Brooks/Cole, 1980.

Schlesinger, L. E., & Frank, D. From demonstration to dissemination: Gateways to employment for epileptics. *Rehabilitation Literature*, 1974, *35*, 98–106, 109.

Steger, J. C., & Brockway, J. A. Sexual enhancement in spinal cord injured patients: Behavioral group treatment. *Sexuality and Disability*, 1980, *3*, 84–96.

Tanaka, T. *Economic security for the disabled*. Unpublished paper.

Threlkeld, R. The use of client planning groups in vocational rehabilitation: An alternative service approach. *Rehabilitation Literature*, 1979, *40*, 146–148, 153.

Trieschmann, R. *Spinal cord injuries: Psychological, social, and vocational adjustment*. New York: Pergamon Press, 1980.

VanStone, W., & Gilbert, R. Peer confrontation groups—What, why, and whether. *American Journal of Psychiatry*, 1972, *129*, 583–589.

Vineberg, S., & Willems, E. Observation and analysis of patient behavior in the rehabilitation hospital. *Archives of Physical Medicine and Rehabilitation*, 1979, *52*, 8–14.

Wagner, N. The sexual adjustment of cardiac patients. *British Journal of Sexual Medicine*, 1974, *1*, 17–22.

Weidman, C. D., & Freehafer, A. A. Vocational outcome in patients with spinal cord injury. *Journal of Rehabilitation*, 1981, *47*, 63–65.

Weinberg, N. Social stereotyping of the physically handicapped. *Rehabilitation Psychology*, 1976, *23*, 115–124.

Weiss, A., & Diamond, M. Sexual adjustment, identification, and attitudes of patients with myelopathy. *Archives of Physical Medicine and Rehabilitation*, 1966, *47*, 245–250.

Wiig, E. H. Counseling the adult aphasic for sexual readjustment. *Rehabilitation Counseling Bulletin*, 1973, *17*, 111–119.

Willems, E. Interface of the hospital environment and patient behavior. *Archives of Physical Medicine and Rehabilitation*, 1972, *53*, 115–122.

Willems, E. Behavioral ecology, health status, and health care: Applications to the rehabilitation setting. In I. Altman & J. Wohlwill (Eds.), *Human behavior and environment*. New York: Plenum, 1976.

Wright, B. *Physical disability: A psychological approach*. New York: Harper & Row, 1960.

Zadny, J. J., & James, L. F. *Another view of placement: State of the art 1976*. Studies in Placement Monograph No. 1. Portland, Maine: Portland State University, Regional Rehabilitation Institute, 1976.

9 Apart and A Part: Family Issues for Young Adults with Chronic Illness and Disability

Henry T. Ireys and Carolyn Keith Burr

Although there is a strong clinical consensus that families play a major role in the care of chronically ill or disabled young adults, theory and research in this area remain weak. Attention to the psychological life of the ill or disabled individual has far exceeded attention to the relationship between the disabled young adult and "the family," whoever that might include. Furthermore, there has been no systematic consideration of the community influences on the ability of a family to care for an ill or disabled young adult—or on ways that health care providers might promote social and community supports for those in caretaking roles.

In this chapter we seek to redress this lack of attention (1) by clarifying the types of living arrangements of young adults in general and the types of families in which chronically ill or disabled young adults are likely to live; (2) by reviewing the literature on family tasks common to the developmental stage of young adulthood; (3) by discussing a variety of empirical findings and conceptual issues regarding the relationship between the disabled young adult and the particular type of family in which he or she lives; (4) by examining treatment strategies that will take into account not only specific concerns of families that care for young adults, but also the larger domain of community support; and (5) by pinpointing questions of special urgency that deserve further study.

Our lamentations about the paucity of good research on family issues for chronically disabled young adults will be loud. The dearth of research—even of basic, large-sample descriptive studies of the living arrangements of chronically disabled young adults—is extraordinary. Furthermore, as many of the authors in this volume have noted, the available literature on adult chronic disability or illness rarely divides subjects into age-groups consonant with a developmental life-span perspective. For this reason, many of our conclusions represent quite tentative hypotheses.

Review of the Literature

To provide a foundation for examining family issues facing chronically disabled young adults, we present a discussion of two quite separate literatures: (1) research on demographic characteristics of American families and (2) theoretical speculations on family developmental tasks for young adults in general. On the basis of this review, we make several distinctions that we believe will promote an understanding of and an appropriate response to the special family problems of chronically ill or disabled young adults in particular. These distinctions include the *types of families* in which a chronically disabled young adult is likely to live and the *specific familial issues* that most chronically ill or disabled young adults are likely to face.

Family Structure

The family life histories of chronically disabled young adults will necessarily occur in the context of family life for America's young adult as a whole. It is useful, therefore, to be cognizant of the ways in which the American family is changing. Three aspects of these changes are of particular import for chronically disabled young adults.

First, compared with the last four decades, a greater proportion of young adults are leaving the family of origin soon after adolescence. In 1940, for example, 12.4 percent of the population of male children and 9.6 percent of female children living in a family household were aged twenty to twenty-five; 5.5 percent of male children and 4.4 percent of female children were aged twenty-five to twenty-nine. By 1970, only 6.1 percent of male children and 5.3 percent of female children living in a household were aged twenty to twenty-four; 1.9 percent of males and 1.4 percent of females were aged twenty-five to twenty-nine (U.S. Bureau of the Census, 1943, 1973). These figures indicate clearly that young adults who acquire a chronic disability will have almost certainly left their family of origin.

The second aspect of the changing American family that is particularly relevant to chronic disability is the population of never-married young adults. It is likely that by 1990, the proportion of young adults who have never married will be quite high: for both sexes aged twenty to twenty-nine, 53.5 percent will have never married. Furthermore, almost 10 percent of both sexes in this age-group will be divorced or separated from a spouse. These projections underscore the fact that an increasing percentage of the nation's population will remain unmarried or become single through their twenties (Masnick & Bane, 1980).

This observation relates to the third aspect of family demography that is of importance to chronically ill young adults: the considerable increase in the percentage of small households. Since 1940, the percentage of one- and two-person households has increased from 31.9 to 52.7; large households (over five persons) have been almost halved during the same time (e.g., U.S. Bureau of the Census, 1979). Masnick and Bane (1980) conclude that this change results from the increase in the number of young adults living alone and from the increase in unmarried young adults (both male and female) heading a household with only one other dependent member (child, parent, or other dependent). In particular, the increase in households headed by unmarried females has been substantial: in 1990, this proportion is projected to reach 29 percent of all households. But households headed by unmarried males have also increased: in 1960, male-headed households comprised 8.1 percent of all households; in 1990, this figure is projected to be about 16 percent (Masnick & Bane, 1980, pp. 49–50). Wilkie's (1981) figures on delayed parenthood further support the overall decrease in size of families.

From this information on the current structure of the American family, we tentatively draw several conclusions:

1. Virtually all young adults who acquire a chronic disability will have already left their family of origin.
2. Many (perhaps most) young adults who acquire a chronic disability will not be married.
3. For those males and females who do not live alone and who are unmarried or married without the spouse present, the other person or persons in the household will be dependents (i.e., persons unable to assume the burden of care).
4. Married young adults who acquire a chronic disability or illness will be living in small families (i.e., families that are likely to have one or two children).

These conclusions, of course, represent hypotheses waiting to be tested through a fairly comprehensive survey of young adults with different types of chronic disability—a survey that has yet to be accomplished. At this point, a variety of published case studies present individuals who conform to the characteristics implicit in our conclusions (Aadalen & Stroebel-Kahn, 1981, Caywood, 1977; Cohen, 1977; Hudson, 1976; Kane, 1981).

If these four conclusions are true, however, they lead to a fifth:

5. If a chronically ill or disabled young adult is to live in a family environment, this family environment will be either of two types: (1) the family of origin, comprising the parents (who are likely to

> be in their mid-forties or older) and any siblings that remain at home; or (2) "the family of commitment," defined as a spouse and the couple's children.

In either case, the family that provides the care is likely to be a small one; unlike earlier decades, where large families would provide many hands to share the burden of care, family members who care for disabled young adults must now assume such burdens knowing that there are few others in the family to help with this task. Because of this dilemma, we believe strongly that families of either type need consistent and appropriate support from the community or the health care system, or both. Only with this ongoing support will the families be able to sustain the burdens of care over time.

While these two types of family environments for the chronically ill or disabled young adult are similar in some respects (e.g., both types of families are likely to be small), they are very different in many other respects. Indeed, as we will discuss below, the issues involved when a disabled young adult returns to the family of origin are quite different than if he or she returns to a family of commitment. At this point, we would emphasize the importance, for both research and practice, of making the distinction between a chronically ill or disabled young adult's family of origin and his or her family of commitment. Too often, research reports speak of "the family" without making this distinction—a particularly important one for this population.

Family Tasks for Young Adults

As life-stage developmental theory has grown, so, too, has the diversity in the conceptualization of life-stage tasks. Thus, young adulthood now includes different challenges than those originally proposed by Erikson (1963), depending on whom one consults. Pertinent issues range from individual tasks (e.g., develop an ethical sense, form and pursue youthful aspirations) to family tasks (e.g., start a family, gain emancipation from parental control) to larger social tasks (e.g., assume civic responsibilities, establish a niche in society). While these conceptualizations are useful in pinpointing major concerns for this age, they are not independent of one another: individual, family, and societal tasks are inherently inseparable. For example, many young adults seek a sense of independence from the family of origin by entering marriage and establishing a family of their own; many others establish families because everyone in their peer group is doing so and it is, therefore, a familiar "niche."

Rather than simply listing "family tasks," a list that is bound to obscure the reciprocal relationship between individual, family, and society, we believe that a more fruitful approach to defining "family issues" for young adults is to consider the complementary processes of individuation and integration (Giele, 1980; Napier & Whitaker, 1978). Like other stages, young adulthood demands that a person not only act independently—establishing one's own source of income, forming coherent values, and so on—but also to act in concert with others—developing intimacy, establishing a social network, and so on. But unlike other ages, young adulthood represents the first proving ground beyond the family of origin. Thus, for many young adults, individuation efforts are those that lead to an initial emancipation from the family of origin; integration efforts are those that lead to the first consistently intimate bond with another adult or with a group of adults or both. In this complementary working of two separate processes, the young adult reaches a definition of self. Or, as Giele (1980, p. 157) says, "It is . . . in the dialectic between differentiation and integration that the larger organization of life is formed."

Table 9.1 selects six concepts, identifying them as most relevant to "family issues" and grouping them into categories of individuating tasks and integrating tasks. As we will show, the occurrence of a chronic disability in young adulthood can affect both sets of tasks dramatically, though in somewhat different ways depending on whether the chronically disabled young adult returns to a family of commitment or to a family of origin. Before proceeding, however, two caveats are necessary: one dealing with the specific effects of income on developmental tasks; the other dealing with the general effects of social forces on family functioning.

Fiske (1980) has shown that the potential for growth and change among middle- and lower-middle income adults may be considerably

Table 9.1. Family Tasks for Young Adults

Individuating Tasks

1. Emancipating oneself from parental controls (Meyer, 1973)
2. Modify existing relationship with parents (Levinson, 1978, 1980)
3. Shifting of center of gravity from family of origin to a new home base (Levinson, 1978, 1980)

Integrating Tasks

1. Developing the capacity for intimacy, for mutual loving, and for living with a partner (Erikson, 1963; Havighurst, 1972; Meyer, 1973; Sheehy, 1974)
2. Sustaining illusions about intimacy with others in order to gain experience in living (Sheehy, 1974)
3. Establishing a niche in society (Levinson, 1978)

diminished in comparison to those in higher income brackets. Her work suggests strongly that income potential may, to a significant extent, influence the types of family issues with which a young adult might struggle. Out of sheer necessity, for example, the son of a blue-collar worker may follow in his father's footsteps without having much opportunity to be concerned about emancipation or the development of a "life structure." His concerns would be focused on maintaining his job and on his position as family breadwinner. Similarly, an unemployed, unmarried twenty-one-year-old woman, receiving Aid to Families with Dependent Children (AFDC) payments for her two children, might live in an extended family environment with her mother, siblings, and possibly other children. In this instance, the struggle to meet basic needs might again preclude attention to any of the family tasks that we have listed. In general, then, the family tasks that we have outlined in Table 9.1 represent relatively higher-order needs in Maslow's (1968) scheme; unless basic needs are met, individuals are not going to face these types of family developmental tasks.

Fiske's research on the effect of income has direct bearing on disabled young adults, whose earning power is often severely curtailed by the disability or the illness (Lonnquist, 1979). We know, for example, that in all age-groups those who do not work full-time bring in less than half the salary of those who do work full-time, and that the difference is greater for men than for women (Masnick & Bane, 1980). Since many illnesses and disabilities prohibit the individual from working full-time, the earning power of such an individual is decreased substantially. Thus, aside from the issues of response to the illness, lower earning levels might themselves decrease the potential for continued intellectual growth and change or for sustained attention to family developmental tasks.

The second caveat concerns the role of larger social forces on family functioning. Several reports have underscored (1) the ways in which community and legislative supports can enable parents to care more productively for their children (Keniston, 1977) and (2) the relationship between community and marital functioning (Holman, 1981). Other researchers and theorists (e.g., Bronfenbrenner, 1979) have convincingly argued that events independent of any one family can have profound effects on that family's functioning. An example of this phenomenon—and one that is particularly germane to families who care for chronically disabled young adults—is the segregating effects of stigma. Community perceptions of disability can increase the stress and isolation of families with a disabled member: friends stop coming by; home care, while parents or spouse go on vacation or even go out for a night, can be expensive or unavailable; family members might not want to be seen in the community out of fear of ridicule or embarrassment. This research leads us to conclude that family developmental tasks are not solely the province of the family. Community and social values can have a profound effect on how families grow and change as their members age.

As a whole, then, the literature on normal developmental family issues enables us to identify two types of tasks: individuating and integrating tasks. Other literatures provide insight into the possible constraints on the negotiation of these tasks, constraints that include income potential and community support.

Empirical Research on Families Who Care for Young Adults with Chronic Illness or Disability

Having identified the current family patterns and family developmental tasks of young adulthood in general, we turn to the implications of these findings for chronically ill and disabled young adults in particular. We approach our discussion by focusing first on the dilemmas arising when a chronically ill or disabled young adult returns to his or her family of origin and then by examining those that arise when a chronically ill or disabled young adult returns to a family of commitment. Much of our discussion must remain tentative because there are few research studies on family issues facing this population. We know little, for example, about the actual proportion of chronically ill or disabled young adults who live with their parents as opposed to their spouse. Other variables, such as extent of functional disability, course of illness or disability, sex, socioeconomic status, education, and cultural background, are likely to be major factors but, again, there is no available study that incorporates these variables, that considers this specific age-group, and that also moves beyond a focus on the individual. Furthermore, virtually no research efforts have considered social factors that influence families who care for chronically ill or disabled young adults.

Taken as a whole, however, the literature offers compelling anecdotal and empirical evidence that families of all sorts—if they provide a supportive environment—can be of enormous benefit to any chronically ill or disabled adult. Adams and Lindeman (1974), for example, present case studies of adolescent patients disabled because of accidents. One of these patients had a family who responded to the accident by mobilizing many strengths and redefining their hopes and aspirations realistically. Though many factors influenced this patient's successful coping, the authors note the supportive role played by the family.

Other researchers have demonstrated positive effects of social and family support with a variety of different adult chronically ill or disabled populations. For dialysis patients, O'Brien (1980) found significant positive correlations between patients' perceived expectations for support from family and close friends and the patients' social functioning. Diamond (1979) also found that better adjustment among dialysis patients, as indicated by fewer changes in social functioning, was significantly associated with greater helpfulness and supportive behavior from family, with increased spouse involvement, and with the availability of a confidant.

With respect to rehabilitation after spinal cord injury, Rogers and Figone (1979) studied thirty-five persons ranging in age from seventeen to fifty-two and noted that "the results illustrate the interplay of significant persons in creating an environment conducive to adaptation, with the family playing a prominent role" (p. 437). Earlier, Kemp and Vash (1971) had found that paraplegics and quadriplegics who received a high degree of social support did not differ on productivity measures; however, among those receiving less support, quadriplegics were less productive than paraplegics. Several studies have reported that hospital and rehabilitation staff give better ratings on a variety of dimensions (e.g., motivation, physical state, improvement) to those patients who report a high level of social support in comparison to patients reporting low levels (Hyman, 1972; Litman, 1966). Finally, a study of facial disfigurement summarizes well the nurturing role that families can play:

> The supporting influence of family and friends provides a secure base to which the patient can return, physically and emotionally, when the strain in the outside world becomes too great [Nordlicht, 1979, p. 1382].

Though these findings point to the importance of family support for all disabled adults, they fail to identify the particular family challenges generated by the onset of a chronic illness or disability in *young* adulthood. In particular, they fail to distinguish between the types of concerns that arise when a chronically ill or disabled young adult returns to a family of origin and those that arise when he or she returns to a small and relatively new family of commitment. We turn now to these specifics.

Returning to Families of Origin

For the parent and siblings who must resume the burdens of care, as well as for the patient, the onset of a disability in young adulthood interrupts many developmental trends. To prevent this interruption from becoming permanent, the family of origin and the young adult must successfully resolve two challenges: they must overcome the daily problems of the disability itself *and* they must do this in such a way that everyone involved and the family as a whole can continue on their developmental road. In essence, these two goals require the reconstituted family to develop new patterns of relating, patterns that are not simply repetitions of those developed when the disabled young adult was a child or adolescent. To illustrate the dilemmas that arise in this situation, we present a description of one of our patients. We present this particular case study because we have been unable to find reports that both focus specifically on chronically ill or disabled young adults who return for care to the family of origin and that also address family issues.

Chuck was twenty-five years old at the time of a motorcycle accident that left him hemiplegic and dysphonic. Though he was not a "biker" in the sense of being in a motorcycle gang, he had many friends who also had motorcycles. During the few years prior to his accident, he had lived with several roommates in an apartment fairly near the factory where he worked, but recently a roommate had moved out and Chuck was in the apartment alone.

Both his friends and his family knew Chuck as somewhat irresponsible but generous; he worked consistently, if not hard, and was a "fun-loving guy." According to his father, "Chuck always thought that he was put on this earth to have fun. The accident was a terrible thing, but if he hadn't been such a hot-dog, it never would have happened. It taught him a lesson he needed to learn."

At the time of his accident—he was driving too fast on a wet road—he had been dating a girl, Rickie, for several months. They had once talked about possibly living together. Chuck's parents owned and operated two small markets and lived in a nearby suburb with Chuck's younger siblings: Susie (twenty years old) and Billy (seventeen years old).

Chuck's accident occurred on New Year's Day and he remained in the hospital for three months. On discharge, he moved back in with his parents, sharing a room with his brother. Hospital staff had arranged for Chuck to receive speech and physical rehabilitation services three days a week from a rehabilitation center about ten miles away from the family's home. Despite fairly close contact between hospital staff and the family, neither Chuck, his siblings, his parents, his friends, his girlfriend, his parents' customers, his siblings' friends, nor his girlfriend's friends accurately anticipated the numerous problems generated by Chuck's return: Chuck was no longer a "fun-loving guy." Instead, he was withdrawn, sullen, and often deliberately mean-spirited.

For Chuck's parents, this change in their son had many implications: "We always had a good time together," said his mother, "and now it seems that he hates us"; and his father once confided to the mother some disappointment about the future: "You know, I always hoped that Chuck would marry Rickie. I would have liked her and she would have made a good daughter-in-law."

One of the major problems in the family concerned the bedroom situation. Billy had always admired his older brother and was looking forward to his returning home, largely because he assumed that his brother would leave the hospital only when he was well. Billy was shocked when Chuck came home with a severe speech deficit and relatively little motor control, even in a wheelchair. Billy also realized quickly that his friends did not want to stop by to listen to music in his room anymore because, as one friend put it, "I know Chuck's your brother, but he gives me the creeps." Furthermore, though he could admit it only much later, Chuck hated having his brother see his disabilities. Chuck said about a year after he had moved back, "I'd be struggling to get dressed and Billy would look at me: disappointment and pity, that's what his eyes were full of. It made me sick."

Billy's understandable response to the disability was not the only source of Chuck's anger and bitterness. The parents' genuine desire to make Chuck feel as comfortable as possible initially led to their "infantilizing" their son. For example, Chuck's mother often forgot to wait for Chuck to answer a question; she would answer it for him while he was orienting himself to speak.

One of the major problems for Chuck's peer group was his girlfriend's reaction to Chuck's disability. The hospital staff had been unable to dissuade Chuck from refusing to see Rickie, but his parents, when he got home, thought that it would do him good for them to talk. So they invited her over one night without telling him. Since she had had no contact with him for four months and had not seen him in the hospital setting, she was unprepared for the extent of his disability. As one of her close friends recalled, "She came over later that night, completely flipped out and shaking. Chuck didn't want to see her and didn't say anything. She blew the rest of that semester at school because Chuck's parents kept asking her to come over. Afterwards, she'd come here or to Sally's, flipped out bad every time."

Chuck later admitted that he wanted to see Rickie, but he was so outraged that his parents had not consulted him that he would not respond. "That was the way it always was—they always made decisions for me. They treated me like a kid again for a long time."

A major problem for the parents was the effect of Chuck's care on their business. Several of their friends, recognizing the new financial burdens on the family, mounted a neighborhood campaign to urge everyone in the community to use the family's two markets instead of the big supermarket in the new mall. For several months, the campaign was quite successful; business perked up considerably. Unfortunately, this sudden increase caught the father by surprise and he often did not have enough stock; by the time he started ordering more, business had fallen back to its usual levels, leaving him with a considerable amount of stock that went unsold. Furthermore, the increased business had put a strain on both parents to keep the stores open and fully staffed when they really wanted and needed to help Chuck with his physical and speech rehabilitation. In essence, the generous neighborhood response backfired, leaving the family somewhat reproachful.

Other problems arose during the first six months of home care: the mother's angina worsened considerably; the daughter quit school; many of the parents' friends stopped inviting them over because they never came when they were asked. These problems so exacerbated difficulties in rehabilitation efforts at the day treatment program that the staff realized that some very active family and community intervention was necessary. First steps included encouraging the daughter to establish a separate residence (which she wanted to do anyway), moving Chuck into the daughter's room, and arranging more appropriate community support in the form of respite care. The parents eventually were able to leave the business with their employees long enough to take a small vacation.

This case study illustrates many of the difficulties that might face a chronically disabled young adult and the family of origin during the initial stages of adaptation to the disability. Within the family, the parents and siblings had to alter many of their expectations and beliefs in response to the loss that the disability represented. For these parents, their son's disability meant the loss of a source of present and future joy. For the brother, Chuck's disability meant the loss of a major role model. Cleveland (1979) and others have noted that these kinds of losses can be associated with a wide variety of physical and emotional responses, such as fear, anger, guilt, anxiety, and emotional numbness. The family evidenced many of these feelings, with an accompanying puzzlement about how to express them constructively.

The parents also had to struggle with their initial impulses "to do things the way we did them before." But eventually, for example, the husband realized that he would have to stay home more, to assume some of the tasks that he had always left to his wife. Chuck's own feelings of "being like a child" and his subsequent rage further slowed the process of adaptation and reorganization.

This case illustration provides an example of a chronic disability. To some extent, however, the issues would be different if Chuck had returned home with a diagnosis of a rare chronic illness. The father's anger and bitterness at Chuck's "sloppy driving," for example, might have been replaced by a more generalized anger at "fate." Overall, the nature of the family's response will depend on many factors, including the ages of the parents, the presence of siblings, the nature of the disability or illness, and the economic status of the family.

As this case illustrates, just as Chuck had many tasks to resolve in respect to his family and friends, so, too, did the family have many tasks to resolve with respect to Chuck and to the community. These tasks are, of course, practically inseparable, but the distinction between individuating and integrating tasks is a useful one here. For Chuck, the individuating tasks which he had largely accomplished had to be worked through once again. As for the integrating tasks, even after a year of rehabilitation, Chuck had taken relatively few steps in resolving them.

Returning to Families of Commitment

The specific family struggles in developing a sense of identity and independence are quite different for those disabled young adults who return not to a family of origin but to a family of commitment—to a spouse and possibly young children. In this situation, the primary challenge for both spouses is to continue to resolve the integrating tasks of young adulthood (1) in the context of a relationship that is likely to be less than five years old and (2) where the ill or disabled adult is likely to be substantially dependent on the spouse in ways unanticipated at the start of the marriage. For the able-bodied spouse the vows, "for better or for worse, in sickness and in health," have surprising implications in the context of a chronic illness or disability that appears early in a marriage. Thus, the central task in this situation is either to renegotiate a marriage contract in which mutuality is reassured or to abandon the marriage contract in a way that is not destructive of either spouse's integrity.

Empirical research on the effect of physical disability on marital functioning has documented the general increase in marital stress as a result of physical disability and the mediating effects of several variables, including: sex, marital role expectations, role intactness, role flexibility, extent of cognitive and intellectual impairment, and socioeconomic factors (Peterson, 1979).

Unfortunately, the articles reviewed in Peterson fail to account systematically for the age of the marriage and ages of the spouses. Many of the articles tend to focus on issues more relevant to the mid-life stage (e.g., Skipper, Fink, & Hallenbeck, 1977; Zahn, 1973). Thus, while the empirical literature provides some important leads in defining concepts and variables, it is not very useful in pinpointing the particular family challenges that face disabled *young* adults and their new families.

Anecdotal reports and case studies, however, provide important clues. Aadalen and Stroebel-Kahn (1981), for example, describe the experiences of a woman who married in her early thirties and had an accident within a few years after the marriage. She was seven months pregnant at the time of the accident, which left her a quadriplegic with a tracheostomy, and which led to the premature birth and subsequent death of her infant. Though somewhat older than a young adult, the dilemmas that she faced with her husband throughout the rehabilitation process illustrate the problems that arise when a chronically disabled young adult returns to a spouse.

She notes that her "inability to actively hold my husband, to actively love him, deeply affected my perception of our sexual relationship. . . . I compared our life before the accident to what it was now." The relationship between this woman and her husband was strong and close, yet the requirements for care at home—the full-time attendants, the mobility limitations, and the total dependence for all personal care—took its toll: four years after the accident, the couple divorced. The woman notes that her husband was finally able "to acknowledge that there was no way he could live with me and have his needs met" (Aadalen & Stroebel-Kahn, p. 1477). A month after the divorce was final, the husband remarried, "devastating" his former wife.

Although there are no empirical findings to support our observation, we believe that divorce rates are particularly high when one spouse acquires a chronic illness or disability. It has been our experience that disabled young adults who are divorced by their able-bodied spouses frequently remarry other disabled individuals. If these patterns are true, it underscores the difficulty that able-bodied and disabled spouses have in sharing experiences. The disabled individual has a whole set of experiences—hospitalization, struggling with adaptive equipment, facing strangers' curiosity—which the able-bodied spouse does not have. Furthermore, the disabled individual may not be able to return caring in tangible ways; "I could not hold my husband and meet his need" is an example of this imbalance in sharing. It is our impression, therefore, that when a disabled person returns to his or her spouse, the two most difficult tasks are (1) discovering a means for the spouses to develop "mutuality" and (2) enabling the disabled person to express caring in tangible ways.

The specific types of problems that arise when a disabled young adult returns to a spouse depend also on the nature of the disability. Kane (1981) describes a twenty-nine-year-old man, married and with two young children, coming to terms with a diagnosis of mesothelioma (cancer of the tissue which lines the outside of the body's organs). She notes that his major concern, as the sole source of family income, was the effect of the illness on his ability to support his family financially. In many ways, Kane suggests, being the breadwinner was the primary means by which the man identified himself. Because cancer affected this role, it altered completely his sense of identity and self-definition.

The social and community support which a spouse is able to mobilize can be a critical factor in the family's adaptation. The presence of an external support system for the spouse is particularly important since he or she must provide so much support, both physical and emotional, to the disabled spouse and may, initially at least, receive little support in return.

The case reports described above point out the many types of family tasks that face a chronically ill or disabled young adult who returns to a family of commitment. For the individuals in these articles, the individuating tasks were difficult but the major challenges lay in becoming reintegrated into family life.

A Summary

To summarize the various issues raised in this section, Table 9.2 redefines the family tasks listed in Table 9.1 for the population of chronically ill or disabled young adults. The case studies and anecdotal reports illustrate these tasks. For example, Chuck and his family struggled to redefine their roles in relation to each other, attempting to ensure that Chuck would not be treated like a child even though he needed much care; the marriage described in Aadalen and Stroebel-Kahn (1981) dissolved partly because the spouses were not able to redefine their roles.

Similarly, chronically ill or disabled individuals need to recreate illusions about intimacy in order to be truly reintegrated into a community or a home. Sheehy (1974) writes of the powerful illusions that young adults often have about close relationships and marriage, illusions such as "if we work together we can solve everything" or "I'll make him a better person by loving him." A disability or an illness can shatter these illusions or beliefs; the couple must resurrect them if they are to sustain an interest in intimacy. Chuck, for example, took many months to believe again that he had something to offer not only his family but his girlfriend. The resurrection of his beliefs that he could be a giving person aided his entrance back to the world of his peers.

Finally, it is important to note that different living arrangements can have substantially different effects on these two sets of tasks. Returning to

Table 9.2. Family Tasks for Chronically Ill or Disabled Young Adults

Individuating Tasks

1. Redefining a role in the family or with a spouse
2. Maximizing control over daily tasks and choices (i.e., maximizing independence from parents, spouse, or caretakers)
3. Finding a "home" of one's own

Integrating Tasks

1. Recreating illusions about intimacy
2. Developing the ability to return care
3. Establishing a niche in society

a family of origin, for example, may indeed make the tasks of individuation more difficult than if a person returns to a spouse. In either case, however, the achievement of these family tasks will not proceed in any linear fashion. Rather, they will be achieved as the caretaker and the individual move through stages in their response to a chronic disability or illness. We turn now to the examination of these issues in the context of appropriate treatment strategies.

Treatment Issues: Applications and Strategies

Health professionals working with chronically ill or disabled young adults and their families can have a decisive influence on the adaptive process of the family. Sensitivity to the needs of family members, as well as to those of the young adult patient, provides the opportunity to promote the healthy adaptation and appropriate achievement of developmental tasks for all concerned. Because the disability creates a crisis in the family, it may, in fact, enhance the opportunity for promoting positive change.

In order to intervene effectively, the health professional must first be aware of the stages of adaptation that family members face. Second, as we pointed out in the previous section, the adaptive process will encompass very different tasks for members of the family of origin and members of the family of commitment—the spouse and children. The unique composition of the family and the strengths and pitfalls inherent in that structure must be kept in mind if the health professional is to work effectively with the family.

Various authors have developed models of adaptation to severe or chronic illness (Mailick, 1979; Lawrence & Lawrence, 1979) similar to those developed for other family crises (Kübler-Ross, 1969; Drotar, Baskiewicz, Irvin, Kennell, & Klaus, 1975). The stages of adaptation identified in these models provide a framework for viewing the professional's role with families. However, these stages are not discrete time periods. Adaptation is a dynamic process, and family members may need to go back and rework a task many times even though they have apparently moved beyond that "stage" (Mailick, 1979). Also, families often do not proceed through adaptive stages as a unit. The disability of a young adult will affect a spouse, a parent, or a sibling very differently. The meaning of the disability for each and, thus, the ability to adapt and the rate at which adaptation occurs, are related to the individual's own developmental stage as well as to his or her role in the young adult's family. Professionals' failure to recognize these differences among family members can lead to added stress for the family and confusion for the professionals.

Onset of Disability

The initial adaptive stage occurs at the time of the diagnosis or accident and is marked by shock and disbelief. As families move through this stage, they must begin to cope with their grief and begin to mobilize their strengths toward adaptation.

Health professionals can be of great assistance to family members by helping them identify their loss and by providing them the opportunity to speak of their own grief. Family members need a respite from "being strong" and "keeping up a good front" for the patient and other family members.

White (1974) identified three critical factors necessary for adaptive behavior. Families with a severely ill or injured member must take on these tasks during the initial stage of the adaptive process (Mailick, 1979). The tasks are: (1) the regulation and utilization of information, (2) the maintenance of autonomy or freedom of movement, and (3) the maintenance of satisfactory internal balance for action and for processing information.

Processing information, the first task, is difficult in a time of crisis. The family often finds itself caught up in a high technology medical setting where multiple interventions are being carried out to save the life of the patient or to initiate treatment. The young adults—patient or spouse—have likely had few encounters with the health care system and this may be the first instance in which they are viewed as responsible adults. In order to begin to cope with the medical setting as well as with the diagnosis and its implications, the family must have access to information—information that the health care providers must give repeatedly and in a language that parents, spouse, and patient can understand. Often either the information or the appropriate timing are lacking, impeding the family's progress toward adaptation.

Research in other areas of health care has shown that communication between health care providers and patients and their families is often of poor quality (Korsch, Freeman, & Negrete, 1971). Clear, sensitive communication, however, has been found to be positively related to patients' satisfaction with care (Ware & Snyder, 1975), problem resolution (Starfield, Wray, Hess, Gross, Birk, & D'Lugoff, 1981), patient compliance (Hulka, Cassel, Kupper, & Burdett, 1976; Francis, Korsch, & Morris, 1969), and family understanding and acceptance (Power & Sax, 1978). Thus, adequate communication between the patient and family and the providers can have a positive impact on patients' and families' adherence to therapeutic plans as well as to their overall adaptation. Systematic approaches to providing information to families need to be incorporated into medical and rehabilitation plans for disabled young adults (Rohrer, Adelman, Puckett, Toomay, Tabert, & Johnson, 1980).

Maintaining a sense of autonomy, the second factor in adaptive behavior, will be a struggle for family members in this situation. Complex decisions about medical management and rehabilitation are often made by health personnel without giving the patient or the family enough information or a real opportunity to participate in the decision. Family members feel powerless. For example, a young spouse may find her developing role as confidant and helpmate to the patient seriously undermined. Parents, in an effort to maintain their own sense of autonomy, may be tempted to take over decision making for the young adult, and professionals may inadvertently encourage this by relating to the parents rather than the patient. Health professionals must make a genuine effort to involve the young adult and family members in decision making in order to maintain their sense of autonomy.

The maintenance of internal organization by individuals and the family unit, the third factor, can also be problematic. Mailick (1979) points out that blame, guilt, and shame as well as anxiety and depression brought about by the illness or injury must be confronted if this task is to be accomplished. The patient's spouse and family of origin need to be able to communicate and work together but may have little history of doing so.

Patterns of communication in the family may temporarily change. Cleveland (1979) describes a family's adjustment to the spinal cord injury of their late adolescent son. In this family, each member felt it was important to protect others by coping with his or her grief alone. However, "this adaptive pattern of protection solidified and unfortunately kept the family members separated from each other, clearly interfering with honest communication among them" (Cleveland, 1979, p. 462).

Professionals need to facilitate communication among family members. Family conferences with patient, family, and professionals are one type of intervention. In some cases, some form of family therapy may be necessary to improve family function. The family that is able to gather information and maintain both a sense of autonomy and an internal organization which allows for action and information processing can begin to carry out behaviors which allow the family and its individual members to begin to adapt to the young adult's disability.

Finally, the onset of a chronic illness or disability in young adulthood can provoke intense feelings in a health care team, particularly if some of the providers are young adults themselves. From one perspective, the health care team is the young adult's family during the initial period of diagnosis and care. For this reason, regular consultation to or support for the "health care family" can often be of enormous benefit in helping the providers to communicate with and support the patient's actual family.

Adaptation to Disability

A growing awareness of the implications of the disability occurs for the young adult as the physical condition persists, symptoms do not diminish, or function does not return. Patient and family during this stage often become angry, and this anger, turned inward because it is unacceptable to express it, can become depression (Lawrence & Lawrence, 1979).

The anger is directed at anyone connected with the disability. The young adult may express his anger to family and staff both verbally and by refusing to participate in his care. Family members may feel anger toward the young adult ("How could you let this happen?" "Why are you doing this to me?"). These feelings may be more pronounced in instances of attempted suicides or accidents, but also occur with illnesses where there is no question of "fault."

Because family members often will not or cannot express their anger at the young adult, they lash out at those providing his care. They may also be justifiably angry at being excluded from the decision-making process surrounding the patient's care.

One of the skills that families must develop in this stage is learning how to interact with physicians and other health personnel in order to gain the information they need and to combat their feelings of powerlessness (Mailick, 1979). Young adults' inexperience with the health care system and with an advocate role exaggerates this problem. Expressing dissatisfaction and anger to those who control the care of one's loved one is difficult to do. Health personnel need to understand the reasons for the family's anger and respond appropriately by changing their own behavior when necessary and by trying to facilitate openness and trust in communication with the family.

Family members may need help in understanding that both anger and depression are parts of the grieving process (Bray, 1980). They may try to protect each other from their own and others' depression and anger. "When carried to an extreme, protection from depression yields an intra-family relationship structure which isolates the protector from the protected, which builds barriers to communication, and which invests the state of depression with an excessive amount of power" (Cleveland, 1979, p. 468). This inhibition of communication can substantially slow the adaptation to disability.

Another task central to adaptation of the family is the shifting of roles within the family. Other family members must take over some of the previous functions of the young adult without shutting him out (Bruhn, 1977; Cleveland, 1979; Mailick 1979). The young adult's loss of his or her role as an employed person, for example, means a financial dependency on family, spouse, or government assistance that is often accompanied by loss of self-esteem for the individual and economic hardship for the family (Kane, 1981; Valentine, 1978). Intervention by social services to help the family identify sources of financial assistance and support services is essential.

One family member may assume the role of caregiver to the disabled young adult. This role is particularly difficult because one must balance meeting the young adult's need for assistance with promoting his or her independent functioning whenever possible. Parents may have particular problems promoting independence (Cleveland, 1979). A conference with the young adult, the family members, and the health professional can have a twofold function. On the one hand, the conference can provide the young adult with the opportunity to identify for the family his or her capabilities with the support of the staff. The staff, on the other hand, may need to point out to the young adult and to family members the areas in which the young adult can and should function independently. Dressing, for example, can be a lengthy process for a spinal cord injured patient, and one which the caregiver may be tempted to take over.

Health professionals can facilitate shifting of roles by encouraging open discussion of task division. For the disabled young adult and spouse, reassessment of roles may be more difficult if "traditional" sex-role divisions previously determined task assignment. Helping the couple to view the whole range of tasks as valuable to the family can be an important step in the adaptive process. A paraplegic young man can no longer mow the lawn but can competently provide child care. A chronically ill young woman might no longer be able to do housekeeping but could manage the family's financial affairs. "Roles must be changed and reallocated in ways which minimize a sense of personal loss and prevent the ill person's social and psychological withdrawal from the family" (Bruhn, 1977, p. 1057).

The needs of other family members often receive little attention during the initial crisis. They resurface when the medical situation has stabilized, but the family may still not feel it is appropriate to direct their energy toward meeting these needs. The impact of inattention to the needs of the children or younger siblings of the patient may be the most noticeable if regression in behavior or acting out occurs. Continued inattention to the needs of adult family members can also result in mental or physical health problems. "The family must find a way of balancing the demands made upon them for rearranging their lives, so as to be able to provide special care to the patient . . . and to advocate for the other needs of family members for continued growth and differentiation" (Mailick, 1979, p. 124).

This process can be helped by providing opportunities for staff, family, and young adults to discuss these issues openly. A trusting relationship with a psychologist, nurse, physician, social worker, or therapist can provide the basis for this discussion.

Picking Up the Pieces

The third stage of adaptation will take different forms depending on the nature of the disability. For a chronic illness, such as cancer or arthritis, the family must deal with remission and the uncertainty of that state. The family must regulate its hopefulness and "balance its image of the patient as presently well, but eventually ill again. It must allow the patient back in its midst, facilitating the reacquisition of as many of the old roles and responsibilities by the patient as possible" (Mailick, 1979, p. 126).

For young adults with permanent disabilities and for their families, the third period of adaptation involves resolving the loss (Lawrence & Lawrence, 1979). The losses are often great—physical health, independent functioning, valued roles in family and community. The young adult must find new roles and form new relationships, and the family members must rework their relationship with the young adult in a way that accepts and accommodates the disability while promoting the young adult's autonomy.

This process of resolution requires changes of values for both the young adult and the family members (Adams & Lindeman, 1974). Dramatic change may be necessary to continue to view oneself or a loved one as a worthy human being (Carlson, 1979). In light of the difficulty of changing one's value system, the enormity of this task cannot be overestimated.

Health professionals must be acutely sensitive to the demands for intrapsychic and interpersonal change that a chronic disability makes on a young adult and on the significant other people in his or her life. The family helps to shape and is shaped by the young adult's adaptation. Professionals caring for disabled young adults need not only a sensitivity to family members and to their role in adaptation but also a structure for providing care that acknowledges the family's role and that systematically provides for inclusion of the family in that care.

Future Trends

For the future, we believe that two matters press for sustained attention. The first concerns basic epidemiological research; the second concerns the development of a long-term perspective on the family life of disabled young adults. Attention to these matters would certainly result in a more accurate understanding of the patterns of family life experiences for this population. Equally important, such attention would also lay the foundation for a fruitful relationship between health care providers and those community institutions that are involved with chronically ill or disabled young adults and their families. It is in this area that the future holds great promise.

References

Aadalen, S. P., & Stroebel-Kahn, F. Coping with quadriplegia. *American Journal of Nursing*, 1981, *81*, 1471–1478.

Adams, J. E., & Lindemann, E. Coping with long-term disability. In G. V. Coelho, D. A. Hamburg, & J. E. Adams (Eds.), *Coping and adaptation*. New York: Basic Books, 1974.

Bray, G. P. Reactive patterns in families of the severely disabled. In P. W. Power & A. E. Dell Orto (Eds.), *Role of the family in the rehabilitation of the physically disabled*. Baltimore, Md.: University Park Press, 1980.

Bronfenbrenner, U. *The ecology of human development*. Cambridge, Mass.: Harvard University Press, 1979.

Bruhn, J. G. Effects of chronic illness on the family. *The Journal of Family Practice*, 1977, *4*, 1057–1060.

Carlson, C. E. Conceptual style and life satisfaction following spinal cord injury. *Archives of Physical Medicine and Rehabilitation*, 1979, *60*, 346–352.

Caywood, T. A quadriplegic young man looks at treatment. In J. Stubbins (Ed.), *Social and psychological aspects of disability*. Baltimore, Md.: University Park Press, 1977.

Cleveland, M. Family adaptation to the traumatic spinal cord injury of a son or daughter. *Social Work in Health Care*, 1979, *4*, 459–471.

Cohen, S. *Special people*. Englewood Cliffs, N.J.: Prentice-Hall, 1977.

Diamond, M. Social support and adaptation to chronic illness: The case of maintenance hemodialysis. *Research in Nursing and Health*, 1979, *2*, 101–108.

Drotar, D., Baskiewicz, A., Irvin, N., Kennell, J., & Klaus, M. The adaptation of parents to the birth of an infant with congenital malformation: A hypothetical model. *Pediatrics*, 1975, *56*, 710–717.

Erikson, E. *Childhood and society*. New York: Norton, 1963.

Fiske, M. Changing hierarchies of commitment in adulthood. In N. Smelser & E. Erikson (Eds.), *Themes of work and love in adulthood*. Cambridge, Mass.: Harvard University Press, 1980.

Francis, V., Korsch, B. M., & Morris, M. J. Gaps in doctor–patient communication: Patients' response to medical advice. *New England Journal of Medicine*, 1969, *280*, 535–540.

Giele, J. Adulthood as transcendence of age and sex. In N. Smelser & E. Erikson (Eds.), *Themes of work and love in adulthood*. Cambridge, Mass.: Harvard University Press, 1980.

Havinghurst, R. *Developmental tasks and education* (3rd ed.). New York: David McKay, 1972.

Holman, T. The influence of community involvement on marital quality. *Journal of Marriage and Family*, 1981, *43*(1), 143–149.

Hudson, M. She's 22 and dealing with a catastrophic illness. *American Journal of Nursing*, 1976, *76*(8), 1273.

Hulka, B., Cassel, J., Kupper, L., & Burdett, J. Communication, compliance, and concordance between physicians and patients with prescribed medication. *American Journal of Public Health*, 1976, *66*, 847–853.

Hyman, M. Social isolation and peer performance in rehabilitation. *Journal of Chronic Diseases*, 1972, *25*, 85–97.

Kane, N. E. The young adult with cancer: a developmental approach. *Oncology Nursing Forum*, 1981, *8*, 16–19.

Kemp, B. J., & Vash, C. L. Productivity after injury in a sample of spinal cord injured persons: A pilot study. *Journal of Chronic Diseases*, 1971, *24*, 259–275.

Keniston, K. *All our children: The American family under pressure*. New York: Harcourt, Brace, Jovanovich, 1977.

Korsch, B. M., Freeman, B., & Negrete, F. Practical implications of doctor–patient interaction analysis for pediatric practice. *American Journal of Diseases of Children*, 1971, *121*, 110–114.

Kübler-Ross, E. *On death and dying*. New York: Macmillan, 1969.

Lawrence, S. A., & Lawrence, R. M. A model of adaptation to the stress of chronic illness. *Nursing Forum*, 1979, *28*, 33–42.

Levinson, D., with Darrow, C., Klein, E., Levinson, M., & McKee, B. *The seasons of a man's life*. New York: Knopf, 1978.

Levinson, D. Toward a conception of the adult life course. In N. Smelser & E. Erikson (Eds.), *Themes of work and love in adulthood*. Cambridge, Mass.: Harvard University Press, 1980.

Litman, T. The family and physical rehabilitation. *Journal of Chronic Disease*, 1966, *19*, 211–217.

Lonnquist, D. Employment rates among severely physically disabled and nondisabled college graduates and dropouts. *Journal of Applied Rehabilitation Counseling*, 1979, *10*(1), 24–27.

Mailick, M. The impact of severe illness on the individual and family: An overview. *Social Work in Health Care*, 1979, *5*, 117–128.

Maslow, A. *Toward a psychology of being*. New York: Van Nostrand, 1968.

Masnick, G., & Bane, M. *The nation's families: 1960–1990*. Boston: Auburn House, 1980.

Meyer, V. The psychology of the young adult. *Nursing Clinics of North America*, 1973, *8*, 5–17.

Napier, A., & Whitaker, C. *The family crucible*. New York: Harper & Row, 1978.

Nordlicht, S. Facial disfigurement and psychiatric sequelae. *New York State Journal of Medicine*, 1979, *79*(9), 1382–1384.

O'Brien, M. E. Hemodialysis regimen compliance and social environment: A panel analysis. *Nursing Research*, 1980, *29*, 250–255.

Peterson, Y. The impact of physical disability on marital adjustment: A literature review. *The Family Coordinator*, 1979, *28*, 47–51.

Power, P., & Sax, D. The communication of information to the neurological patient: Some implications for family coping. *Journal of Chronic Disease*, 1978, *31*, 57–65.

Rogers, J. C., & Figone, J. J. Psychosocial parameters in treating the person with quadriplegia. *American Journal of Occupational Therapy*, 1979, *33*, 432–439.

Rohrer, K., Adelman, B., Puckett, J., Toomey, B., Tabert, D., & Johnson, E. Rehabilitation in spinal cord injury: Use of a patient–family group. *Archives of Physical Medicine and Rehabilitation*, 1980, *61*, 225–229.

Sheehy, G. *Passages: Predictable crises of adult life*. New York: E. P. Dutton, 1974.

Skipper, J. K., Fink, S. L., & Hallenbeck, P. H. Physical disability among married women: Problems in husband–wife relationship. In J. Stubbins (Ed.), *Social and psychological aspects of disability*. Baltimore, Md.: University Park Press, 1977.

Starfield, B., Wray, C., Hess, K., Gross, R., Birk, P., & D'Lugoff, B. The influence of patient–practitioner agreement on outcome of care. *American Journal of Public Health*, 1981, *71*, 127–131.

U.S. Bureau of the Census. *Sixteenth Census of the United States: 1940*. "Characteristics by Age," Vol. 4:1, U.S. Summary. Washington, D.C.: U.S. Government Printing Office, 1943.

U.S. Bureau of the Census. *U.S. Census of the Population: 1970*. Characteristics of the population. Vol. 1:1, Sec. 2. U.S. Summary. Washington, D.C.: U.S. Government Printing Office, 1973.

U.S. Bureau of the Census. *1979 Census of the United States*. Washington, D.C.: U.S. Government Printing Office, 1979.

Valentine, A. S. Caring for the young adult with cancer. *Cancer Nursing*, 1978, *1*, 385–389.

Ware, J. E., & Snyder, M. K. Dimensions of patient attitudes regarding doctors and medical care services. *Medical Care*, 1975, *13*, 669–682.

White, R. H. Strategies of adaptation: An attempt at systematic description. In G. V. Coelho, D. A. Hamburg, & J. E. Adams (Eds.)., *Coping and adaptation*. New York: Basic Books, 1974.

Wilkie, J. The trend toward delayed parenthood. *Journal of Marriage and the Family*, 1981, *43*(3), 583–591.

Zahn, M. Incapacity, impotence, and invisible impairment: Their effects upon interpersonal relations. *Journal of Health and Social Behavior*, 1973, *14*, 115–123.

V

Middle Age

10 Personal Impact of Myocardial Infarction: A Model for Coping with Physical Disability in Middle Age

Andrew R. Block, Sara L. Boyer, and Cheryl Imes

Introduction

When an individual reaches adulthood, the possibility that he or she may be suddenly afflicted with a physically disabling condition may seem very remote. Yet illness, accident, or disease combine to produce physical disabilities with surprising frequency during middle age. Wright (1980), for example, states that approximately 30 percent of all individuals aged fifty-five to sixty-four have some form of physical disability.

While it is not pleasant to contemplate falling victim to any circumstance which might lead to protracted physical disability, one particular event, myocardial infarction (MI), seems to inspire exceptional fear. As with many disability engendering events, MI often strikes unpredictably and without warning, since predisposing factors (e. g., hypertension, high cholesterol, high blood pressure) likely go unnoticed. Once the MI strikes, the victim is no longer able to influence his or her chances for survival. Instead, while constantly on the brink of death during the first hours and days post-MI, the patient is totally dependent for survival on the split-second actions of others. This experience, during the initial post-MI period, of total helplessness in the face of death adds to the traumatic nature of coronary disease. Ultimately, however, the most traumatic aspect of this disease is its tremendously high mortality rate: 40 percent of MI victims will be dead within twenty-eight days (Peel & Semple, 1972).

Fortunately, of the approximately 1,300,000 individuals who experience an MI each year, about 625,000 will survive (Second Report, 1975). The devastation associated with MI, however, cannot be indexed merely by death rates, for the physical capacity and psychosocial functioning of its victims may be altered in ways which are profound and protracted. Even if physical capacity is restored, emotional and psychosocial status may remain affected for extended periods.

It is the purpose of this paper to consider: (1) data on the long-term psychosocial and affective adjustment of post-MI patients and (2) implications these data have for treatment. In reviewing the literature the present paper will consider only those studies which are of a well-controlled scientific nature and in which patients have been examined at least twelve weeks post-MI.

There are several reasons why a focus on the post-MI patient may be of value. First, since there are a great number of post-MI patients seeking rehabilitation services, it is important for the rehabilitation specialist to become familiar with the problems and needs of these individuals. Second, rehabilitation techniques can produce very significant results in helping the patient recover functioning. Third, the large body of well-conducted research focused on this population allows one to draw relatively confident conclusions about the long-term impact of MI. In the final section of this paper, we will present means by which findings on the impact of MI can be related to data on the impact of other physical disabilities.

Literature Review

Psychosocial Functioning

The aspects of psychosocial functioning which have been investigated in post-MI patients can be divided into two broad areas: (1) economic disruptions, including return to work status and changes in income; and (2) interpersonal behavior, physical activity, and sexuality.

Return to Work. All patients experience at least a transient disruption in their employment and economic status in the first year post-MI. Many do eventually return to work, however, with some surveys reporting that over 90 percent of patients return to work after a heart attack (Croog & Levine, 1977; Mayou, Foster & Willimason, 1978; Shapiro, Weinblatt, & Frank, 1972) and others reporting rates as low as 50 percent (Wishnie, Hackett & Cassem, 1971). Any simple report of reemployment rate must be accepted with some caution, however, for as many as two-thirds of the patients who return to work in the first year post-MI are forced to alter their level of physical activity at work (Mayou et al., 1978). Such an alteration in activity may adversely affect employment experience. In one study (Croog & Levine, 1977), 44.9 percent stated that their heart attack had affected their work, with 29.8 percent reporting that it had a negative effect on promotion or opportunity for advancement and 12.9 percent stating that it had affected their relationships with employers and co-workers. Further, Mayou et al. (1978) state that, of the 33 percent of patients who reported that they were dissatisfied with the quality of their work experiences at one year after an MI, most had had "to modify their jobs considerably or change altogether" (p. 449). Thus, simply returning to work may not provide a great deal of encouragement to the recovering MI patient. The quality of the work experience must be examined also.

Further, it should be noted that return to work may not provide a highly accurate index of the physical recovery process for there is not a simple relationship between the extent of tissue damage sustained in the MI and the probability of return to work. Wishnie et al. (1971) reported that the amount of tissue damage evident in post-MI patients who eventually returned to full-time work, as measured by the Peel Prognostic Index (Peel & Semple, 1972), was only slightly lower than that evident in patients who eventually returned to part-time work. Further, Nagle, Morgan, and Bird (1976) demonstrated that the degree of psychopathology was equally effective in predicting return to work after an MI as was the experience of cardiac symptoms. This theme of an inconsistent relationship between cardiac status on the one hand and psychosocial or affective impairment on the other hand is one which will be repeated frequently throughout this chapter.

Interpersonal Relationships and Physical Activity. While one of the after-effects of an MI may be a change in employment status, perhaps a more profound effect, as far as the quality of the patient's life is concerned, involves changes in the family interaction. Ability to participate in household chores, responsibilities in childrearing, recreational activities, and sexual behavior all may be altered during the long-term recovery phase with the patient developing a new and less energetic role in the family.

Perhaps the most commonly reported change is in the area of sexual relations. Hellerstein and Friedman (1969), in the first well-controlled investigation examining this area, reported a 24 percent decline in sexual activity in the period after an MI. Other investigators have reported even higher rates of decline, nearing 50 percent (Bloch, Maeder, & Haissly, 1975; Mayou et al., 1978). The reasons for such a decline in sexual activity, however, are not at all clear.

The physiological effects of intercourse on the recovering cardiac patient have been reviewed in several places (Hellerstein & Friedman, 1969; Wagner, 1976) with all reviewers agreeing that, while intercourse is indeed a stressful activity (as measured by heart rate increases), it is no more stressful than some other activities commonly engaged in by the same patients, such as brisk walks (Hellerstein & Friedman, 1969). Furthermore, the energy requirements involved in sexual intercourse have been shown not to exceed the cardiac capacity of a patient recovering from an uncomplicated MI.

Tuttle, Cook, and Fitch (1964) have implicated the role of inappropriate expectations in mediating a decline in sexual activity. They suggested that it was misinformation more than the experience of cardiac symptomatology which led to such declines. The authors concluded that "having received little or no advice from their physicians, these patients set their own patterns which represented a considerable deviation from their previous activity" (p. 143). If Tuttle and Cook's suggestion is correct, it implies that failure to attempt sexual behavior, rather than the experience of cardiac symptoms during intercourse, is an important factor responsible for such decreases.

As was noted earlier, many areas of the post-MI patient's family life other than sexual behavior may remain disrupted for an extended period of time. Wishnie et al. (1971) noted that, of the twenty-four patients examined at three months post-MI, seventeen reported spending most of their time puttering around the house or watching TV, and twenty-three reported being frustrated at their inactivity during this period. Mayou et al. (1978) also noted that a large number of patients (61.4 percent) reported decreases in domestic chores and responsibilities at one year post-MI. Once again, the factors leading to such decreases in general activity around the home are probably complex and not attributable solely to pathophysiology, since Croog & Levine (1977) have found that of the 73.4 percent of patients who did not return to pre-illness activity around the home at one year post-MI, 64.6 percent were judged by physicians, using a multiple-criteria rating system, to have made a full recovery by this time.

Affective Responses

Several studies which have examined the affective status of patients at three or more months post-MI most often find that patients report an affective state which can best be characterized as dysphoria, with the most frequently reported feelings being those of depression and anxiety. In these studies the percentage of patients reporting feelings of depression ranges from 21 percent (Dorossiev, Paskova, & Zachariev, 1976) to 73 percent (Acker, 1978) with an average around 50 percent (Croog & Levine, 1977; Mayou et al., 1978). Similar results are found for report of feelings of anxiety, although all studies which assessed such feelings found rates of reported anxiety in the 60–70 percent range (Dorossiev et al., 1976; Mayou et al., 1978). As can be seen from the results of the Wishnie et al. (1971) study, these feelings of depression and anxiety are often of sufficient intensity that the patient may require a tranquilizer or antidepressant medication.

As stated above, behavioral changes in the post-MI patient frequently bear no more than a moderate correlation with indices of actual tissue damage sustained in the MI (Peel & Semple, 1972). The relationship between affective status and tissue damage or cardiac symptomatology is also of only a moderate degree. Croog and Levine (1977) noted that depression was highly positively correlated with symptom frequency and negatively correlated with return to work status. These findings suggest that the cause of depression in many patients might be a failure to return to work or other normal activities, mediated by the experience of cardiac symptoms, such as angina, on exertion. After all, failure to return to normal levels of activity certainly could lead to decreased self-esteem, a finding commonly reported in connection with recovering post-MI patients (Acker, 1978). The experience of cardiac symptoms on exertion, then, would cause the patient to maintain minimal levels of activity and therefore could account for the behavioral deficits, negative affective states, and decreased self-esteem displayed by many patients.

Several lines of evidence argue against this simple proposition that the experience of cardiac symptoms mediates widespread behavioral and affective deficits in post-MI patients. First, it is well known that patients experiencing depression have an increased tendency toward somatic complaints (Blumer & Heilbronn, 1982). Depression, as noted above, is a widely reported affective state in the post-MI patient. Depressed post-MI patients, therefore, ought to be more likely to experience cardiac symptoms. Second, the experience of angina is not necessarily directly related to cardiac ischemia. Ockene, Slay, Alpert, Weiner, and Dalen (1980) found that in approximately 10 percent of patients referred for coronary angiography with major complaints of chest pain, there was no evidence of heart disease. Despite this finding, however, at approximately sixteen months post-catheterrization, 47 percent of these patients described their activity as limited by chest pain and 51 percent were unable to work. Leaman, Brower, Meester, Serruys, and Van Den Brand (1981) found that the severity of narrowing in coronary arteries was unrelated to frequency and severity of angina episodes. Finally, Schang and Pepine (1977) obtained continuous ten-hour electrocardiographic recordings accompanied by daily diaries of cardiac symptoms from men with documented coronary artery disease. In 2,826 hours of recording, they found evidence of 411 episodes of cardiac ischemia (as indexed by ST segment depression), but only 101 episodes were associated with angina. Since angina may not be experienced during ischemic episodes and may be experienced during periods when no ischemia occurs, any speculation as to the role of angina in mediating affective difficulties must be highly suspect. Further, since both those post-MI patients judged to have made adequate affective and psychosocial recovery and those whose adjustment has not been so adequate report chest pain and moderate breathlessness on exertion (Mayou et al. 1978), symptomatology alone cannot account for variations in affective adjustment.

Implications for Rehabilitation

The present review has noted that the course of rehabilitation after an MI is far from uniform. Some patients display fairly rapid recovery of function and show almost no psychosocial or affective impairment within several months. For other patients, however, adverse effects are both protracted and widespread. Fortunately, major advances have been made recently in cardiac rehabilitation, and many hospitals now begin such efforts soon after the MI (cf. Schiller, 1972; Task Force on Cardiovascular Rehabilitation of the National Heart, Lung and Blood Institute, 1976). These rehabilitation efforts, most often focusing upon reduction of risk factors such as obesity, smoking, or cholesterol and upon patient education, have proven to be fairly successful (Wenger & Gilbert, 1980). A description of the many components of a successful cardiac rehabilitation program is beyond the scope of this chapter. By focusing on the psychosocial and affective sequelae of MI, however, a few suggestions are obtained which may be applied to current rehabilitation efforts.

Physical Exercise. Although physical exercise is not appropriate for all post-MI patients (see Gilbert, 1978, for contraindications), when used appropriately, its value may be great. Many of the psychosocial difficulties displayed by post-MI patients (such as failure to return to work, decrease in household chores, decline in sexual activity), while not solely attributable to a decrease in the functional capacity of the heart, must bear some relationship to cardiac status. Fortunately, regular physical exercise increases cardiac performance by (1) reducing the "double product" (heart rate times systolic blood pressure) obtained in performing any specific task (Detry & Bruce, 1971; Redwood, Rosing, & Epstein, 1972), and (2) increasing aerobic capacity (VO_2 max: Hartung & Rangel, 1981). Thus, many patients will experience fewer cardiac symptoms on exertion and have increased endurance as a result of physical exercise training. Additional hemodynamic changes resulting from exercise training include bradycardia at rest and alterations in peripheral circulation (Froelicher, 1973).

Further, physical exercise training may have significant effects in relieving the depression experienced by many patients. Work with both post-MI patients (Naughton, Bruhn, & Lategola, 1968) and other populations (Folkins & Sime, 1981) demonstrates a significant antidepressant and antianxiety affect of exercise (see Ransford, 1982, for a review).

There are, however, some difficulties involved in the application of physical training for post-MI patients. The major difficulty stems from lack of compliance. Several studies have suggested a number of factors which may negatively influence the extent to which patients engage in prescribed physical exercise. For example, Andrew, Oldridge, Parker, Cunningham, Rechnitzer, Jones, Buck, Kavanaugh, Shepard, Sutton, and McDonald (1981) noted that in a group of 728 post-MI patients, 44.6 percent dropped out of the exercise program. The authors found a number of factors which were predictive of dropping out, including difficulty attending sessions, interference with daily activities, and a negative perception of staff members. The factor which most distinguished noncompliers from compliers, however, was a perception of lack of spouse support for the program. This points to a second implication for treatment.

Involvement of Spouse and Family Members. As many chapters in the present volume indicate, all members of a family are affected when one member becomes afflicted with a disability. Nowhere is this more true than with disabilities acquired by middle-age individuals, especially those experiencing MI. For example, Mohamed, Weisz, and Waring (1978) found that spouses of depressed chronic pain patients were more likely to develop pain problems themselves than were depressed non-pain patients. Additionally, in this study the spouses of depressed chronic pain patients had extremely low scores on the Locke-Wallace scale of marital adjustment, indicating dissatisfaction with their marriages.

Involvement of the spouse in rehabilitation efforts may be hypothesized to be one of the critical variables which influence long-term rehabilitation efforts. Any gains which the post-MI patient makes in rehabilitation during hospitalization may be undercut if spouses are nonsupportive or actually act in opposition to the patient's efforts. For example, many spouses, worried about the patient "pushing himself too hard," may discourage physical exercise, sexual activity, and the like. Unfortunately, the effect of such overprotective actions is to reward low levels of activity, making it unlikely that the patient will regain functional status (Block, Kremer, & Gaylor, 1980; Fordyce, 1976). Further, many actions by the spouse, while not directly countertherapeutic, may make it difficult for the patient to comply with treatment recommendations. Croog and Richards (1977), for example, found that wives of post-MI patients were unlikely to decrease their smoking behavior once the patient was discharged from the hospital. One might expect that patients would have difficulty complying with recommendations to cease smoking if their spouses continue to smoke at high rates.

Several factors seem to be of significance in involving spouses in rehabilitation of disabled patients in general and the post-MI patient in particular (Fordyce, 1976). The first involves education of the spouse about the disability process and the basis of the rehabilitation regimen. Helping the spouse to understand the patient's illness and agree to participate in treatment ought to enhance a sense of "social support" (Cobb, 1976), a factor which has been found to lessen the impact of stressful events upon the individual. Next, spouses must be taught to recognize and anticipate countertherapeutic responses, such as attending to the patient only when he complains of symptoms (Fordyce, 1976). Finally, since the quality of the marital relationship as perceived by the spouse has been found to significantly influence spousal responses toward disabled patients (Block, 1982), one ought to consider marital counseling as an adjunct in the rehabilitation process.

Vocational Evaluation and Retraining. No amount of physical exercise training, even if supported by the spouse, will help the post-MI patient to work if he perceives his job as too physically taxing, if he lacks employment skills, or if he does not want to return to his premorbid employment. Even though it was seen that the majority of patients eventually returned to work, it is true that blue-collar workers do not stand as good a chance of regaining employment. Croog and Levine (1977) reported that one year after the first MI more professional and high level executives were employed full time (91.4 percent) than were semiskilled workers (62.2 percent). (See also Schiller & Baker, 1976.) Thus, blue-collar workers, in particular, may need vocational retraining for positions involving lower levels of physical activity. Since, for middle-aged individuals, employment in addition to its financial benefits significantly influences self-esteem, one should consider evaluation of employable skills, perhaps through work simulation (Weitz & Adler, 1973) and employment retraining before deciding on retirement.

Group Intervention. A number of investigations have reported that "group therapy" sessions can provide significant benefits to the post-MI patient (Bilodeau & Hackett, 1971; Ibrahim, Feldman, Sultz, Staiman, Young, & Dean, 1974; cf. Karasu, 1979, for review). In the study by Ibrahim et al., one group of post-MI patients was given a one-year trial of group psychotherapy, while a control was given no such therapy. At the end of one year, group therapy patients were found to have dropped significantly in competitiveness and not to have increased in social alienation, whereas controls showed significant increases in alienation and no change in competitiveness. Further,

> The one-year survival rate was 10 percent higher among treatment patients than among the controls. Most of the difference resulted from the differences

> among the more severely affected patients. One-year survival among the more severely ill experimental patients was 93 percent contrasted to 74 percent among the control ill patients [p. 264].

Although the nature of the group therapy sessions is difficult to describe precisely, Ibrahim et al. (1974) state that the sessions focused on "questions of medication usage, diet regimen and degree of physical activity," with patients "spend[ing] many hours discussing ways to make more constructive use of leisure time in an effort to eliminate stress and to reduce the seriousness with which they undertook job and home responsibilities" (p. 255). Thus, although it is difficult to determine whether group therapy results in an increased sense of social support, greater information about the disease process, or specific information for coping with the disability, this intervention may be useful, especially for the patient who appears to be progressing exceptionally slowly in rehabilitation.

Directions for Future Research

The present review found rather widespread long-term psychosocial and affective effects of MI. Such consequences, as has frequently been noted, cannot be solely attributable to tissue damage sustained in the MI nor to the presence of cardiac symptoms experienced upon exertion by the post-MI patient. Such an inconsistent relationship between the pathophysiology and behavior leads one to search for psychological factors which may mediate the rehabilitation process. There are several levels of psychological factors which may prove useful in future investigations:

Cognitive Factors. Beck (1974) has pointed to the importance of thought processes in depression. Certain forms of illogical thinking, particularly with regard to self-deprecation and self-blame, seem particularly connected with depression. Such cognitive distortion has also been found in chronic pain patients (Lefevbre, 1981). Since many post-MI patients exhibit depression, one may expect to find that they display cognitive distortion or other cognitive difficulties—for example, deficits associated with learned helplessness (Abramson, Seligman, & Teasdale, 1978). Such maladaptive cognitive patterns may engender other psychological or affective difficulties.

Behavioral Factors. The patient may not learn appropriate behaviors necessary for improvement or, as noted above, may be discouraged from having functional improvement. Further, certain behavior patterns, such as Type A behavior (Friedman & Rosenman, 1974), may put the patient at risk for further coronary events.

Personality Factors. Croog and Levine (1977), as well as Schiller and Baker (1972), noted that certain premorbid personality patterns or post-history of psychopathology predict poorer adjustment. Cromwell, Butterfield, Brayfield, and Curry (1977) examined the influence of a trait known as locus of control (Rotter, 1966) on recovery from MI. Locus of control essentially refers to the belief that one has control over the events which occur to him or her (internal locus of control) versus the belief that one's outcomes are independent of one's action (external locus of control). Cromwell et al. (1977) found that internals showed greatest improvement if allowed to control and set the pace of recovery, whereas externals showed greatest improvement if treatment were dictated to them by staff.

Interpersonal Factors. The response of the patients' "significant others," health care providers, and employers has been shown to greatly influence the rehabilitation process. However, much research is needed to delineate the most beneficial, as well as the most countertherapeutic, responses by each of these groups of individuals.

Finally, it must be noted that this review has focused upon only one form of disability acquired in middle age. Many of the problems experienced by the post-MI patient may not be experienced by other populations. For example, while amputation is traumatic, once an amputee has recovered from surgery, his or her disability does not constitute a threat to existence, as does a weakened heart. Further, the post-MI patient has what Wright (1980) has termed a "hidden disability" (i.e., one which is not visible). In some ways, the adjustment to "hidden disability" is more difficult, for the individual does not have the patent explanation for functional limitations which is evident in the case of more visible disabilities such as amputation. On the other hand, the post-MI patient is not subject to the stigmatization which often accompanies obvious physical deformity.

In considering the impact of various disabilities upon the middle-aged individual, it is valuable to consider that disabilities may be classified along several dimensions. First, as suggested by Wright (1980), some disabilities are associated with obvious indications of the individual's condition (e.g., spinal-cord injury, Parkinson's disease) whereas other disabilities are "hidden" (e.g., post-MI, diabetes). We prefer the term *patency* for this dimension. Second, disabilities vary in *threat*—the possibility that the condition will increase in scope or severity or be prone to unexpected exacerbations (e.g., asthma, post-MI, Huntington's chorea) versus a stable, nonprogressive condition (e.g., traumatic amputation, blindness). Finally, disabilities vary in the extent to which the underlying medical condition limits the individual's behavior—a dimension we term *limitations*. Some disabilities may severely limit activities (e.g., quadriplegia); some may not limit activities to a great extent (e.g., epilepsy); whereas some disabilities may be associated with a wide range of limitations (e.g., chronic low back pain). It may be possible to find consistencies in the psychosocial and affective impact of varying disabilities by considering such commonalities between conditions. Thus, the difficulties displayed by post-MI patients may be seen as part of a general pattern of adjustment to disabilities having similar characteristics.

References

Abramson, L. Y., Seligman, M. E., & Teasdale, J. D. Learned helplessness in humans: Critique and reformulation. *Journal of Abnormal Psychology*, 1978, *87*, 49–74.

Acker, J. E. Psychological aspects of cardiac rehabilitation: Assessment and approach to treatment. *Advances in Cardiology*, 1978, *24*, 116–119.

Andrew, G. M., Oldridge, N. B., Parker, J. O., Cunningham, D. A., Rechnitzer, P. A., Jones, N. J., Buck, C., Kavanaugh, T., Shepard, R. J., Sutton, J. R., & McDonald, W. Reasons for dropout from exercise programs in post-coronary patients. *Medicine and Science in Sports and Exercise*, 1981, *13*, 164–168.

Beck, A. I. The development of depression: A cognitive approach. In R. J. Friedman & M. M. Katz (Eds.), *The psychology of depression: Contemporary theory and research*. Washington: V. H. Winston, 1974.

Bilodeau, C. B., & Hacket, T. P. Issues raised in a group setting by patients recovery from MI. *American Journal of Psychiatry*, 1971, *28*, 73–78.

Bloch, A., Maeder, J., & Haissly, J. Sexual problems after myocardial infarction. *American Heart Journal*, 1975, *90*, 536.

Block, A. R. An investigation of the response of the spouse to chronic pain behavior. *Psychosomatic Medicine*, 1982, *43*, 415–422.

Block, A. R., Kremer, E. F., & Gaylor, M. Behavioral treatment of chronic pain: The spouse as a discriminative cue for pain behavior. *Pain*, 1980, *9*, 243–252.

Blumer, D., & Heilbronn, M. Chronic pain as a variant of depressive disease. The pain-prone disorder. *The Journal of Nervous and Mental Disease*, 1982, *170*, 381.

Cobb, S. Social support as a moderator of life stress. *Psychosomatic Medicine*, 1976, *38*, 300–314.

Cromwell, R. L., Butterfield, E. C., Brayfield, F. R., & Curry, J. L. *Acute myocardial infarction: Reaction and recovery*. St. Louis: Mosby, 1977.

Croog, S. H., & Levine, S. *The heart patient recovers: Social and psychological factors*. New York: Human Sciences Press, 1977.

Croog, S. H., & Richards, N. P. Health beliefs and smoking patterns in heart patients and their wives: A longitudinal study. *American Journal of Public Health*, 1977, *67*, 921–930.

Detry, J. M., & Bruce, R. A. Effects of physical training on exertional S-T segment depression in coronary heart disease. *Circulation*, 1971, *44*, 390–396.

Dorossiev, D., Paskova, V., & Zachariev, Z. Psychological problems of cardiac rehabilitation. In U. Stocksmeier (Ed.), *Psychological approach to the rehabilitation of coronary patients*. New York: Springer, 1976.

Folkins, C. H., & Sime, W. E. Physical fitness training and mental health. *American Psychologist*, 1981, *36*, 373–389.

Fordyce, W. E. *Behavioral methods for chronic pain and illness*. St. Louis: Mosby, 1976.

Friedman, M., & Rosenman, R. H. *Type A behavior and your heart*. New York: Knopf, 1974.

Froelicher, V. F., Jr. The hemodynamic effects of physical conditioning in healthy, young and middle-aged individuals and in coronary heart disease patients. In J. Naughton & H. K. Hellerstein (Eds.), *Exercise testing and training in coronary heart disease*. New York: Academic Press, 1973.

Gilbert, C. A. Exercise testing of cardiac function. In J. W. Hurst, R. B. Logue, R. C. Schlant, & N. K. Wenger (Eds.), *The heart*. New York: McGraw-Hill, 1978.

Hartung, G. H., & Rangel, R. Exercise training in post-myocardial infarction patients: Comparison of results with high risk coronary and post-bypass patients. *Archives of Physical Medicine and Rehabilitation*, 1981, *62*, 34–38.

Hellerstein, H. K., & Friedman, E. H. Sexual activity and the post-coronary patient. *Medical Apsects of Human Sexuality*, 1969, *3*, 70–83.

Ibrahim, M. A., Feldman, J. G., Sultz, H. A., Staimen, M. G., Young, L. V., & Dean, D. Management after myocardial infarction: A controlled trial of the effect of group psychotherapy. *International Journal of Psychology in Medicine*, 1974, *5*, 253–268.

Karasu, T. B. Psychotherapy of the medically ill. *American Journal of Psychiatry*, 1979, *136*, 1–11.

Leaman, D. M., Brower, R. W., Meester, G. T., Serruys, P., & Van Den Brand, M. Coronary artery atherosclerosis: Severity of the disease, severity of angina pectoris and compromised left ventricular function. *Circulation*, 1981, *63*, 285–292.

Lefevbre, M. Cognitive distortion and cognitive errors in depressed psychiatric and low back pain patients. *Journal of Consulting and Clinical Psychology*, 1981, *32*, 234–238.

Mayou, R., Foster, A., & Williamson, B. Psychosocial adjustment in patients one year after MI. *Journal of Psychosomatic Research*, 1978, *22*, 447–453.

Mohamed, S. N., Weisz, G. M., & Waring, E. M. The relationship of chronic pain to depression, marital adjustment and family dynamics. *Pain*, 1978, *5*, 282–292.

Nagle, R., Morgan, D., & Bird, J. Interaction between physical and psychological abnormalities after myocardial infarction. In U. Stocksmeier (Ed.), *Psychological approach to the rehabilitation of coronary patients*. New York: Springer, 1976.

Naughton, J., Bruhn, J. G., & Lategola, M. T. Effects of physical training on physiologic and behavioral characteristics of cardiac patients. *Archives of Physical Medicine and Rehabilitation*, 1968, *49*, 131.

Ockene, I. S., Shay, M. J., Alpert, J. S., Weiner, B. H., & Dalen, J. E. Unexplained chest pain in patients with normal coronary arteriograms. *The New England Journal of Medicine*, 1980, *303*, 1249–1252.

Peel, A. A. F., & Semple, T. Immediate prognosis in acute myocardial infarction. In L. E. Meltzer & A. J. Dunning (Eds.), *Textbook of coronary care*. Philadelphia: Charles Press, 1972.

Ransford, C. P. A role for amines in the antidepressant effect of exercise: A review. *Medicine and Science in Sports and Exercise*, 1982, *14*, 1–10.

Redwood, D. R., Rosing, D. R., & Epstein, S. E. Circulatory and symptomatic effects of physical training in patients with coronary artery disease and angina pectoris. *New England Journal of Medicine*, 1972, *286*, 959–965.

Rotter, J. B. Generalized expectancies for internal versus external control of reinforcement. *Psychological Monographs*, 1966, *80* (whole No. 609).

Schang, S. L., & Pepine, C. J. Transient asymptomatic S-T segment depression during daily activity. *American Journal of Cardiology*, 1977, *38*, 396.

Schiller, E. Cardiac Rehabilitation: Its potential in the early prevention of disability after MI. *The Medical Journal of Australia*, 1972, *2*, 751–757.

Schiller, E., & Baker, J. Return to work after an MI: Evaluation of planned rehabilitation and of a predictive rating scale. *The Medical Journal of Australia*, 1972, *1*, 859–862.

Second Report of the Director of the National Heart and Lung Institute. DHEW Publication No. (NIH) 75–748. U.S. Government Printing Office: Washington, D.C., 1975.

Shapiro, S., Weinblatt, E., & Frank, C. W. Return to work after myocardial infarction. *Archives of Environmental Health*, 1972, *24*, 17.

Task Force on Cardiovascular Rehabilitation of the National Heart, Lung and Blood Institute. Needs and opportunities for rehabilitating the coronary heart disease patient. DHEW Publication No. (NIH) 76–750. U.S. Government Printing Office: Washington, D.C., 1976.

Tuttle, W. B., Cook, W. L., Jr., & Fitch, E. Sexual behavior in post-myocardial infarction patients. *American Journal of Cardiology*, 1964, *13*, 140.

Wagner, N. Some sexual aspects of the rehabilitation of cardiac patients. In U. Stocksmeier (Ed.), *Psychological approach to the rehabilitation of coronary patients*. New York: Springer, 1976.

Weitz, J., & Adler, S. The optimal use of simulation. *Journal of Applied Psychology*, 1973, *58*, 219–224.

Wenger, N. K., & Gilbert, C. A. Rehabilitation of the myocardial infarction patient. In J. W. Hurst, R. B. Logue, R. C. Schlant, & J. W. Purks (Eds.), *The heart*. New York: McGraw-Hill, 1980.

Wishnie, H. A., Hackett, T. P., & Cassem, N. H. Psychological hazards of convalescence following myocardial infarction. *Journal of the American Medical Association*, 1971, *215*, 1292–1296.

Wright, G. N. *Total rehabilitation*. Boston: Little, Brown, 1980.

11 Family Adjustment to Chronic Illness and Disability in Mid-Life

Lynne C. Rustad

Normative Tasks and Challenges in Mid-Life

Any consideration of the effects of chronic illness and disability on families in mid-life must rest on some understanding of the normal developmental tasks and challenges associated with this portion of the life span. Jung (1933, 1966), Havighurst (1948), and Erikson (1950) were among the first to devote attention to the mid-life phase from a theoretical perspective and in so doing exerted a significant influence on the thinking of later workers in the field. Unfortunately, as Chiriboga (1981) and Neugarten (1977) have pointed out, this pivotal phase of life remains relatively neglected in terms of empirical studies.

While differing in details of conceptualization, Jung, Havighurst, and Erikson shared the view that not only youth but the whole of the life span is developmental, with specific tasks to be accomplished at given stages. Jung (1933, 1966) viewed the task of the later half of life as being one of bringing into harmony opposing elements of personality, some of which are suppressed earlier in life in the interest of accomplishing tasks specific to the earlier stages. Erikson (1950) saw the essential task of mid-life as "generativity," that is, concern for others and care, nurturance, and guidance of the younger generation. Havighurst (1948) was more specific about the nature of mid-life tasks. They included:

1. Assisting teenage children to become responsible and happy adults,
2. Developing adult leisure time activities,
3. Relating to one's spouse as a person,
4. Accepting and adjusting to the physiological changes of middle age,
5. Adjusting to aging parents.

Both Erikson and Havighurst clearly saw the tasks of middle age as being intimately associated with the family—relationships to children, spouse, and parents.

There is some empirical evidence in support of Jung's theory that mid-life is a time of transition, with shifts in interests and goals reflecting expression of personality characteristics suppressed earlier in life. These shifts appear to be in different directions for men and women and to occur independent of socioeconomic or racial group membership. The changes from a cross-cultural perspective have been well summarized by Gutmann (1977). Neugarten and Gutmann (1968) and Chiriboga and Thurnher (1975) found in their studies that both middle-class and lower-middle-class men in early mid-life tend to be concerned with mastery and skill and have a sense of control and confidence. In the postparental years there is a trend away from this orientation and toward heightened emotional sensitivity, sensuality, and concern for interpersonal relationships. A similar trend was found in groups of both black and white men, who shared increased "familistic" values as they aged (Youmans, Grigsby, & King, 1969).

In contrast, the women in the first two studies seemed to move from a less confident and more nurturant, dependent, and family-centered orientation to one of increased assertiveness, mastery, and self-confidence and to be more accepting of their own aggressiveness and self-centered interests. Neugarten (1977) suggests that this "balancing" of suppressed aspects of the personality may be facilitated by the release from childrearing responsibilities and the division of labor it requires.

The results of several studies suggest that the childrearing years, up to and including the time of launching children from the parental home, are a relatively stressful period for the marital relationship. Investigating the differential weighting of stress during adulthood, Chiriboga and Cutler (1980) found that middle-aged individuals report greater life change in a negative direction than young people and this change is particularly associated with family functioning. Other life-span studies suggest that marital satisfaction decreases as children enter school and is lowest during the years of adolescence and launching (Burr, 1970; Chilman, 1968; Glenn, 1975; Rollins & Feldman, 1970). Men in the Rollins and Feldman study reported less variability in satisfaction over the life-span than did women. The authors hypothesize that this difference may be related to the men's greater investment in careers outside the home while women have the greater responsibility for childrearing. However, distress associated with separation of children from the parental home, the "empty nest syndrome" (Deykin, Jacobson, Klerman, & Solomon, 1966), may be as severe for fathers as it is for mothers (Lewis, Freneau, & Roberts, 1979).

The postparental years appear to be a time of decreasing stress and increased marital satisfaction. Chiriboga and Cutler (1980) found that individuals at this stage report greatest change in a positive direction, and the results of other studies indicate that there is an increase in marital satisfaction in the postparental group (Burr, 1970; Rollins & Feldman, 1970).

Retirement at the end of the mid-life phase, or earlier if illness or economic factors intervene, can bring new stresses and challenges. How stressful, or successful, retirement is seems to depend on a number of factors including: social class (Simpson, Back, McKinney, 1966; Stokes & Maddox, 1967), economic status (Eisdorfer, 1972; Osborne, 1971; Pollman, 1971), preparation, (Coelho & Adams, 1974), whether it is voluntary or forced (Paykel, Prusoff, & Uhlenhuth, 1971), and whether or not the family is accepting and supportive of retirement (Heyman & Jeffers, 1968). Chiriboga and Cutler (1980) found that individuals at this stage of life report the least change in a positive direction while Rollins and Feldman's study (1970) suggests that marital satisfaction increases after retirement.

One of the changes experienced by the mid-life couple is declining sexual activity. While it may result in part from the physiological effects of aging, social and psychological determinants also appear to be very important. Pfeiffer, Verwoerdt, and Davis (1972) in their study of sexuality in middle- and upper-middle-class individuals found that the sharpest decrease in sexual activity occurs between the ages of forty-five and fifty. Among individuals who had ceased having sexual intercourse by age fifty (49 percent of men and 58 percent of women in their study), husbands and wives were in agreement that the husband had been primarily responsible for cessation of activity. Inability to perform sexually (for men), illness of the husband, and death of the spouse (for women) were the most common reasons given.

In view of the many challenges faced by the mid-life couple, it is not surprising that many marriages do not survive and that stress-related disorders appear. The incidence of divorce in this group appears to be increasing. United States Bureau of Census figures (1979) indicate that the divorce rate for individuals between the ages of forty-five and sixty-four rose by 83 percent between 1960 and 1978. The development of psychiatric illness during mid-life is also common. Depression, alcoholism, and suicide are the most prevalent psychiatric disorders between the ages of forty-five and sixty (Boyd & Weissman, 1981). For some individuals, stress may contribute to the development of physical illnesses, or the onset of illness may add to the normative strains of mid-life. Bracht's survey (1979) of U.S. Government statistics indicates that approximately 14 percent of adults in the age range of forty-five to sixty-five years have some form of chronic illness—heart disease, hypertension, emphysema, and arthritis being the most prevalent. Activity-limiting chronic conditions appear to be disproportionately great among financially disadvantaged people, perhaps in part because of poorer health care. Heart disease, cancer, and stroke are the major causes of death in individuals over the age of forty-five, with heart disease accounting for 40 percent of these deaths.

While mid-life clearly brings changes and often in a negative direction, Neugarten (1977) has suggested that expected, age-appropriate life change may not be sufficient to cause a crisis in adaptation. Rather, it is the non-normative or "off-time" event which is likely to precipitate a crisis. The onset of severe, chronic illness or disability, especially in early mid-life, is one of the serious "off-time" events with which some families must cope.

Effects of Illness and Disability on the Spouse

Although there has been a traditional bias in clinical research toward the study of the "patient" with relative inattention to the implications of illness for the family, there is now a growing body of clinical and research data which suggests that chronic disease and disability may have profound effects on the able-bodied spouse. Some examples: Skelton and Dominian (1973), studying wives of men who had had myocardial infarctions, found that one year post-MI more than one-half of the wives manifested some degree of emotional disturbance and in one-quarter the degree was severe. Spouses of patients treated with home hemodialysis for chronic renal failure demonstrated a high incidence of emotional problems even when they were performing the home dialysis procedure adequately (Shambaugh, Hampters, Bailey, Snyder, & Merrill, 1967). Spouses of patients with chronic pain reported significantly decreased marital adjustment following onset of pain (Toshihiko, Osborne, Swanson, & Halling, 1981). Finally, bereaved spouses of patients who die after a lengthy chronic illness appear to adjust less well than spouses of patients who die after a shorter chronic illness (Gerber, Rusalem, Hannon, Batten, & Arkin, 1975).

The wife of the disabled person must often adjust to significant changes in role and life-style. If she was dependent prior to the onset of her husband's illness and tended to see him in a strong, dominant, and protective role, the reversal brought about by illness which suddenly places her in the position of caretaker may severely challenge her ability to cope. On the other hand, the wife forced, with some resentment, into a dependent, passive role before illness may welcome the opportunity to gain control and "take charge" even when this is detrimental to her husband's rehabilitation and self-esteem. Czaczkes and De-Nour (1978) have suggested that dependence–dominance conflicts arising from illness may play a central role in family disruption.

When the husband's disability leads to his temporary or permanent unemployment, the housewife may be forced to seek work outside the home and assume the breadwinner role, thus facing increased job and domestic responsibilities. For the wife who has successfully discharged many family responsibilities including the rearing of children and the provision of emotional support to her husband during the earlier stages of his career, this transition may be bearable and she may even welcome the chance to pursue her own career, provided she has help with domestic chores. The earlier mid-life wife with children still at home or the individual who has little interest in a career may see this unwelcome role reversal as a violation of the implied marital "contract" (Nadelson, Polonsky, & Mathews, 1978, 1979; Sager, 1976). Such changes in contract which challenge implied or explicit assumptions may cause serious disruption of the relationship. It is of interest in this respect that Crewe, Athelstan, and Krumberger (1979) in a study of pre- and post-spinal cord injury marriages found that marriages which took place after injury were happier than those which occurred before the trauma. These authors postulate that marriages occurring after injury involved free choice, thus leading to better adjustment and less resentment than found in marriages where the disability was an unexpected imposition.

The wife of the disabled individual must also cope with anxiety about her spouse's health, and she may live in constant fear that she will do something that will harm him (Block, Maeder, & Haissly, 1975; Skelton & Dominian, 1973). She may even be afraid to express anger or her own feelings of helplessness, lest she upset her husband.

Changes in sexual functioning following illness or disability may further threaten the integrity of the relationship and, for the mid-life couple, illness of the husband appears to be an important factor in decreased sexual activity (Pfeiffer, et al., 1972). Sexual dysfunction in this context may be of organic, psychogenic, or, most commonly, mixed etiology. Problems such as spinal cord injury (Comarr, 1970) and multiple sclerosis (Liluis, Valtonen, & Wikstrom, 1976) may lead to physiologic disruption of normal sexual response. Surgery for peripheral vascular disease (Weistein & Machleder, 1975) and drugs used to treat high blood pressure may also cause impotence or ejaculatory dysfunction. As high as 80 percent of treated male hypertensive patients may be affected in this way (Laver, 1974).

Sexual problems accompanying many disorders, however, appear to be primarily functional and related to anxiety or depression in the patient or spouse or to more general disruption of the marital relationship. At least one-half of men who have suffered MIs experience decreased sexual activity following infarction (Kavanagh & Shephard, 1977; Klein, Dean, Wilson, & Bogdonoff, 1965, Block et al., 1975; Hellerstein & Friedman, 1969) and wives of MI patients may avoid intimacy because they fear that sexual activity will cause another heart attack or even death (Adsett & Bruhn, 1968; Wishnie, Hackett, & Cassem, 1971). In spite of patients' and spouses' concerns about diminished libido and fears of death during intercourse, they may be reluctant to discuss these issues with the physician and the physician may avoid dealing with them in a direct manner (Bilodeau & Hackett, 1971). Loss of sexual desire may also occur in up to 30 percent of individuals who have had a stroke (Kalliomaki, Markkanen, & Mustonen, 1961), and Wiig (1973) reports that some women who have suffered a CVA may fear orgasm because the sensations involved remind them of those accompanying their strokes or subsequent seizures.

Often it is not the sexual dysfunction, per se, that disrupts the couple's relationship but their response to it. If the husband copes with his sexual problems by withdrawing and maintaining emotional and physical distance (often on the grounds of "not wanting to start something I can't finish"), the wife may interpret his withdrawal as a sign of disinterest or rejection. It is not uncommon in clinical practice to hear wives complain that it is not so much the "sex" they miss as the lack of warmth, affection, and physical intimacy.

The husband of the disabled woman has been relatively neglected by clinicians and researchers alike. In part this may be a function of the fact that potentially disabling illnesses such as heart disease, stroke, and emphysema are more likely to strike mid-life men than women and disabilities caused by trauma, such as spinal cord injury, are more common among men. It is also possible that husbands with disabled spouses are less vocal about the problems they encounter and less likely to seek professional advice and help than their opposite sex counterparts. In addition, changes required in traditional roles may not be as great when the wife rather than the husband is disabled. The lack of attention paid to these men is disturbing since they, too, may experience significant life-style disruption and stress.

In addition to continuing to perform his usual work, the husband whose wife becomes disabled may be expected to assume additional responsibilities in the home. He may have to devote significantly more time to the physical and emotional care of their children as well as assisting with homemaking tasks. Hospital and nursing care bills can pose a severe financial burden. The recently disabled wife may also make increased demands on his time and emotional resources. This can be especially stressful for the husband in early mid-life who is strongly committed to developing his career. For the postparental husband, the stresses may be less significant since childcare is no longer an issue, his job or career is often secure, and caring for his wife may be gratifying if he has experienced the shift toward a more nurturant orientation which has been noted to occur in men at this stage of life. The couple's sexual relationship may be disrupted if the husband finds her less attractive as a result of disability or perceives her as fragile, or if the disability is severe enough to make sexual activity difficult or painful. The wife may also withdraw because of concerns about loss of attractiveness or femininity.

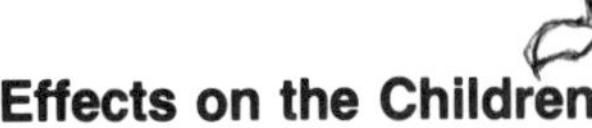

Effects on the Children

Children of disabled parents appear to suffer from the same relative lack of professional attention as husbands with disabled wives. This is particularly unfortunate since identification of the nature, prevalence, and severity of illness-related problems in these children has important implications for appropriate intervention and long-term adjustment. That parental disability, per se, need not be detrimental is supported by Buck and Hohmann's study (1981) of children whose fathers became paralyzed as a result of spinal cord injury. On a variety of measures of personality and adjustment, these children did not differ significantly from those in a control group whose parents were able-bodied. As the authors note, however, care must be taken in generalizing the results of this study. Children in their study were raised from the age of two or younger with the disabled parent, and criteria for selection of subjects tended to bias the sample toward the inclusion of stable, intact families.

Clinical experience suggests that regardless of the stability of the family, the period immediately following onset of severe illness and disability is stressful and children may be especially vulnerable. Hospitalization of the ill parent not only deprives children of that parent's physical presence. The healthy parent may be so absorbed by concerns about his or her spouse and the implications of the illness that the children are effectively deprived of the emotional support and physical presence of both parents and left to weather the crisis as best they can. Younger children, especially, may not understand what has happened, and parents may deliberately withhold information in an effort to protect them. As a result, the children are forced to rely on fantasies, which may be far more grim than reality. Older children may have a more adequate grasp of the situation, but this does not prevent their experiencing anxiety about the short- and long-term consequences of the illness. Realistically, the longer term consequences can include for them sigificantly increased responsibility, a lower standard of living, and basic changes in the role structure of the family.

Children who are about to leave or have already left the parental home may experience conflict because of their own desire for freedom and

independence and parental demands for physical and emotional support. Essentially, they are placed in the role of "parenting their parents" (Rogers, 1981). While this role tends to be an expected part of adult development at a later age, being thrust into it prematurely may result in anxiety or rebellion.

An added burden is placed on the child of a parent whose disease is inherited or occurs more frequently in certain families. Huntington's chorea, for example, follows an autosomal dominant pattern of inheritance and 50 percent of the children in such a family may be expected to develop the disease. Early onset coronary disease, while following no such clear pattern of inheritance, does tend to occur with increased frequency in some families. Children of parents with such diagnoses must cope not only with the immediate crisis of the parent's illness but with the very real threat to their own well-being and life expectancy and those of their children. One consequence of this type of stress is observed in the "anniversary phenomenon." A patient is admitted to the Coronary Care Unit with severe chest pain but no objective evidence of infarction or, perhaps, of coronary artery disease. On inquiry it is discovered that the patient's father died following a heart attack at about the same age that the patient is now. The patient's expectation, harbored for many years, that he would die as his father did can precipitate symptoms mimicking the actual disease.

Factors Affecting Family Adjustment to Chronic Disease and Disability

While some families are able to cope constructively with the stress of illness and integrate the disabled member into a functional family unit, others are not. In the latter group, although the patient remains at home, he or she is seen as a burden and chronic source of stress. The family often demands frequent and continued intervention by the health care system. In some cases, stress is sufficiently severe or the family's ability to adapt so impaired that permanent disruption occurs. Identification of the variables which distinguish between functional and dysfunctional families has important implications for early recognition of the family at risk and determination of appropriate modes of intervention. Thus far, theories and clinical impressions abound but rigorous studies addressing these issues are few. It is hoped that this section, in addition to providing a summary of relevant literature, will also point to areas where additional research is needed.

Given the stresses imposed on the family by illness and disability, it would appear to be important that the premorbid adjustment of the unit be reasonably stable so that the family can mobilize resources to deal with the crisis. There is some evidence suggesting that often the family is not stable prior to onset of disease, that stress may have played a role in precipitating illness, and that these stressors are most often family-related (marital separation and other family problems, divorce, death of spouse) (Groen, 1976; Holmes & Rahe, 1967). Groen found that the most common emotionally laden areas prior to heart attack centered around work conflict and family problems. Other studies of patients with heart disease suggest that premorbid personality factors may be involved. In a prospective study of individuals developing coronary artery disease, particularly with angina (Ostfield, Lebovitz, Shekelle, & Paul, 1964), it was found that anxiety and neuroticism scales were higher in individuals who developed the disease than in those who did not. Following development of the disease, the degree of anxiety increased further (Lebovitz, Shekelle, Ostfield, & Oglesby, 1967). The Type A personality, marked by aggressiveness, competitiveness, time urgency, and hostility, appears to be associated particularly with early-onset heart disease (Rosenman, 1974).

That premorbid personality problems may have consequences for adjustment to disease as well as onset is suggested by a prospective study of coronary artery bypass surgery patients (Rustad, 1979). In this group of individuals, both symptom relief and positive rehabilitation outcome were significantly related to the absence of clinical evidence of chronic psychological problems preoperatively. Given the apparent relationship between some personality types, onset of disease, and consequent adjustment to it, it would seem that further investigation of the role of such personality variables in family adjustment to disease is warranted.

While rehabilitation professionals often appear to think in terms of some optimal or ideal family adjustment to disability, there is little evidence that such exists. Just as families tend to differ in their patterns of interaction under normal circumstances, they are likely to differ in the way they adjust to the crisis of disability, and more than one mode may be functional. Czaczkes and De-Nour's observations (1978) would seem to support this hypothesis, which requires further testing. They looked at marital adjustment to chronic hemodialysis in terms of dominance–dependency relationships in the dyad and whether the dominant or dependent status of each spouse was selected (voluntary) or enforced. More than one variety of dominance–dependency relationship appeared to be compatible with adequate adjustment to dialysis. The authors caution professionals about overzealousness in treating patients and trying to make them more "active." In some dyads, this might lead to disruption of the relationship.

There is some evidence that role rigidity may be an important variable in family adjustment to disease. Streltzer, Finkelstein, Feigenbaum, Kitsen, and Cohn (1976) have noted that spouses highly dependent on their partners prior to onset of renal failure may not be able to accept the increased responsibility necessitated by home dialysis or they may need significant professional support to make this transition. Overs and Healy (1973) found that rigid role definitions interfere with family adjustment following stroke and that greater rigidity appeared to be associated with older age and lower educational level. In contrast, role flexibility appears to be related to ease in adjustment. In a study of families with disabled husbands still intact two to five years following onset of disability, Carpenter (1974) found that there was little stress associated with changed roles, with disabled husbands of working wives assuming more responsibility for housework and cooking than those with nonworking wives. Christopherson (1960) noted that some of the most disabled homemakers in his study had among the most smoothly functioning households. He attributed their success as disabled homemakers to their appropriate role modifications and creative approach to adapting their environment so that they could function effectively. Aldous (1974) has stated that the making of new roles requires flexibility, interpersonal sensitivity, self-esteem, and some sense of personal control of destiny. Empirical support for these and other possible determinants of role flexibility is needed as well as information about the ways in which, and the extent to which, professionals can assist in role modification.

Communication patterns within the family may also be related to success in coping with disability. In a study of the relationship between family communication and success in adjusting to home dialysis (Pentecost, Zwerenz, & Manuel, 1976), it was found that transmission of accurate and explicit information within the family, with members taking personal responsibility for transmission ("intrafamily identity"), was related to success. Postlaryngectomy patients were found to develop higher quality esophogeal speech and in a shorter period of time when spouses were more likely to disagree verbally and asked questions which encouraged long answers (Gibbs & Achterberg-Lawlis, 1979).

Although the role of intelligence in successful adjustment to disability in mid-life has not been addressed directly, Livson and Peskin's study (1980) suggests that intellectual competence and wide interests in adolescence are good predictors of healthy mid-life adjustment in general. Certainly, cognitive resources would appear to be helpful to the family in understanding the disease and treatment regimens and in solving problems that arise in the course of adjustment. In addition, intelligence may be an important element in the role flexibility and communication patterns discussed above as well as being related to variables such as vocational and financial status which have important implications for adjustment to disability.

Numerous studies have found that rehabilitation outcome, including return to work, shows little relationship to degree of disability (Benesch, Neuhaus, Rivas-Martin, & Loogen, 1979; Blümchen, Scharf-Bornhofen,

Brandt, van den Bergh, & Bierck, 1979; Brown & Rawlinson, 1975; Christopherson, 1960; Rustad, 1979). Occupational level at time of disease onset does appear to be related to return to work. White-collar workers and professionals are more likely to be employed following disability than laborers (Benesch et al., 1979; Blümchen et al., 1979; Rustad, 1979). The physically demanding nature of the blue-collar worker's job and the employer's reluctance to hire a disabled worker probably contribute to this difference. Disability benefits, which can act as employment disincentives, may also play a role. If the labor can earn almost as much money by remaining at home as by working, motivation to return to work is reduced. This is unfortunate since retirement has important consequences for the family, especially if the husband is a blue-collar worker.

Simpson and co-workers (1966) suggest that while professionals are the least anxious to retire, they have the best postretirement experience, while those in mid- or lower-level jobs who are generally anxious to retire or passively accepting of it have the least satisfying experience. Low morale appears to be associated with low postretirement income (Osborne, 1971; Pollman, 1971). Poor financial status can also contribute to the family's difficulties in adjusting to disability. Hospitalization and rehabilitation may impose severe financial burdens on them and, where disability is severe, they are unlikely to be able to pay for home nursing care or homemaking services which could spare family members from physical and emotional exhaustion.

Since empirical studies, where they exist, tend to be limited in scope to the consideration of a specific disease or disability, little is understood about how the *nature* of the disease or disability affects the family's ability to adapt. Studies investigating the relative stresses imposed on families by a variety of illnesses are needed. There would appear to be differences between disorders such as spinal cord injury, in which, following the early stages, the individual often attains some degree of medical stability and multiple sclerosis, in which the course is frequently marked by exacerbations and remissions. Similarly, one might expect the family to be affected differently if the disabled member is relatively hospital independent as opposed to hospital dependent as tends to be true of patients on chronic hemodialysis.

Intervention

Since the family as well as the patient is affected by the onset of chronic illness and disability, it is important that family needs, too, be addressed in treatment. Among the authors who have recognized this is Minuchin (1974), who suggests that facilitation of adjustment to chronic illness requires modification of the patient's extrapsychic as well as intrapsychic environment; modification of the extrapsychic environment includes minimizing family pathology. Minuchin is particularly concerned with enmeshment, overprotection, rigidity, and lack of conflict resolution in the family. Strain and Beallor (cited in Strain, 1978) set as goals for family adaptation to an ill member the following: (1) family acceptance of physical and mental regression, (2) the ability to help the patient ward off stresses secondary to illness, (3) the ability to tolerate the patient's expression of fears and feelings, (4) the ability to enlist the patient's trust yet support autonomous function, and (5) the ability to mobilize outside support.

In contrast to the psychodynamic literature, which is primarily concerned with the effects of pathological defenses on adjustment, the rehabilitation literature tends to stress coping in adaptation to illness (Mailick, 1979). Wright (1960), for example, has suggested the following rehabilitation goals: (1) enlarging the scope of values, (2) subordinating physique, (3) containing disability effects, (4) arriving at asset values, (5) reordering priorities, (6) sharing the load, and (7) encouraging an enabling role.

How one reaches such goals, and whether or not they are attainable, is often unclear to the professional working with the patient and family. In this section, an attempt will be made to offer specific suggestions for intervention based on clinical experience as well as the current literature.

Perhaps the first step in providing appropriate intervention for the family with a seriously ill or disabled member is recognition by involved professionals of the often profound and pervasive consequences which the disability may have for the family. It is not unusual for professionals confronted with severe disease to use denial or other protective devices in regard to the consequences of disability lest they themselves feel overwhelmed and powerless (Rustad, 1980). This is regrettable. For the family in crisis, attempting to cope with often chaotic feelings, what they may need first from professionals is recognition and acceptance of their feelings and reassurance that theirs is not an unusual reaction to threatened disruption of the family's life-style and well-being.

Since it is not unusual for the family to have a poor understanding of the course, duration, prognosis, and life-style of the disease or disability (Finlayson & McEwen, 1977; Overs & Healy, 1973), to the extent that it is possible they should be provided with this information at an early stage. The family's level of intelligence, education, and medical sophistication should be considered so they can be informed in an appropriate and comprehensible manner. In a crisis situation, even the most sophisticated families may not process information as readily as under less stressful circumstances. For this reason, repeated explanations may be necessary. Professionals need not assume that persistent and repeated questioning by the family is a reflection of the family's ignorance or the professional's failure to provide adequate explanations. Obviously, there are times when caregivers must be tentative about the patient's long-term course and prognosis, and this may prove frustrating to the family looking for definite answers. In such cases, it is often helpful to give them concrete time limits within which the answers to specific questions should be known and to assure them that contact will be maintained.

In addition to providing the family with information about the disability, per se, it is also important they they understand the treatment plan, its rationale, and any medical regimen for which they and the patient will share responsibility upon returning home. The treatment team should include at least one person who can act as a resource to help the family cope with problems as they arise and who can provide liaison to other members of the team. Careful assessment at this stage of the family's life-style, resources, patterns of interaction, and concerns can be useful in anticipating future problems so that early intervention can be planned. Younger children should not be neglected (Romano, 1976).

Some future problems may be alleviated if the family is assisted in mobilizing intra- and extrafamilial resources. In addition to those available within the acute or rehabilitation setting, these include members of the extended family, friends, and community agencies and support groups. If it is expected that the patient will be able to return to work but not to his or her former job, referral to federal, state, or private agencies for vocational counseling should be initiated as soon as the patient is medically and psychologically stable. There is some evidence that failure to return to work is related to the length of time unemployed following disability onset (Rustad, 1979). If the patient will not be able to return to work and his spouse who has been a full-time homemaker must find a job, family counseling may be helpful to assist them in making necessary role modifications.

While the need for vocational counseling and retraining is sometimes recognized, the need for avocational counseling is usually ignored. This is unfortunate since major family problems may arise if the disabled individual is suddenly faced with abundant leisure time which he or she cannot use in a satisfying and productive manner. Particularly if the disability leads to early or "off-time retirement," or if the individual is a blue-collar worker, he may have few resources for coping with leisure time. Assessment of the disabled individual's strengths, interests, and flexibility may reveal new options for using his energy and skills. These options may include increased involvement in care of the home and children (especially helpful if the former homemaker must find work outside of the home), volunteer work, or development of craft and technical skills which might be used to supplement income.

Financial-aid resources should be identified for the family if assessment indicates that they do not have adequate funds to cope with the financial burden of the illness. Aid in mobilizing community resources such as visiting nurse and home health aide services may allow the family to remain intact and functional rather than removing the disabled member to a nursing home or having the able-bodied spouse risk physical and emotional exhaustion. When disability is severe and the family elects to take responsibility for extensive nursing care in the home, periodic "vacations" for the family during which the disabled individual spends short periods with other family members or in a nursing home can help to maintain the family's physical and emotional health.

The extent to which the family subscribes to cultural norms which place high value on youth, physical strength, and traditional roles can indicate a need for reassessment of attitudes, values, and priorities. The extent to which the family sees the disabled individual as helpless, shameful, fragile, or in need of constant care and protection may indicate the amount of assistance needed to reach an adequate adjustment to disability. Family attitudes toward the disabled individual can have important consequences for rehabilitation (Deutsch & Goldston, 1960).

Counseling or psychotherapy, especially of the cognitive restructuring or rational emotive type (Oliver, 1977), may be useful at this stage to help the family replace destructive attitudes and beliefs with more adaptive ones. Modeling, too, may prove beneficial whether it is provided by professional staff in their interactions with the patient or by individuals and families who have made an adequate adjustment to disability. If the family views the effect of disability as a "violation of contract," the specifics of the often implicit and unspoken contract and expectations must be made explicit. This is a necessary first step in the process of renegotiating a new and more adaptive "contract" or, where differences are irreconcilable, ending the contract (Sager, 1976).

The disparate and strong needs of the patient and the family during the process of adjustment may bring them into serious conflict and, as Minuchin (1974) has pointed out, resolution of these conflicts can be important if an adequate adjustment is to be reached. Unfortunately, even families who maintained relationships reasonably well premorbidly may find they lack the skills needed to deal with the conflicts and problems which arise as an outgrowth of the disability. Where there is commitment to the relationship and some desire and capacity for change, new skills may be taught in the process of family or group therapy.

Frequently, conflicts arise—and fail to be resolved—because of problems in communication among family members. They may be quite vocal in expressing their own displeasure but unable to really attend to the concerns of other members. Some may express their needs and concerns in indirect ways, which are ignored or misinterpreted by others. Still other patients and family members attempt to hide their emotional or physical discomfort completely at the expense of mounting resentment and psychophysiological disorders. A first step in resolving the conflicts that arise is open acknowledgment and discussion of the conflicts in an atmosphere of mutual acceptance. The professional treating the family can aid by "permitting" the family members to have feelings which they may consider socially unacceptable and help them to express these feelings in a supportive and accepting atmosphere.

Use of assertiveness training techniques (Epstein, 1981; Lange & Jakubowski, 1976) can be very helpful in teaching family members to express themselves in ways that are not damaging to other members. Where communication problems are exacerbated by cognitive or speech deficits (e.g., following CVA or head trauma), family intervention by the speech therapist (Wiig, 1973) or neuropsychologist can be helpful. Deficits can be explained and the patient and family provided with techniques to minimize deficits and cope more adequately with residual problems. Problem-solving skills may also be taught in the course of counseling and therapy with the family (Epstein & Williams, 1981). Frequently, conflicts are resistant to solution because family members fail to see or consider available options. Helping them to investigate alternatives which they may not have considered and to negotiate compromises can be effective.

Thus far, we have discussed intervention with the individual patient and family by one or more professionals. Recent literature suggests that group approaches are increasingly popular and that they have been used to assist in coping with adjustment to a variety of disabilities. Groups may be conducted by professionals in the hospital or outpatient setting, independently or as part of a comprehensive rehabilitation program. Self-help groups are usually led by individuals who have coped successfully with adjustment to a specific disease or disability. Some programs for post-MI patients and families utilize both separate and combined groups for patients and spouses (Granger, 1974; Segev & Schlesinger, 1981). Others have only separate patient and wives groups (Adsett & Bruhn, 1968). Separate groups have also been used for counseling wives of renal dialysis patients (D'Afflitti & Swanson, 1975; Shambaugh & Kanter, 1969). Where sexual dysfunction and its implications for the relationship are a major concern, as they are in spinal cord injury, groups may be designed to address these issues (Eisenberg & Rustad, 1976; Romano & Lassiter, 1972). Community groups and local chapters of national organizations also sponsor educational and support groups. Examples are educational programs for family caregivers sponsored by the Multiple Sclerosis Society, support and education groups sponsored by the Kidney Foundation, and self-help groups such as "Reach to Recovery" (for postmastectomy patients) and "Cardiac Clubs."

The group approach may have significant advantages over individual counseling in some situations. It can provide an opportunity for patients and families to express fears and concerns in a mutually supportive and understanding atmosphere since experiences and concerns are shared. This sharing of experiences and feelings also helps to reassure the family that they are not strange or unique, a common problem following onset of disability. They may also be encouraged about eventual outcome and their own ability to cope with the adjustment process by observing people who have negotiated rehabilitation successfully. Patients and families who have made an adequate adjustment are also less likely to be sympathetic to a "sick-role" adjustment and challenge those who use illness as an excuse for avoiding responsibility. For individuals well along in the rehabilitation process, the opportunity to serve as a model and to help others can yield significant benefits in terms of increased self-esteem and feelings of productiveness.

While the recent literature reflects increased professional interest in the family with a disabled member, much remains to be learned. The effects of parental disability on children, particularly, is an area that bears further investigation as well as modes of intervention designed to meet identified needs. Empirical data are also needed to assist professionals in the early identification of families at high risk for disruption following onset of illness, so that intensive intervention can be instituted at an early stage. Professional training must be reevaluated and changes instituted so that curricula will reflect the need for intervention with the whole family unit rather than being patient focused as it tends to be currently. Finally, disability may strike at any point in the life span. The differing needs of the family at various developmental stages must be identified more clearly and appropriate modes of intervention developed to meet these needs.

References

Adsett, C. A., & Bruhn, J. G. Short-term group psychotherapy for post-myocardial infarction patients and their wives. *Canadian Medical Association Journal*, 1968, *99*, 577–584.

Aldous, J. The making of family roles and family change. *Family Coordinator*, 1974, *23*, 231–235.

Benesch, L., Neuhaus, K. L., Rivas-Martin, J., & Loogen, F. Clinical results and return to work after coronary heart surgery. In H. Roskamm & M. Schmuziger (Eds.), *Coronary heart surgery*. New York: Springer-Verlag, 1979.

Bilodeau, C. B., & Hackett, T. P. Issues raised in a group setting by patients recovering from myocardial infarction. *American Journal of Psychiatry*, 1971, *128*, 105–110.

Block, A., Maeder, J. P., & Haissly, J. C. Sexual problems after myocardial infarction. *American Heart Journal*, 1975, *90*, 536–537.

Blümchen, G., Scharf-Bornhofen, E., Brandt, D., van den Bergh, C., & Bierck, G. Clinical results and social implications in patients after coronary bypass surgery. In H. Roskamm & M. Schmuziger (Eds.), *Coronary heart surgery*. New York: Springer-Verlag, 1979.

Boyd, J. H. & Weissman, M. M. The epidemiology of psychiatric disorders of middle age: Depression, alcoholism, and suicide. In J. G. Howells (Ed.), *Modern perspectives in the psychiatry of middle age*. New York: Brunner/Mazel, 1981.

Bracht, N. F. The social nature of chronic disease and disability. *Social Work in Health Care*, 1979, *5*, 129–144.

Brown, J. S., & Rawlinson, M. Relinquishing the sick role following open-heart surgery. *Journal of Health and Social Behavior*, 1975, *16*, 12–27.

Buck, F. M., & Hohmann, G. W. Personality, behavior, values and family relations of children of fathers with spinal cord injury. *Archives of Physical Medicine and Rehabilitation*, 1981, *62*, 432–438.

Burr, W. R. Satisfaction with various aspects of marriage over the life cycle: A random middle class sample. *Journal of Marriage and the Family*, 1970, *32*, 29–37.

Carpenter, J. O. Changing roles and disagreement in families with disabled husbands. *Archives of Physical Medicine and Rehabilitation*, 1974, *55*, 272–274.

Chilman, C. Families in development at midstage of the family life cycle. *The Family Coordinator*, 1968, *17*, 297–312.

Chiriboga, D. A. The developmental psychology of middle age. In J. G. Howells (Ed.), *Modern perspectives in the psychiatry of middle age*. New York: Brunner/Mazel, 1981.

Chiriboga, D. A., & Cutler, L. Stress and adaptation: Life span perspectives. In L. Poon (Ed.), *Aging in the 1980's: Selected contemporary issues in the psychology of aging*. Washington, D.C.: American Psychological Association, 1980.

Chiriboga, D. A., & Thurnher, M. Concept of self. In M. F. Lowenthal, M. Thurnher, D. Chiriboga, & Associates (Eds.), *Four stages of life: A comparative study of women and men facing transitions*. San Francisco: Jossey-Bass, 1975.

Christopherson, V. A. Role modifications of the handicapped homemaker. *Rehabilitation Literature*, 1960, *21*, 110–117.

Coelho, G. V., & Adams, J. E. Introduction. In G. V. Coelho, D. A. Hamburg, & J. E. Adams (Eds.), *Coping and adaptation*. New York: Basic Books, 1974.

Comarr, A. E. Sexual function among patients with spinal cord injury. *Urologia Internationalis*, 1970, *25*, 134–168.

Crewe, N. M., Athelstan, G. T., & Krumberger, B. A. Spinal cord injury: A comparison of pre-injury and post-injury marriages. *Archives of Physical Medicine and Rehabilitation*, 1979, *60*, 252–256.

Czaczkes, J. W., & De-Nour, A. K. *Chronic hemodialysis as a way of life*. New York: Brunner/Mazel, 1978.

D'Afflitti, G. D., & Swanson, D. Group sessions for the wives of home-hemodialysis patients. *American Journal of Nursing*, 1975, *75*, 633–635.

Deutsch, C. P., & Goldston, J. A. Family factors in home adjustment of the severely disabled. *Journal of Marriage and the Family*, 1960, *22*, 312–316.

Deykin, E. Y., Jacobson, S., Klerman, G., & Solomon, M. The empty nest: Psychosocial aspects of conflict between depressed women and their grown children. *American Journal of Psychiatry*, 1966, *122*, 1422–1426.

Eisdorfer, C. Adaptation to loss of work. In F. M. Carp (Ed.), *Retirement*. New York: Behavioral Publications, 1972.

Eisenberg, M. G., & Rustad, L. C. Sex education and counseling program on a spinal cord injury service. *Archives of Physical Medicine and Rehabilitation*, 1976, *57*, 135–140.

Epstein, N. Assertiveness training in marital treatment. In G. P. Sholevar (Ed.), *The handbook of marriage and marital therapy*. New York: Spectrum Publications, 1981.

Epstein, N., & Williams, A. M. Behavioral approaches to the treatment of marital discord. In G. P. Sholevar (Ed.), *The handbook of marriage and marital therapy*. New York: Spectrum Publications, 1981.

Erickson, E. *Childhood and society*. New York: Norton, 1950.

Finlayson, A., & McEwen, J. *Coronary heart disease and patterns of living*. New York: Prodist, 1977.

Gerber, I., Rusalem, R., Hannon, N., Batten, D., & Arkin, A. Anticipatory grief and aged widows and widowers. *Journal of Gerontology*, 1975, *30*, 225–229.

Gibbs, H. W., & Achterberg-Lawlis, J. The spouse as facilitator for esophageal speech: A research perspective. *Journal of Surgical Oncology*, 1979, *11*, 89–94.

Glenn, N. D. Psychological well being in the postparental stage: Evidence from national surveys. *Journal of Marriage and the Family*, 1975, *37*, 105–110.

Granger, J. W. Full recovery from myocardial infarction: Psychosocial factors. *Heart and Lung*, 1974, *3*, 600–610.

Groen, J. J. Psychosomatic aspects of ischaemic (coronary) heart disease. In O. Hill (Ed.), *Modern trends in psychosomatic medicine* (3rd ed.). London, Boston: Butterworths, 1976.

Gutmann, D. The cross-cultural perspective: Notes toward a psychology of aging. In J. E. Birren & K. W. Schaie (Eds.), *Handbook of the psychology of aging*. New York: Van Nostrand Reinhold, 1977.

Havighurst, R. J. *Developmental tasks and education*. New York: David McKay, 1948.

Hellerstein, H. K., & Friedman, E. H. Sexual activity and the post-coronary patient. *Medical Aspects of Human Sexuality*, 1969, *3*, 70–96.

Heyman, D. K., & Jeffers, F. Wives and retirement: A pilot study. *Journal of Gerontology*, 1968, *23*, 488–496.

Holmes, T. H., & Rahe, R. H. The social readjustment rating scale. *Journal of Psychosomatic Research*, 1967, *11*, 213–218.

Jung, C. G. *Modern man in search of a soul*. New York: Wiley, 1933.

Jung, C. G. *Collected works* (Vol. 7), *Two essays on analytic psychology*, Princeton, N.J.: Princeton University Press, 1966.

Kalliomaki, J. L., Markkanen, T. K., & Mustonen, V. A. Sexual behavior after cerebral vascular accident. *Fertility and Sterility*, 1961, *12*, 156–158.

Kavanagh, T., & Shephard, R. J. Sexual activity after myocardial infarction. *Canadian Medical Association Journal*, 1977, *116*, 1250–1253.

Klein, R. F., Dean, A., Wilson, L. M., & Bogdonoff, M. D. The physician and postmyocardial infarction invalidism. *Journal of the American Medical Association*, 1965, *194*, 123–128.

Lange, A. J., & Jakubowski, P. *Responsible assertive behavior: Cognitive/behavioral procedures for trainers*. Champaign, Ill.: Research Press, 1976.

Laver, M. C. Sexual behavior patterns in male hypertensives. *Australian and New Zealand Journal of Medicine*, 1974, *4*, 29–31.

Lebovitz, B. Z., Shekelle, R. B., Ostfield, A. M., & Oglesby, P. Prospective and retrospective psychological studies of coronary heart disease. *Psychosomatic Medicine*, 1967, *29*, 265–272.

Lewis, R. A., Freneau, P. J., & Roberts, C. L. Fathers and the postparental transition. *Family Coordinator*, 1979, *28*, 514–520.

Lilius, H. G., Valtonen, E. J., & Wilstrom, J. Sexual problems in patients suffering from multiple sclerosis. *Journal of Chronic Disease*, 1976, *29*, 643–647.

Livson, N., & Peskin, H. Psychological health at age 40: Prediction from adolescent personality. In D. Eichorn, P. Mussen, J. Clausen, N. Haan, & M. Honzik (Eds.), *Present and past in middle life*. New York: Academic Press, 1980.

Mailick, M. The impact of severe illness on the individual and family: An overview. *Social Work in Health Care*, 1979, *5*, 117–128.

Minuchin, S. *Families and family therapy*. Cambridge: Harvard University Press, 1974.

Nadelson, C. C., Polonsky, D. C., & Mathews, M. A. Marital stress and symptom formation in midlife. *Psychiatric Opinion*, 1978, *15*, 29–33.

Nadelson, C. C., Polonsky, D. C., & Mathews, M. A. Marriage and midlife: The impact of social change. *Journal of Clinical Psychiatry*, 1979, *40*, 292–315, 298–321.

Neugarten, B. L. Personality and aging. In J. E. Birren & K. W. Schaie (Eds.), *Handbook of the psychology of aging*. New York: Van Nostrand Reinhold, 1977.

Neugarten, B. L., & Gutmann, D. L. Age-sex roles and personality in middle age: A thematic apperception study. In B. L. Neugarten (Ed.), *Middle age and aging: A reader in social psychology*. Chicago, Ill.: Univeristy of Chicago Press, 1968.

Oliver, R. The "empty nest syndrome" as a focus of depression: A cognitive treatment model, based on Rational Emotive Therapy. *Psychotherapy: Theory, Research and Practice*, 1977, *14*, 87–94.

Osborn, R. W. Social and economic factors in reported chronic morbidity. *Journal of Gerontology*, 1971, *26*, 217–223.

Ostfield, A. M., Lebovitz, B. Z., Shekelle, R. B., & Paul, O. A prospective study of the relationship between personality and coronary heart disease. *Journal of Chronic Diseases*, 1964, *17*, 265–276.

Overs, R. P., & Healy, J. R. Stroke patients: Their spouses, families and the community. In A. B. Cobb (Ed.), *Medical and psychological aspects of disability*, Springfield, Ill.: Charles C. Thomas, 1973.

Paykel, E. S., Prusoff, B. A., & Uhlenhuth, E. H. Scaling of life events. *Archives of General Psychiatry,* 1971, *25,* 340–347.

Pentecost, R. L., Zwerenz, B., & Manuel, J. W. Intrafamily identity and home dialysis success. *Nephron,* 1976, *17,* 88–103.

Pfeiffer, E., Verwoerdt, A., & Davis, G. C. Sexual behavior in middle life. *American Journal of Psychiatry,* 1972, *128,* 1262–1267.

Pollman, A. W. Early retirement: A comparison of poor health to other retirement factors. *Journal of Gerontology,* 1971, *26,* 41–45.

Rogers, R. R. On parenting one's elderly parent. In J. G. Howells (Ed.), *Modern perspectives in the psychiatry of middle age*. New York: Brunner/Mazel, 1981.

Rollins, B. C., & Feldman, H. Marital satisfaction over the family life cycle. *Journal of Marriage and the Family,* 1970, *32,* 20–28.

Romano, M. D. Preparing children for parental disability. *Social Work Health Care,* 1976, *1,* 309–315.

Romano, M., & Lassiter, R. E. Sexual counseling with spinal-cord injured. *Archives of Physical Medicine and Rehabilitation,* 1972, *53,* 568–572.

Rosenman, R. H. The role of behavior patterns and neurogenic factors in the pathogenesis of coronary heart disease. In R. S. Eliot (Ed.), *Stress and the heart*. New York: Futura, 1974.

Rustad, L. C. Heart surgery: A clinical view. Paper presented at the 86th Annual Convention of the American Psychological Association, New York, N.Y., 1979.

Rustad, L. C. Facilitating communications: An aid to effective treatment on the renal dialysis unit. In M. G. Eisenberg, J. Falconer, & L. Sutkin (Eds.), *Communications in a health care setting*. Springfield, Ill.: Charles C. Thomas, 1980.

Sager, C. J. *Marriage contracts and couple therapy—Hidden forces in intimate relationships*. New York: Brunner/Mazel, 1976.

Segev, U., & Schlesinger, Z. Rehabilitation of patients after acute myocardial infarction—an interdisciplinary, family-oriented program. *Heart & Lung,* 1981, *10,* 841–847.

Shambaugh, P. W., Hampters, C. L., Bailey, G. L., Snyder, D., & Merrill, J. P. Hemodialysis in the home—emotional impact on the spouse. *Transactions of the American Society for Artificial Internal Organs,* 1967, *13,* 41–45.

Shambaugh, P. W., & Kanter, S. S. Spouses under stress: Group meetings with spouses of patients on hemodialysis. *American Journal of Psychiatry,* 1969, *125,* 928–936.

Simpson, I. H., Back, K. W., & McKinney, J. C. Attributes of work involvement in society and self-evaluation in retirement. In I. H. Simpson & J. C. McKinney (Eds.), *Social aspects of aging*. Durham, N.C.: Duke University Press, 1966.

Skelton, M., & Dominian, J. Psychological stress in wives of patients with myocardial infarction. *British Medical Journal,* 1973, *2,* 101–103.

Stokes, R. G., & Maddox, G. L. Some social factors on retirement adaptation. *Journal of Gerontology,* 1967, *22,* 329–33.

Strain, J. J. *Psychological interventions in medical practice*. New York: Appleton-Century-Crofts, 1978.

Streltzer, J., Finkelstein, F., Feigenbaum, H., Kitsen, J., & Cohn, G. L. The spouse's role in home dialysis. *Archives of General Psychiatry*, 1976, *33*, 55–58.

Toshihiko, M., Osborne, D., Swanson, D. W., & Halling, J. M. Chronic pain patients and spouses: Marital and sexual adjustment. *Mayo Clinic Proceedings*, 1981, *56*, 307–310.

United States Bureau of the Census. Marital status and living arrangements. Current Population Reports, Series P-20, No. 388:3. Washington, D.C.: U.S. Government Printing Office, 1979.

Weinstein, M. H., & Machleder, H. I. Sexual function after aorto-iliac surgery. *Annals of Surgery*, 1975, *181*, 787–790.

Wiig, E. H. Counseling the adult aphasic for sexual readjustment. *Rehabilitation Counseling Bulletin*, 1973, *17*, 110–119.

Wishnie, H. A., Hackett, T. P., & Cassem, N. H. Psychological hazards of convalescence following myocardial infarction. *Journal of the American Medical Association*, 1971, *215*, 1292–1296.

Wright, B. A. *Physical disability—A psychological approach*. New York: Harper Brothers, 1960.

Youmans, E., Grigsby, S., & King, M. Social change, generation and race. *Rural Sociology*, 1969, *34*, 305–312.

VI

Old Age

12 Clinical Intervention with Older Adults

Donald R. Schienle and John M. Eiler

Literature Review and Empirical Findings

In a discussion of the stereotypes surrounding aging, the first director of the National Institute on Aging, Robert Butler (1974), describes the myth of serenity, which portrays old age as "a time of relative peace and serenity when people can relax and enjoy the fruits of their labors after the storms of life are over." The true picture for the majority of aged Americans stands in stark contrast to this rocking chair image. In reality, older adults experience at least as many stresses as any other age-group, stresses which can often either cause or result from chronic disability.

In general, these stresses may be framed as the necessity for adaptation to losses in later life (Burnside, 1970; Gaitz & Varner, 1980; Pfeiffer, 1977). While losses can certainly occur at any age, as people age their losses occur more frequently and with a cumulative effect. Losses can be construed as affecting three areas of well-being: physical, social, and psychological. These should not be considered, however, as independent factors; physical, social, and psychological stressors have an interactive effect on the functional ability of the older adult. One of the major tasks of later life is adaptation to these losses.

Physical Stress

Eight-five percent of the elderly suffer from at least one chronic physical condition (Wilder, 1971). If the definition of "chronic condition" is restricted to include only those disorders that impose some limitation on the person having them, then 53 percent of older men and 41 percent of older women are limited in activity to some extent by chronic disabling conditions. About 41 percent of the older population are severely limited by chronic disabling conditions.

Heart disease, cancer, cerebrovascular disease, and respiratory disease are the most prevalent physical diseases of old age, limiting daily functioning and eventually leading to death. Arthritis, rheumatism, and sensory impairments (such as loss of vision and hearing) are also responsible for limiting the activities of well over 25 percent of older adults (Wilder, 1971).

In addition to these physical disabilities, approximately 5 percent of older adults suffer some type of organic damage to the brain that can result in chronic impairment of cognitive functioning (Busse, 1973). This damage may result from a specific disease process such as arteriosclerosis, heart disease, or a cerebrovascular accident (stroke). In other cases, such as senile dementia of the Alzheimer's type, damage results from brain cell death of unknown etiology.

All of the above physical disorders are the result of pathological processes that occur with increased frequency in older adults. Each of these disease entities can result directly in chronic disabilities such as reduced activity, mobility, or cognitive ability. In contrast to these diseases are another set of normative changes in physiological systems that occur to some degree in all persons as they age. These include normal sensory system changes in vision and hearing, endocrine system changes affecting drives of hunger and sex, autoimmune system changes reducing resistance and recovery from disease, and central nervous system changes resulting, for example, in slowed reaction time and alterations in sleep patterns (Birren & Schaie, 1977; Finch & Hayflick, 1977).

These normative physiological changes do not necessarily result in chronic disabilities, as do most of the pathological changes mentioned above. In the absence of unusual stress, the aging individual can typically function adequately despite these changes. These normative changes may severely reduce an older adult's potential to respond adaptively to a stressful state, however, leading to an increased probability of chronic disability given other exacerbating conditions. For example, the normal aging brain may have limited capacity to respond to stress, allowing an older adult to "look organic" under certain stressful situations, yet appear normal when the stress fades (Gaitz & Varner, 1980).

Social Stress

Ageism. Butler (1969) coined the term *ageism* to describe the widespread prejudice against the aged. "Ageism can be seen as a process of systematic stereotyping of and discriminating against people because they are old, just as racism and sexism can accomplish this with skin color and gender. Old people are categorized as senile, rigid in thought and manner, old-fashioned in morality and skills" (p. 243). Not only do these negative attitudes allow younger generations to see older people as different and somehow less human than themselves, but older adults themselves may begin to accept many of these stereotypes and behave accordingly. What factors are responsible for fostering these attitudes?

Rosow (1974) has analyzed changes in our basic social organizations that relegate the aged to a position of devalued social status. These include the rapid rate of technological change that makes an older adult's knowledge "obsolete," a flooded labor market that devalues the older worker, the reduction of property ownership among the elderly, and movement away from traditional religious, community, and kinship networks. Wigdor (1980) emphasizes our industrialized culture's emphasis on competitiveness and achievement, with the result of low esteem for individuals who don't behave in achievement-related patterns. Society offers few achievement-oriented goals or roles for older adults; most goals and roles are maintenance oriented. This incongruity between what is expected and what is acutally offered presents a severe social stressor, affecting the self-esteem of the elderly.

An attempt to explain these role changes was offered by Cumming and Henry (1961) in their theory of disengagement. This was originally framed as a gradual but inevitable process whereby the aging individual withdraws or disengages from active middle-aged roles, toward ever-increasing concern with self and decreased interaction with others in the social situation. More recently, other researchers (Hoschschild, 1975; Streib & Schneider, 1971) have pointed out flaws in accepting disengagement as an inevitably occurring natural process for older individuals. Neugarten (1977) found that high life satisfaction ratings were more often present in older persons who were socially active and involved. Disengagement from some previous roles may be one possible response to aging, but substituting continued activity in certain roles appears to be critical in maintaining morale.

Disengagement theory may, however, appropriately explain the withdrawal of the elderly at a societal, rather than individual, level (Newell, 1961). Occupational institutions retain stability over time by gradually and constantly phasing older people out and young people in. While beneficial to the continuity of the social institution, this does not necessarily reflect the older individual's desires, as indicated by current debate over mandatory retirement requirements. Forced disengagement of this type represents a serious social stress; if the work role is not replaced with an acceptable alternate role, a variety of adjustment disorders may result.

Perhaps the bottom line in indexing the status of the aged in the United States is their relative financial security. In 1975, half of the families with heads of household aged 65 or over earned $8,000 or less annually, while the median income of younger families was approximately

$15,000. This dismal financial picture is compounded by the precipitous increase in medical expenditures in the elderly, about three-and-one-half times those of the young. The prospect of government relief in this situation is also unlikely. Although one-fifth of our 1980 fiscal budget provided services to the elderly, nearly seven million of these individuals still exist below the poverty line (Botwinick, 1978).

Social Networks. In addition to broad societal stress on older adults, a person's social relationships and informal support networks can also be expected to undergo radical changes in late life. Loss of spouse and the reduction of social networks through death of friends, children moving away, retirement, and limited mobility stress the aged and threaten them with isolation and loneliness.

Bereavement following the death of a spouse has long been recognized as a crisis point, with well documented reports of greatly increased morbidity (in both physical and mental health) and mortality in the postbereavement period (Parkes, 1970). The bereaved tend to experience a great deal of painful social isolation and frequently encounter major problems in their attempts to reintegrate themselves into society. Factors such as additional crisis situations, the mode of death and preparation for it, preexisting marital interactions (such as extreme dependence or ambivalence), and, most critically, the quality of support from the social network immediately following the death of a spouse all contribute to resolution of the bereavement crisis (Maddison & Raphael, 1975).

A variety of late life events that limit social networks were mentioned above as stressors that may result in isolation and loneliness. But is isolation or loneliness the crucial social factor in precipitating disability? Busse and Pfeiffer (1969) note that "solitude need not be experienced as loneliness, while loneliness can be felt in the presence of other people" (p. 71). For example, Lowenthal (1964) noted that isolation did not appear to lead to mental illness, but instead may be a consequence of mental illness. Botwinick (1978) tentatively concludes that loneliness is the key stressing variable, rather than isolation per se, and that social loss is responsible for loneliness.

Psychological Stress

An estimated 10 to 20 percent of noninstitutionalized persons over age sixty-five are in need of mental health services, based on a summary of seven epidemiological studies of prevalence rates (Kramer, Taube, & Redick, 1973). Although the reliability of psychiatric diagnoses in these community studies has been questioned, these studies certainly signal the need for concern about the psychological well-being of older adults.

The incidence of various stressful conditions typically undergoes a cumulative increase in late life, as discussed above. The relation between the number of stressful life events and the actual stress perceived by the individual may not be a simple linear model, however, as early theorists assumed. The early influential work on life events by Holmes and Rahe (1967) presented a ranked hierarchy of events (the Schedule of Recent Events) with psychometrically derived weights to assess the degree of life change for each event. Although the stress ranking of these events appears to be consistent across various groups, the weights assigned for specific events did show great variability according to culture and age (Harmon, Masuda, & Holmes, 1970; Masuda & Holmes, 1978). In addition, many of the major life events of late life are not included on this scale (Amster & Krauss, 1974). The important theoretical point, however, is that the individual's psychological perception or appraisal of the amount of stress in a given situation is the crucial variable in determining their reaction to the event (Lazarus & Weinberg, 1980). This cognitive appraisal may vary considerably among various individuals and during a person's life.

Individual differences in the cognitive appraisal of stressful situations are dependent, to a large extent, on a person's style of coping with or adapting to stress (Horowitz & Wilner, 1980). In other words, to predict the effects of the physical and social stressors listed above, an older adult's life-span patterns of coping with stress must be evaluated.

Late Life Psychological Disorders

There are currently no epidemiological studies that offer a breakdown of the frequencies of various psychological disorders in older adults. There is, however, considerable agreement among clinical practitioners on the most frequently seen disturbances. It should be reemphasized that these disorders are not unavoidable reactions to stress. The diagnosis and treatment of these psychopathologies must be evaluated in the life-span context of an older adult's previous psychological functioning and adaptive style.

Depression. Depression is such a common symptom in the aged that it is often considered a characteristic of old age. Its prevalence is thought often to stem from the older adult's feelings of helplessness in adjusting to the various physical and social losses outlined above.

Features of depression are a dysphoric mood and loss of interest or pleasure in most usual activities. Depression is relatively persistent and is associated with other symptoms including appetite disturbance, change in weight, sleep disturbance, psychomotor agitation or retardation, decreased energy, feelings of worthlessness or guilt, difficulty in concentrating, thinking, or making decisions, and thoughts of death or suicide. Common associated features include tearfulness, anxiety, irritability, fear, brooding, excessive concern with physical health, panic attacks, and phobias, as defined in the *Diagnostic and Statistical Manual of Mental Disorders—DSM III* (American Psychiatric Association, 1980).

Severely depressed patients can show signs of cognitive impairment, such as disorientation, distractability, difficulty in concentration, as well as memory loss. For this reason, depression may be misdiagnosed as dementia. Miller (1977) suggests that it would be favorable to err on the side of depression rather than dementia, allowing for attempts at treatment. Diagnosis of depression is further complicated by physical symptoms which may mask depression in the elderly. Goldfarb (1974) describes depressive equivalents as physical symptoms such as back pain, headaches, or neckaches which patients tend to complain about rather than sadness or depression.

A serious danger in major depression is the risk of suicide. Older adults account for roughly 25 percent of reported suicides in the United States each year, with the highest rates in elderly males (Butler & Lewis, 1977). It is crucial to evaluate the suicide risk of depressed older adults, often by carefully probing for suicidal thoughts or plans. Typically, however, older suicide victims tend not to make threats, but simply kill themselves. Because of this, staff working closely with patients must be keenly alert to subtle clues (i.e., writing of notes or wills, giving away possessions, saying a formal good-bye to friends and relatives, or contacting acquaintances from their past). Often the suicidal act will occur just when the depression appears to be lifting and the patient seems to be getting better, possibly because a decision to commit suicide alters the sense of helplessness. Suicide will occur even with the proper evaluation and seemingly correct treatment, and the occurrence needs to be evaluated by the caregivers without guilt or self-condemnation.

Paranoia. The essential features of paranoia are persistent persecutory delusions such as being conspired against, cheated, spied upon, followed, poisoned, maliciously maligned, harassed, or obstructed in the pursuit of goals. Small slights may be exaggerated and become the focus of the delusional system. Common associated features include resentment and anger, which may lead to violence, grandiosity, social isolation, seclusiveness, eccentricities of behavior, and suspiciousness (APA, 1980). Paranoid individuals rarely seek treatment and are usually brought for treatment by relatives or governmental agencies as a result of angry disruptive behavior.

As discussed above, physical and social losses can exacerbate a predisposition to a psychological disorder. Hearing loss, for example, decreases effective communication and social interaction and can accentuate suspiciousness or paranoid tendencies, often leading to a late life paranoia (Corso, 1977). Recognition of ageist attitudes in society, coupled with a declining social network, can also foster persecutory delusions in some older persons.

Hypochondriasis. Hypochondriasis is an unrealistic interpretation of physical signs or sensations as abnormal, leading to preoccupation with the fear of having a serious disease. Physical evaluation does not support the individual's unrealistic interpretation of the physical disorder. The preoccupation may be with bodily functions such as heartbeat, sweating, or breathing, or with minor physical abnormalities such as a small sore or occasional cough. The paranoid individual interprets these sensations or signs as evidence of serious disease. There may be a preoccupation with an individual organ, such as in "cardiac nervosis" in which an individual believes he has heart disease (APA, 1980).

These patients often present their medical history in great detail. They have a history of "doctor shopping" and poor doctor–patient relationships commonly resulting with anger and frustration on both sides. The physical complaints may be used to exert control over relationships with family and friends. Anxiety, depressed mood, and compulsive personality traits are often associated with hypochondriasis.

Given the dramatic increase in the prevalence of pathological physical conditions in the elderly and the inevitable normative physiological changes that accompany aging, an increased preoccupation with bodily function in older adults is difficult to define as unrealistic. The lack of available information about these physical changes for most older adults can certainly increase fears about serious diseases when they do detect a change in bodily functions. Diagnosing hypochrondriasis in the aged should not depend on the presence of a physical preoccupation of fear, per se. Instead, diagnosis should be based on evidence of functional impairment, such as decreased mobility or interpersonal difficulties, resulting from this preoccupation with bodily functioning.

Adjustment Disorder. Adjustment disorders are defined as maladaptive reactions to identifiable physical or psychosocial stresses. The maladaptive reactions include depressed or anxious moods, anger, conduct outside of societal norms, or withdrawal (APA, 1980). The physical and psychosocial stressors that accumulate in later life have been discussed above; the potential for increase in adjustment disorders of late life is evident. Adjustment disorders are characterized by their short-term, temporary nature, and the cessation of symptoms when the stressor is removed. Adjustment disorders evolve into chronic disabilities, however, if the stressor is not removed or if effective coping mechanisms are not employed.

Treatment Issues: Applications and Strategies

Having described the primary disabling conditions prevalent in the elderly, and discussed their causes, we now turn to treatment of these chronic disabilities. In parallel with our conceptualization of psychological, physical, and social components of stress, we will describe three models of treatment: psychotherapy, physical rehabilitation, and community intervention. This is a somewhat artificial division; older adults do not necessarily select one treatment model to the exclusion of others, but may instead utilize some combination of treatments to effectively manage a complex disability. These models may present somewhat different approaches in specific goals, methods of treatment, and professional training, yet they share the same overriding goal: improving the quality of life for chronically disabled older adults.

Psychotherapy

Stigma against Treating the Aged. Gatz, Smyer, and Lawton (1980) suggest that the underutilization of mental health services by older adults results from attitudes both in the providers of mental health services and within the elderly themselves. Storandt (1977) estimated that fewer than 100 professionals had received formal training in clinical psychology and aging. In a national survey of clinical psychologists, Dye (1978) identified fewer than 400 who were seeing older clients. Similarly, Mills, Wellner, and VandenBos (1979) found that only 28 of the 25,510 psychologists listed in the 1976 edition of the *National Register of Health Service Providers* reported that over 75 percent of their clientele were age 65 or older, and that these 28 practitioners were significantly older than other groups of psychologists. The reason often given for not providing service to the aged is that it is too late for them to be helped. This idea can be traced back to Freud, who felt that it was a waste of time to work with the aged because their defenses were too rigid.

A report by the Group for the Advancement of Psychiatry (1971) describes some of the negative attitudes toward treating the elderly, as follows: (1) the therapists' fear of their own old age and conflict about their parents' aging; (2) the belief that growing old means inevitable decline; (3) the view that the therapist's skills will be wasted because the older patient is near death and does not deserve treatment; (4) feeling that the therapist's sense of importance and the respect of his colleagues will decline as a result of his treating older patients. Storandt (1977) points out that frequently there is an expectation of being stuck with a depressed, anguished patient, which will result in personal distress and very little gratification. Feifel (1959) points out that there is a special association between the aged and death, which arouses the clinician's own anxieties.

A useful concept in facing the stigma or bias against treating the aged is Carl Rogers' (1961) notion of "unconditional positive regard." This describes an attitude of total acceptance of the older client. Instead of blaming the elderly for not being good candidates for psychotherapy, the therapist must understand that the older adult is doing the best he can in his present situation, given individual and cohort differences in attitudes, beliefs, and points of view. The therapist's approach must be based on respect for aged clients: that their problems are real to them, that they have the ability to understand them better, and that they can, in fact, change. The assertion that older adults cannot benefit from psychotherapy usually stems from the therapist's lack of understanding and respect for the elderly client.

Bias of Older Clients against Receiving Psychotherapy. In a study on utilization, the aged represented only 7 percent of inpatient services and 3 percent of outpatient services in community mental health centers (Kramer, 1973). Older people may resist mental health treatment for various reasons: desire for independence, suspiciousness based on past experiences, fear of being institutionalized, resistance to change, a feeling that most "helping" programs are inadequate, and clumsy, insensitive, or patronizing techniques on the part of mental health professionals (Butler & Lewis, 1977).

Current services in both the mental health and aging sectors appear to fail to focus on the major concerns of the elderly (Lawton, 1979). Older adults who are the consumers of community service programs have little input into the programs designed for them (Weber, 1977). Some elderly people have incorporated the negative cultural view of themselves, which leads to low self-esteem and discouragement about the possibilities of treatment.

In order to overcome the resistance of the elderly to mental health programs a number of steps need to be taken: (1) developing trust by including the elderly in the planning and development of programs designed for them; (2) setting of goals which are congruent with the needs of the elderly; (3) open discussions about ageism to counter the negative views held by both the elderly and the caregivers; and (4) increasing the quality of care through improved training in the field of gerontology.

Life-span Continuity in Psychological Functioning. Is psychological treatment of the older adult necessarily different from the treatment of the younger adult? Kastenbaum (1978) points out that gerontologists and advocates for the elderly often protest that age-grading is relied upon too heavily by our society, yet mental health professionals may inadvertantly contribute to this overemphasis by prescribing a separate psychotherapeutic approach with the elderly. Smyer and Gatz (1979) suggest that "creation of a separate sub-specialty in clinical gero-psychology will not effectively serve older adults" (p. 242). The authors suggest that what is needed is a synthesis of existing expertise in such areas as clinical psychology, life-span development theory, and community and social psychology. This combination of existing skills could provide a conceptual framework for a set of intervention approaches which can form a basis for training programs in mental health and aging.

Kaiser's (1955) work supports the idea of treating the elderly in a similar fashion to younger clients and not trying to create a category of patients with "elderly problems." He would recognize that the problems of the elderly have a unique flavor, but his approach to psychotherapy would not change. Shapiro (1965) describes a system of neurotic disorders based on specific "styles" that persons develop throughout their lifetime. These styles are the accumulation of specific ways of thinking, attitudes, and points of view, and are relatively consistent over a person's life span. Just because a person is classified as aged does not suddenly change his or her character, but instead, personality style in late life is the result of a gradual developmental process.

There is evidence that personality characteristics maintain continuity across the life span (Casady, 1975). For example, if you are immaturely adjusted at thirty, you are likely to stay that way into the seventies, with the reverse also being true. If you have problems of depression, fear, or rigidity when you are young, the tendency is to still experience these problems in later life. A large-scale longitudinal study of the personality development of several hundred San Francisco residents over a period of forty years also indicates that personalities appear to be relatively stable throughout life (Neugarten, 1977).

Instead of viewing older adults as inherently different from young adults and devising separate treatments for them, it appears more productive to assume life-span continuity in psychological style. Although older adults certainly face different issues in late life than when young, their strategies and coping styles are based on psychological resources developed throughout their life and maintained in a consistent fashion.

Group Therapy. The shortage of therapists trained in work with the elderly makes group therapy an expedient mode of treatment. In addition, some elderly patients reject individual therapy, but find it acceptable to attend group therapy. Lazarus and Weinberg (1980) list a variety of possible advantages to group therapy with the elderly, such as enhancing self-esteem and self-worth, encouraging socialization, providing information and suggestions for problem solving, encouraging reality testing and orientation, increasing motivation, renewing former interests and relationships, providing opportunities for the elderly to share and help one another, clarifying diagnoses and prognoses, clarifying and resolving both intrapsychic and interpersonal conflicts, and supplementing the goals of individual psychotherapy.

The principal issues discussed by elderly patients in group therapy include concerns about somatic illness, coping with loss, memories about the past, family conflict, death and dying, and fear and ambivalence about increasing emotional and physical dependency (Lazarus & Weinberg, 1980). The universality of these themes in older adults enhances group cohesion and sharing, providing the elderly client with an atmosphere of acceptance and trust. This can be instrumental in reestablishing feelings of worth and self-esteem and encouraging an interest in involvement with others. In an effort to circumvent the stigma of seeking "therapy," such group sessions are often defined as "rap groups" or educational programs, and are often led by older paraprofessionals with special training in group dynamics.

One problem in conducting group therapy in an outpatient setting is inconsistent attendance. This occurs for a variety of reasons, such as physical illness, depression, social uneasiness, withdrawal, and lack of transportation. If this problem arises, it is an appropriate issue for group discussion. Another potential problem is the therapist's anxiety about discussing such issues as death and sexuality, leading to avoidance of these crucial topics. The therapist must acknowledge and face these anxieties for the group's needs to be appropriately met.

As with individual psychotherapy, little empirical evidence exists concerning the effectiveness of group therapy with people of all ages. There are very few adequately controlled studies in this area. Eisdorfer and Stotsky (1977) conclude that we cannot reliably determine which programs are successful or which factors lead to a successful group experience.

Behavioral Therapy

Behavioral therapy refers to an approach to psychological treatment that emphasizes change in specific, concrete behaviors and situations rather than focusing primarily on alleviating underlying causes of psychological symptoms. The behavior therapist becomes an active agent of change, often functioning as an educator or a case manager. The older client is viewed as capable of learning new skills in order to take positive action in improving the quality of later life.

Behavior therapy demands a detailed assessment of the problems that a particular older adult faces in daily living. Instead of a gerenal focus on such issues as loss or fear of death, behavioral techniques entail an analysis of specific situations (persons, places, times) that result in anxiety, frustration, or inappropriate behaviors. For example, a behavioral treatment for depression would require detailing the specific situations that lead to or alleviate depressed feelings, and devising strategies to help the client to either change or reinterpret his or her behavior in these situations.

Several excellent reviews discuss the application of behavioral treatment with older adults in a variety of settings (Richards & Thorpe, 1978; Rosenstein & Swenson, 1980).

Physical Rehabilitation

As discussed previously, chronic physical disabilities affect a large proportion of older adults, accounting for a significant proportion of national expenditure for health care. The major goal of rehabilitation with the elderly is to establish more independent living skills. Treatment is directed at enhancing the patient's ability to perform activities of daily living, improving physical functioning, and developing social supports and relationships (Melamed & Siegel, 1980). Given the degenerative nature of many late life disabling conditions, continued improvement of function may not always be realistic. In many cases, the maintenance of current levels of functioning should be considered an appropriate and worthwhile goal for rehabilitation. In these cases, it is critical to reward older patients for their work in maintaining an acceptable functional level, instead of discontinuing treatment when improvement stops, thereby ensuring decline in functioning.

A number of assessment devices to measure the Activities of Daily Living (ADL) are available, some of which are appropriate for use with older adults. One such instrument is the Instrumental Activities of Daily Living Scale (IADL), developed by Lawton and Brody (1969). This scale rates competence and independence in a variety of activities relevant to everyday life, ranging from self-care skills (i.e., dressing, bathing, grooming) to instrumental activities (i.e., shopping and handling money). A new ADL scale (Weintraub, Baratz, & Mesulam, 1982) has been developed to assess patients with cognitive deficits that can limit functioning.

Rehabilitation services for the elderly can be provided in a variety of settings. Institutional placements include nursing homes, acute care hospitals, and rehabilitation hospitals. Outpatient settings include clinics for the aged and adult day-care centers. In some cases, in-home rehabilitation services may be available. For some older adults, institutional care is only a temporary stage until they have regained sufficient physical, cognitive, and social skills to return home. Other older patients remain institutionalized either because of more serious impairment or because of the lack of alternative assistance in their care.

The treatment setting appropriate for an older person is not strictly dependent on physical condition. Linn and Gurel (1972) demonstrated that the decision to institutionalize an older adult is more dependent on family attitude and burden than on the actual physical condition of the older adult. Creative discharge planning demands examination of a variety of possible supportive situations that can enable the older person to live in reasonable independence, comfort, and security. Such planning should start at the beginning of treatment and be integrated into the rehabilitation goals.

Inpatient Settings. Just over 4 percent of persons over age sixty-five in the United States are now living in some type of institutional setting, representing a total of about one million chronically impaired older adults (NIMH, 1978). As age increases, however, so does this percentage. For example, 24 percent of those eighty-five years old or older live in institutions (Kovar, 1977). Nine percent of these institutionalized older individuals reside in over 18,000 nursing homes and homes for the aged in the United States, with the remainder living in mental hospitals or chronic disease hospitals (Kovar, 1977). The average length of stay in a nursing home is 1.1 years, and 85 percent of persons who enter a nursing home die there (Butler, 1975). The national cost to provide institutional care for the elderly is currently in the billions of dollars, and rising. These sobering figures demand a concerted examination of the quality of life of these institutionalized older persons.

The majority of the institutionalized elderly have more than one chronic physical condition, and it is estimated that 58 percent of all nursing home residents are considered confused some or most of the time (National Center for Health Statistics, 1977). The main factors precipitating admissions are incontinence, disorientation, confusion, a tendency to wander, and a need for extensive nursing care (Butler, 1975). The decision to institutionalize is typically the result of a series of attempts to cope with a chronic disability and is usually viewed as a last resort.

Key factors in forcing this "last resort decision" are the older adult's previous residential setting and support system. A disruption in long-standing residential circumstances, such as urban renewal or change in apartment ownership, often precipitates institutionalization. Many of the chronically impaired elderly avoid institutionalization if they have relatives or friends to help care for them, or sufficient financial resources to obtain additional help. The elderly who become institutionalized tend not to have had a spouse, and typically lived alone (Atchley, 1980), reflecting limited social supports.

Most older people have a negative view of nursing homes, resulting from a desire to live independently in familiar surroundings, near friends and relatives. Resistance to institutionalization stems from perceived loss of independence and privacy, fear of rejection by their children, and formal proof that death is near (Atchley, 1980).

Kahana (1975) interviewed residents before and after admission to a nursing home. Results suggested that most institutionalized elderly entered nursing homes for health reasons and were encouraged by others to make this step. They viewed themselves as having little or no active part in this decision. Although most reported a neutral attitude toward life in a nursing home (perhaps reflecting passive resignation to an unalterable situation), they did express dissatisfaction with poor food, lack of mental stimulation, and lack of freedom. Other complaints of nursing home residents include loss of money and personal belongings, loss of dignity and personal privacy, restrictive rules, and dissatisfaction with staff attitudes (Burnside, 1970).

A recent survey and field study of ninety-one nursing facilities throughout the United States found the quality of care to be far better than anticipated, at least with regard to medical care and physical facilities (Glasscote, 1976). Widespread problems were noted in mental health care, however. Inadequate diagnosis and treatment of depression and other mental disorders, lack of trained psychosocial and social work staff, and underutilization of family members as a resource were listed as common problems. In addition, many elderly residents were viewed as "over-placed," that is, living in facilities that offer more intensive levels of care than needed.

There is an additional caution in institutionalization that applies more generally to any decision to change the living situation of older adults. Relocation trauma can result in potentially devastating mental and physical consequences for the very old, frail, or cognitively impaired elderly, regardless of the possible benefits from the move. Increased confusion, disorientation, and withdrawal often accompany institutional placement (Lieberman, 1969). While a moderately impaired aged person may have sufficient cognitive resources to function adequately in an overlearned, highly routinized setting, the additional demands necessary in adapting to new places, people, and rules can be overwhelming. Geriatric Reality Orientation programs have been initiated in many nursing homes to assist confused patients, although experimental evaluations of effectiveness are equivocal (Storandt, 1977).

A "natural experiment" involving the transfer of sixty-one aged chronically disabled patients to a new institutional setting resulted in a death rate exactly double that of unrelocated matched control patients (Bourestion & Tars, 1974). The mortality rate was particularly high during the three-month period following the move, but also increased prior to the move, suggesting trauma in anticipation of relocation. Patients who survived the move were less active in the new setting than before relocation.

Specific therapeutic programs to reduce relocation trauma through advance preparation with older adults and their families and group orientation and support sessions following relocation have been successfully demonstrated (Dye & Richards, 1980; Pastalan, 1976).

Outpatient Settings. As we have seen, intervention can be harmful as well as helpful. Although intensive institutional treatment should be available when needed, it is best to follow a policy of "minimal intervention" (Kahn, 1965). The intervention that is least disruptive of usual functioning in the usual setting should be the treatment of choice for the chronically impaired older adult. Minimal intervention is a positive concept that must be differentiated from neglect; careful assessment is necessary to insure that the needs of the elderly are indeed being met.

Brody (1973) criticizes current health care for overemphasizing remedial treatment at the expense of preventive health care. Consistent with the directive of minimal intervention, preventive health care would require attention to periodic health examination, adequate nutrition, accident prevention for frail elderly, proper exercise, and rehabilitation programs to encourage self-sufficiency. Since Medicare and third-party medical insurance rarely reimburse for these services, preventive care currently depends on a concentrated effort in public education, available through private physicians, medical clinics and hospitals, or community agencies such as senior centers.

Geriatric patients with physical or emotional impairments are generally under the care of their primary physician (internist, family or general practitioner), who assumes a crucial role in coordinating the patient's treatment. It is not uncommon for the elderly patient to visit several different physicians for multiple complaints, making coordination of treatment quite difficult. Lack of specialized training in geriatric medicine is an additional problem; only fifteen of ninety-six medical schools surveyed offer geriatric training, although the elderly comprise a large segment of patients in general practice (Zarit, 1980).

Specialized geriatric health care services are becoming available to provide specialized outpatient care for older adults. Some clinics provide health screening coupled with a case management approach to coordinate the necessary treatments. Another approach is the interdisciplinary assessment clinic for treatment and rehabilitation planning (Kemp, in press). This model provides a thorough, integrated evaluation of the impaired older patient at the request of the primary physician, devises a specialized treatment plan, then assists the primary physician in implementing the treatment. In this way, specialized expertise in geriatric rehabilitation is made available to primary physicians, without unduly disrupting their relationship with their older patients.

Some older adults with chronic disabilities may become anxious or even change living arrangements because of fear of life-threatening health emergency situations. The Lifeline telephone emergency alarm system has recently become available to connect frail elderly persons with a central station operator in case of emergency (Lowy, 1980). The signal can be triggered by a portable transmitting device or signal automatically if not reset in twenty-four hours. The operator, typically in a hospital, has lists of nearby friends or relatives to alert for assistance and can send backup services if necessary. This simple intervention may allow some disabled elderly to become more comfortable in independent living situations.

Community Treatment

A third model for the treatment of chronically impaired older adults, the community model, does not exist as an alternative to traditional psychotherapy and medical psychology. Instead, a community treatment approach provides a parallel system of service delivery—a "continuum of care," maintaining the well-being of older adults of varying functional capacities. For example, the elderly widow at a senior center nutrition site, the hemiplegic stroke victim being transported to physical therapy sessions, and the retired worker receiving advice about Social Security and Medicare are all benefiting from a community treatment model.

When demographers pointed out the changing age structure of the United States population, the aged emerged as a growing constituency with special needs. Legislation produced the Social Security Amendments (Medicare and Medicaid) and the Older Americans Act, which established a Federal agency, the Administration on Aging, that is primarily responsible for community care of the elderly by overseeing (1) grants for community service projects, (2) applied research and demonstration programs, and (3) the training of personnel to serve the elderly (Gatz et al., 1980). The community programs developed by the AOA and other government agencies provide social services to large numbers of the elderly, many with chronic disabling conditions.

As we will see, the community treatment model encompasses a wide variety of specific programs. There are, in general, several advantages to this model: (1) many community programs do not carry the stigma of treatment mentioned above, (2) community services are available to economically disadvantaged older adults, (3) community programs link with informal caregiving networks (such as families, neighbors, and church or civic groups) to provide care for disabled elderly, (4) the shortage of professional therapists can be offset by the use of paraprofessionals and trained volunteer workers in community programs, and (5) community treatment, by coordinating parallel services, is sensitive to the complex interplay of physical, psychological, and social variables in treating older adults.

Senior Centers. Multipurpose senior centers serve a clearing-house function for social services to older adults. These centers have proliferated rapidly from 340 in 1966 to 5,000 in 1975, with numbers still increasing (Lowy, 1980). The definition reached by the National Council on Aging (1975) is that a senior center is "a program for older people provided in a designated facility open three or more days a week." This rather loose definition allows for a great deal of variation among facilities, but the typical center offers congregate nutritional programs, delivered meals, transportation, recreational activities, outreach, and information, referral, and screening for medical, legal, and psychosocial services.

The uniqueness of the senior center comes from building an atmosphere of wellness and independence, while encouraging interdependence and supporting unavoidable dependencies (Lowy, 1980). This is accomplished by working *with* older people, instead of *for* them. The senior center can serve as a base for a variety of community programs, some of which will be detailed below.

Paraprofessional Training. As discussed above, older adults are underserved by the mental health profession, given the lack of trained professionals and the stigma of receiving mental health treatment prevalent in many older adults. Using paraprofessional personnel is currently regarded as one way to alleviate these problems.

Since older adults constitute a natural and available resource, many paraprofessional training programs have been developed in which age peers are used as counselors, community outreach workers, and advocates. There appear to be double benefits in paraprofessional programs, namely, the personal benefits reaped by nonprofessionals from working as helpers and the benefits to older adults receiving paraprofessional assistance (Reissman, 1965).

Gatz (1980) demonstrated these benefits in a two-year evaluation of older adults as paraprofessional community workers trained in interviewing and active listening, problem solving, and using formal and informal community resources. Increased knowledge of community services, increased life satisfaction, and an improved sense of personal control were obtained in older community residents and paraprofessional helpers, supporting Reissman's helper-therapy principle.

An interesting variation on paraprofessional support is offered by Project LINC—Living Independently through Neighborhood Cooperation (Kaplan & Fleisher, 1981). This is a self-help, mutual-help neighborhood-based network, in which community members of all ages exchange concrete services (such as grocery shopping and transportation) as well as psychological and emotional support. The goal of this program is to forestall premature institutionalization of frail elderly by increasing neighborhood assistance with the tasks of daily living. It was recognized that many older adults would find it less threatening to their dignity to accept help from their neighbors (rather than from a service agency), particularly if they could also provide some services as well as receive them.

The neighborhood support system was organized by a volunteer corps of residents and co-sponsored by a multipurpose senior center responsible for answering requests for formal supports. This program is still undergoing evaluation, but offers promise as a creative community option for the care of chronically disabled by easing the outreach process to disabled elderly in need of help.

Protective Services. Another community support function is the provision of protective services to take over the affairs of older adults whose chronic disabilities make them incapable of taking care of themselves, yet have no viable support system to assist in their care. This is typically the case in instances of severe mental impairment, yet it is estimated that approximately one in every twenty older people needs some form of protective services due to defective social resources (Atchley, 1980). Protective services involve casework and outreach to provide services, but in many cases legal intervention is necessary to initiate action if all other alternatives have been exhausted.

An example of the difficulties encountered in providing protective services is available from a demonstration project in Cleveland in the mid-1960s (Blenkner, Bloom, & Nielson, 1971). One hundred sixty-four mentally impaired older adults presenting potential danger to themselves or others and living without necessary resources of social supports were assigned for one year either to a group receiving very intensive protective services at the discretion of a caseworker or to a control group receiving standard community aid. The discouraging results of this one-year comparison were that although the intensively managed elderly were more "protected," they experienced an increase in death rate at the end of the year (25 percent vs. 18 percent for controls) and showed decreased functional competence and increased rates of institutionalization. After a five-year follow-up, survival rates were much lower for the group receiving intensive protective services (37 percent vs. 48 percent for controls), and more than three-fifths of this group were institutionalized (61 percent) as compared to less than one-half of the control group. The apparent deleterious effects of this sort of intensive protective services raise some very serious issues for community treatment. Was the intervention too severe, taking over too much responsibility for the impaired older adult's life?

The Dependency Issue. One of the most dreaded role changes for disabled older adults involves dependency: shifting from being an independent adult to a position of physical, mental, or social dependency. Autonomy and self-sufficiency are deeply valued in our society, leading to guilt, anger, frustration, or depression at their loss. The older adult is faced with an unmanageable situation with little opportunity for personal control or influence. Clark and Anderson (1967) found that the primary cause of low morale among older people was dependency, either financial or physical.

There is a clear warning against serving older adults by means that interfere with their independence, yet the need for outside help is realistically necessary for the chronically disabled older adult. The mandate for community care of these persons is to provide the necessary amount of support, *and no more,* stressing the maintenance of individual responsibility and independence despite a disabling condition. This necessitates critical evaluation of a broad array of potential treatments in the "continuum of care" and a clear discussion of the available options with the disabled older adult and those close to him. Providing minimal intervention means (1) relying on existing informal support systems, such as family and neighbors, (2) providing in-home services when needed, such as visiting nurses, homemaker services, and Meals-on-Wheels, and (3) if absolutely necessary, helping the disabled older adult to realistically evaluate and decide about his or her need for some institutional assistance, whether outpatient or inpatient.

Future Trends

A White House Conference on Aging has convened each decade since 1950 in order to develop recommendations that guide or establish programs for older Americans. The 1981 White House Conference on Aging was political to an unprecedented degree, as delegates confronted current Administration policies on limited Federal support for social services. While Social Security was the major issue, many of the nearly 600 recommendations made can be expected to influence the care of chronically impaired elderly (Newman, 1982).

One strong recommendation of the White House Conference was dramatically to increase the research and training budget in gerontology. Of the $140 billion in Federal funds to assist the elderly, approximately $140 million, (1/10 of 1 percent), are currently spent on research and training. Educating students in graduate and professional schools on problems specific to the aged, as a condition for graduation or licensure, would insure attention to the issues of an aging society and help combat the current shortage of professionals trained in geriatrics. Increased research budgets can help alleviate the current dearth of empirical information on treating the problems of the elderly. For example, controlled outcome studies comparing the effectiveness of various types of therapists and treatment techniques on groups of older clients are crucial to planning appropriate interventions.

Recommendations to raise or eliminate current Medicare ceilings on reimbursement for outpatient mental health treatment could have a dramatic effect on the availability of psychotherapy for older adults. If psychological treatment for the elderly became routinely available, the bias against providing and receiving psychotherapy might be greatly reduced. Delegates to the White House Conference also mandated community health centers to allocate special funds and staff for geriatric care in proportion to the percentage of elderly in the community. This could substantially improve outpatient treatment of disabled older adults.

Suggestions were also made for coordinating an interdisciplinary approach among health, social, and mental health professionals in treating the elderly. An important aspect of this recommendation was the inclusion of mental health professionals in long-term care programs, such as nursing homes. Hopefully, a focus on rehabilitation rather than simply custodial care can improve the quality of life for the institutionalized elderly.

Finally, cutbacks in funding for social programs demand the creative use of existing social support networks in meeting the needs of chronically impaired older adults. Current policy forestalls provision of government assistance until the elderly person has depleted all available supports. Bolstering informal supports with partial government assistance may actually prove to be a more cost-effective procedure. For example, a family attempting to care for an impaired older relative in the home does not receive substantial assistance until they exhaust their resources and decide to institutionalize the aged person. Assistance with in-home care is not only in accord with principles of minimal intervention, but may actually cost less than institutionalization.

In conclusion, the growth of the older population into the twenty-first century will create an explosion in the demand for services for impaired older adults. The annual demand for space in acute care hospitals is expected to increase from 79 million bed-days in 1970 to 125 million in the year 2000. Nursing home residents will increase from 720,000 to over 1.3 million. The over 85-year-old population will more than double (Atchley, 1980). Federal and private health insurance cannot pay for services needed now. How can it cope with both inflation and this population explosion of older adults? These policy questions can only begin to be answered with concerned examination of the special needs of the elderly. They will not go away.

References

American Psychiatric Association. *Diagnostic and statistical manual of mental disorders* (3rd ed.). Washington, D.C.: American Psychiatric Association, 1980.

Amster, L. E., & Krauss, H. H. The relationship between life crises and mental deterioration in old age. *International Journal of Aging and Human Development*, 1974, *5*, 51–55.

Atchley, R. *The social forces in later life*. Belmont, Calif.: Wadsworth, 1980.

Birren, J. E. & Schaie, K. W. *The handbook of the psychology of aging*. New York: Van Nostrand Reinhold, 1977.

Blenkner, M., Bloom, M., & Nielsen, M. A research and demonstration project of protective services. *Social Casework*, 1971, *52*, 483–499.

Botwinick, J. *Aging and behavior*. New York: Springer, 1978.

Boureston, J., & Tars, S. Alterations in life patterns following nursing home relocation. *Gerontologist*, 1974, *14*(6), 506–510.

Bordy, E. B. *Social forces and mental illness*. Boston: Little, Brown, 1973.

Burnside, I. M. Loss: A constant theme in group work with the aged. *Hospital and Community Psychiatry*, 1970, *21*(6), 173–177.

Busse, E. W. Mental disorders in later life—organic brain syndromes. In E. W. Busse & E. Pfeiffer (Eds.), *Mental illness in later life*. Washington, D.C.: American Psychiatric Association, 1973.

Busse, E. W., & Pfeiffer, E. Functional psychiatric disorders in old age. In E. W. Busse & E. Pfeiffer (Eds.), *Behavior adaptation in late life*. Boston: Little, Brown, 1969.

Butler, R. N. Age-ism: Another form of bigotry. *Gerontologist*, 1969, 9(4), 243–246.

Butler, R. N. Successful aging and the role of the life review. *Journal of the American Geriatrics Society*, December, 1974, 22(12), 529–535.

Butler, R. N. *Why survive? Being old in America*. New York: Harper & Row, 1975.

Butler, R. N., & Lewis, M. *Aging and mental health*. St. Louis: Mosby, 1977.

Casady, M. Character lasts: If you're active and savvy at 30, you'll be warm and witty at 70. *Psychology Today*, November, 1975, 9, 138.

Clark, M., & Anderson, B. *Culture and aging*. Springfield, Ill.: Charles C. Thomas, 1967.

Corso, F. Auditory perception and communication. In J. E. Birren & K. W. Schaie (Eds.), *Handbook of the psychology of aging*. New York: Van Nostrand Reinhold, 1977.

Cumming, E., & Henry, W. E. *Growing old: The process of disengagement*. New York: Basic Books, 1961.

Dye, C. J., & Richards, C. Facilitating the transition to nursing homes. In S. Stansfeld Sargent (Ed.), *Nontraditional therapy and counseling with the aged*. New York: Springer, 1980.

Eisdorfer, C., & Stotsky, B. A. Intervention, treatment, and rehabilitation of psychiatric disorders. In J. E. Birren & K. W. Schaie (Eds.), *Handbook of the psychology of aging*. New York: Van Nostrand Reinhold, 1977.

Feifel, H. (Ed.). *The meaning of death*. New York: McGraw-Hill, 1959.
Finch, C. E., & Hayflick, L. *The handbook of the biology of aging*. New York: Van Nostrand Reinhold, 1977.
Gaitz, C. M., & Varner, R. V. Adjustment disorders of late life: Stress disorders. In E. W. Busse & D. G. Blazer (Eds.), *Handbook of geriatric psychiatry*. New York: Van Nostrand Reinhold, 1980.
Gatz, M. Enhancement of individual and community competence: The older adult as a community worker. *American Journal of Community Psychology*, 1980.
Gatz, M., Smyer, M. A., & Lawton, M. P. The mental health system and the older adult. In L. W. Poon (Ed.), *Aging in the 1980's*. Washington, D.C.: American Psychological Association, 1980.
Glasscote, R. *Old folks at homes: A field study of nursing and board-and-care homes*. Washington, D.C.: Joint Information Service, 1976.
Goldfarb, A. I. Masked depression in the elderly. In S. Lessee (Ed.), *Masked depression*. New York: Jason Aronson, 1974.
Group for the Advancement of Psychiatry. *The Aged and Community Mental Health: A Guide to Program Development*, 1971, *8*, (Series No. 81).
Harmon, D. K., Masuda, M., & Holmes, T. H. The social readjustment rating scale: A cross-cultural study of Western Europeans and Americans. *Journal of Psychosomatic Research*, 1970, *14*, 391–400.
Hochschild, A. R. Disengagement theory: A critique and proposal. *American Sociological Review*, 1975, *40*(5), 553–569.
Holmes, T. H., & Rahe, R. H. The social readjustment rating scale. *Journal of Psychosomatic Research*, 1967, *11*, 213–218.
Horowitz, M. J., & Wilner, N. Life events, stress, and coping. In L. W. Poon (Ed.), *Aging in the 1980's*. Washington, D.C.: American Psychological Association, 1980.
Kahana, E. Matching environments to needs of the aged: A conceptual scheme. In J. Gubrium (Ed.), *Late life: Recent developments in the sociology of aging*. Springfield, Ill.: Charles C. Thomas, 1975.
Kahn, R. L. Excess disabilities in the aged. From *Mental impairment in the aged*. Philadelphia Geriatric Center, 1965.
Kaiser, H. The problem of responsibility in psychotherapy. *Psychiatry*, 1955, *18*, 205–211.
Kaplan, B. H., & Fleisher, D. Are neighbors a viable support system for the frail elderly? Paper presented at the 34th Annual Meeting of the Gerontological Society, Toronto, Canada, November 8–12, 1981.
Kastenbaum, R. Personality theory, therapeutic approaches, and the elderly client. In M. Storandt, C. Siegler, & M. F. Elias (Eds.), *The clinical psychology of aging*. New York: Plenum Press, 1978.
Kemp, B. Rehabilitation in older adults. In J. E. Birren & K. W. Schaie (Eds.), *Handbook of the psychology of aging* (2nd ed.). New York: Van Nostrand Reinhold (in press).
Kovar, M. G. Health of the elderly and use of health services. *Public Health Reports*, 1977, 92(1), 9–19.
Kramer, M., Taube, C. A., & Redick, R. W. Patterns of use of psychiatric facilities by the aged; past, present, and future. In C. Eisdorfer & M. P. Lawton

(Eds.), *The psychology of adult development and aging*. Washington, D.C.: American Psychological Association, 1973.

Kramer, M. *Historical tables in changes in patterns of the use of psychiatric facilities 1946–1971*. Rockville, Md.: Biometry Branch, NIMH, 1973.

Lawton, M. P. Clinical geropsychology: Problems and prospects. In *Master Lectures on the Psychology of Aging*. Washington, D.C.: American Psychological Association, 1979.

Lawton, M. P., & Brody, E. M. Assessment of older people: Self-maintaining and instrumental activities of daily living. *Gerontologist*, 1969, *9*, 179–188.

Lazarus, L. W., & Weinberg, J. Treatment in the ambulatory care setting. In E. W. Busse & D. G. Blazer (Eds.), *Handbook of geriatric psychiatry*. New York: Van Nostrand Reinhold, 1980.

Leiberman, M. A. Behavioral effects of institutionalization. *Journal of Gerontology*, 1969, *24*, 330–340.

Linn, M. W., & Gurel, L. Family attitude in nursing home placement. *Gerontologist*, 1972, *12*, 220–224.

Lowenthal, M. F. Social isolation and mental illness in old age. *American Sociological Review*, 1964, *29*, 54–70.

Lowy, L. Mental health services in the community. In J. Birren & R. B. Sloane (Eds.), *Handbook of mental health and aging*. Englewood Cliffs, N. J.: Prentice-Hall, 1980.

Maddison, D., & Raphael, B. Conjugal bereavement and the social network. In B. Schoenberg (Ed.), *Bereavement: Its psychosocial aspects*. New York: Columbia University Press, 1975.

Masuda, M., & Holmes, T. H. Life events: Perceptions and frequencies. *Psychosomatic Medicine*, 1978, *40*, 236–261.

Melamed, B. G., & Siegel, L. J. *Behavioral medicine*. New York: Springer, 1980.

Miller, E. *Abnormal ageing*. Chichester: Wiley, 1977.

Mills, D. H., Wellner, A. J., & VandenBos, G. R. The National Register survey: The first comprehensive study of all licensed/certified psychologists. In C. A. Kiesler, N. W. Cummings, & G. R. VandenBos (Eds.), *Psychology and national health insurance: A sourcebook*. Washington, D.C.: American Psychological Association, 1979.

National Center for Health Statistics. Profile of chronic illness in nursing homes. In *Vital and Health Statistics* (Series 13, No. 29), Hyattsville, Md.: U.S. Department of Health, Education and Welfare, 1977.

National Council on Aging. *Directory of senior centers and clubs*. Washington, D.C.: National Council on Aging, 1975.

National Institute of Mental Health. *New view on older lives*. Science Monographs, DHEW Publication No. (ADM), 1978, 78–687.

Neugarten, B. L. Personality and aging. In J. E. Birren & K. W. Schaie (Eds.), *Handbook of the psychology of aging*. New York: Van Nostrand Reinhold, 1977.

Newell, D. S. Social structural evidence for disengagement. In E. Cumming & W. E. Henry (Eds.), *Growing old*. New York: Basic Books, 1961.

Newman, L. Aging conference takes stand on mental health. *APA Monitor*, 1982, *13*, 2.

Parkes, C. M. The first year of bereavement. *Psychiatry*, 1970, *33*, 44.

Pastalan, L. *Report on Pennsylvania nursing home relocation program—Interim research findings*. Ann Arbor: Institute of Gerontology, University of Michigan, 1976.

Pfeiffer, E. Psychopathology and social pathology. In J. E. Birren & K. W. Schaie (Eds.), *Handbook of the psychology of aging*. New York: Van Nostrand Reinhold, 1977.

Reissman, F. The helper-therapy principle. *Social Work*, 1965, *10*, 27–32.

Richards, W. S., & Thorpe, G. Behavioral approaches to the problems of later life. In M. Storandt, I. C. Siegler, & M. F. Elias (Eds.), *The clinical psychology of aging*. New York: Plenum Press, 1978.

Rogers, C. R. *On becoming a person*. Boston: Houghton Mifflin, 1961.

Rosenstein, J. C., & Swenson, E. W. Behavioral approaches to therapy with the elderly. In S. S. Sargent (Eds.), *Nontraditional therapy and counseling with the aged*. New York: Springer, 1980.

Rosow, I. Institutional position of the aged. In *Socialization to old age*. University of California Press: Berkeley, 1974.

Shapiro, D. *Neurotic styles*. New York: Basic Books, 1965.

Smyer, M. A., & Gatz, M. Aging and mental health—business as usual? *American Psychologist*, 1979, *34*, 240–246.

Storandt, M. Graduate education in gerontological psychology: Results of a survey. *Educational Gerontology*, 1977, *2*, 141–146.

Streib, G. F., & Schneider, C. J. *Retirement in American society*. Ithaca, N.Y.: Cornell University Press, 1971.

Weber, R. E. Evaluation research: Community mental health services for the aged. In J. E. O'Brien & G. F. Streib (Eds.), *Evaluative research on social programs for the elderly*. DHEW Publication No. (OHD) 77–20120. Washington, D.C.: U.S. Department of Health, Education and Welfare, 1977.

Weintraub, S., Baratz, R., & Mesulam, M. M. *Assessment of daily living activities in Alzheimer's disease*. In R. Wurtman, J. Growdon, & S. Corkin (Eds.), Memory and aging. New York: Raven Press, 1982.

Wigdor, B. T. Drives and motivations with aging. In J. E. Birren & R. B. Sloane (Eds.), *Handbook of mental health and aging*. Englewood Cliffs, N.J.: Prentice-Hall, 1980.

Wilder, C. S. *Chronic conditions and limitations of activity and mobility: United States, July 1965 to June 1967*. Vital and Health Statistics, Series 10, No. 61, 1971.

Zarit, S. H. *Aging and mental disorders: Psychological approaches to assessment and treatment*. New York: The Free Press, 1980.

13 Psychological Approaches to Families of the Elderly

Steven H. Zarit and Judy M. Zarit

Older people depend on their families. When they are ill or have other major problems, relatives are most likely to provide assistance. For those older people with serious physical and mental impairments, family members generally make the difference between whether they go into nursing homes or are able to stay at home. If relatives are willing and able to provide assistance, nursing home care can be avoided. If, on the other hand, home care is too taxing for the family, or they are not willing to provide assistance, then the older person faces relocating into a nursing home or similar facility.

This chapter will focus on the role of families of older people in providing assistance when there is a chronic disability. Major emphasis will be placed on the special disability of aging: senile dementia. Once thought to be an inevitable part of the aging process, senile dementia is now recognized as the result of degenerative processes of the brain which affect a small proportion of the elderly, perhaps only 5 to 7 percent (Gurland, 1980; Kay, Beamish, & Roth, 1964). But in many ways, it is the most disturbing of the degenerative illnesses of old age; its disabilities place a tremendous burden on family members. Although there are no medical treatments as yet, it is possible to make interventions which lessen the burden on the family, while maintaining the older person in his or her own home. The example of senile dementia also provides a blueprint for assisting families caring for older people with other disabilities.

Aging, Chronic Disability, and Senile Dementia

The image that the general public has of older people is that they are physically and mentally incapacitated, but the acutal conditions of aged persons in this society are quite different. The majority of people over sixty-five are independent, live in the community rather than nursing homes, and are able to take care of themselves fully. Based on community surveys, it has been estimated that only 10 percent of the population over sixty-five have major problems in functioning (Bouvier, Atlee, & McVeigh, 1975; Wilder, 1973). Another 4 to 5 percent reside in nursing homes or similar institutional settings. The most typical pattern is for an older person to be living alone with his or her spouse, to have one or more chronic health problems, but to be fully independent in all or nearly all areas of daily life.

Health problems are the major threat to a satisfying old age (Larson, 1978). Although several disorders can lead to severe disability and loss of independence, senile dementia almost invariably progresses to that point. Senile dementia is associated with a gradual loss of intellectual abilities, especially memory, and can result in changes in personality and deterioration of self-care activities, such as dressing, bathing, or feeding oneself. The senile older person, forgetful and incompetent, has come to represent all of old age to many people, even though it is not an inevitable part of aging.

There are several types of senile dementia, but the two most common are Senile Dementia of the Alzheimer's Type (SDAT) and Multi-infarct Dementia. Alzheimer's disease is a degenerative process of the brain marked by the appearance of abnormal structures peculiar to the disease, senile plaques, neurofibrillary tangles, and granulovacular structures. Restricted cerebral blood flow and other evidence of artery disease are usually not present. Alzheimer's disease was once thought to be a presenile dementia, occurring between the ages forty and fifty-five, but recent investigations have found that this disorder occurs after fifty-five as well, and its prevalence increases with advancing age. Most of these people who were formerly considered "senile" or diagnosed as having "hardening of the arteries" to the brain are now thought to have SDAT. Perhaps as many as 4 percent of all persons over sixty-five have this disorder, or approximately one million people. Multi-infarct dementia, in turn, affects perhaps 1 to 2 percent of the elderly. This dementia is usually identified when the person has suffered a series of small strokes, presumably caused by pieces of plaque on artery walls breaking off and traveling to the brain (Hachinski, Lassen, & Marshall, 1974). Some cases are a mixed type of dementia, with brain pathologies typical of both Alzheimer's and Multi-infarct Dementias. There are also several rarer diseases which can lead to dementia, such as Pick's and Jakob-Creutzfeldt's diseases. Although there are some behavioral differences between the different types of dementia, the overwhelming picture in each is a pattern of gradual deterioration of intellectual functions.

There are various theories about the etiologies of the dementias, such as genetic, viral, biochemical, or trauma-induced (Miller & Cohen, 1981). Multi-infarct dementia is probably related to risk factors associated with other cardiovascular problems, such as diet and exercise. At present, there is inconclusive evidence for these various theories. Medical treatments, including psychoactive drugs, vasodilators, hyperbaric oxygen, and lecithin, have not proven effective in reversing or even stabilizing the disease process (Funkenstein, Hicks, Dysken, & Davis, 1981).

Senile dementia is a major cause of psychiatric hospitalization and nursing home placement for the elderly. Kramer, Taube, and Redick (1973) report that 55 percent of older patients in general hospital psychiatric wards and 68 percent of nursing home samples are diagnosed as senile dementia. Similarly, Pfeiffer (1977) estimates that one-half of all nursing home patients have symptoms of senile dementia. The majority of older people with senile dementia, however, are not hospitalized. Surveys have shown that there are more cases of people with senile dementia living at home than in institutions, and their symptoms are often as severe (Gurland, 1980; Kay et al., 1964; Lowenthal, Berkman & Associates, 1967).

Chronic Disability and the Role of Families

When an older person develops a chronic disability, family members often assume much of the responsibility for assistance. Rather than fading away, as some social scientists predicted at mid-century, the extended family continues to be the most important support network for older people (Shanas, 1979a). Survey estimates by the National Center for Health Statistics show that families provide 80 percent of the health care to older relatives in the community (Kovar, 1977). The majority of older people have supportive relatives who give substantial assistance that ranges from emotional support to transportation to mediating between the older person and institutional bureaucracies (Silverstone, 1978; Sussman, 1976).

Focusing on the homebound elderly, Shanas (1979b) found that the main source of help is the family. The most frequent provider is a spouse, followed in numbers by children. Other relatives such as siblings and friends play a role mainly when the older person has no children or spouse. Compared to the family's role, social services contribute a small amount of home help to homebound elderly. Sainsbury and Grad de Alarcon (1970) also found families to be willing to assume responsibility, even for those older people with severe disabilities.

When families take on the care of a relative, they frequently find it stressful, time-consuming, and disruptive of personal and family life. Several studies have linked breakdowns in the family support system to institutionalizing chronically ill older people. Lowenthal and her associates (1967) reported that institutionalization occurs in a majority of cases when there are changes in a caregiver's ability to provide assistance, rather than as the result of a worsening of the older person's physical or mental condition. They found that caregivers became physically, emotionally, or financially exhausted in their role. Ross and Kedward (1977) found that burden to the family is a major factor leading to institutionalization. Family support is also critical in determining the length of stay in an institution (Bergmann, Foster, Justice & Mathews, 1979). In particular, older people with senile dementia are more likely to remain in the community if they live with relatives, especially a spouse. Early intervention with families that relieves their burden before it becomes excessive has been cited as a crucial part of a program that maintains mentally disabled older people at home (Macmillan, 1958).

Playing a caregiving role takes a toll on family members. Confirming the findings of Lowenthal and her associates (1967) cited above, other researchers have outlined the effects of caregiving. Adams, Caston, and Danis (1979) found that, after a year of caregiving, most families reported changes in daily routine, and over one-third indicated that their health had suffered. Though care provided by the family made it possible for the ill older person to live at home, the detrimental effects on the family were substantial. Sainsbury and Grad de Alarcon (1963a, 1963b) also reported that caregiving has an effect on health. In addition, caregivers in their study reported feelings of anxiety and disruption of home routines and social and recreational activities.

An obvious problem for families is troublesome or disturbing behavior. In a sample, 62 percent of whom had a diagnosis of senile dementia, Sanford (1975) asked family caregivers to rate their tolerance for various behaviors. He found that sleep disturbance was the most difficult to tolerate. Restriction of the caregiver's social life, especially being unable to leave the home for long periods of time, was another factor that was cited often. Sainsbury and Grad de Alarcon (1970) found that families were troubled most when the patient engaged in potentially dangerous behavior, acted oddly, or was restless, troublesome at night, or uncooperative. Similar findings are cited by Lowenthal (1964).

While the changes in behavior manifested by the older person are clearly the precipitants of the family's burden, other factors may mediate their impact. One important consideration is the relationship of the caregiver to the older person. Brody (1979) and Lowenthal and Robinson (1976) have speculated that the burden falls hardest on middle-aged daughters, who are caught between the responsibilities to their own growing children and their aging parents. Hoenig and Hamilton (1969), however, reported subjective burden to be greater among spouses who were caregivers than among children. Reever and Bach-Peterson (1979) partially replicated that finding. Using a quantified measure of burden, they reported no difference between spouses or children serving as caregivers. On a measure of psychiatric symptoms, however, spouses had significantly higher levels of distress.

Whether the well spouse is husband or wife may also make a difference. While quantitative studies are lacking, clinical observations have found that wives complain that husbands with dementia follow them around and are dependent. Husbands also have difficulty giving up activities outside the home, especially driving, which their wives must take over. In contrast, when husbands are the caregivers, they must gradually assume responsibility for the household, often limiting wives from performing activities such as shopping and cooking when they can no longer perform those functions.

The relation of burden to specific behaviors is important, but perhaps not as critical as the overall situation. Lowenthal et al. (1967) found no differences in physical or mental symptoms between samples that had to be institutionalized and those continuing in the community (see also Kay et al., 1964). Similarly, Zarit, Reever, and Bach-Peterson (1980) reported no relation between feelings of burden of caregivers and the extent of behavioral and mental symptoms. Burden was, instead, associated with social support, with caregivers reporting less burden when more family members were visiting the household.

Other possible factors mediating feelings of burden have not been investigated. These include changes in personality of affected persons so that they seem to relatives to be a different person, the quality of the relationship between caregiver and patient prior to the illness, and whether the patients continue to provide positive feedback or gratification, acknowledging the caregiver's efforts in some way (Zarit & Zarit, 1982).

Traditional Approaches: Custodial Care

When an older person is physically or mentally impaired, both family and individual are placed in a difficult dilemma. Families are typically advised by physicians or friends and relatives that they should place their relative in a nursing home, or they will face insurmountable problems. As they have already had some experience with how difficult caring for an impaired relative can be, this advice carries a lot of weight. But nursing homes are a poor alternative, both for the patient and ultimately for the family. They create problems for patients because of their prevailing custodial philosophy of care, and for families because they only shift rather than relieve the sources of burden.

A custodial bias prevails in the management of older people with disabilities. Custodialism refers to a philosophy of care in which there is emphasis on the control and safekeeping of patients, but not on restoring individuals to their previous level of functioning (Kahn, 1975). Because of a person's age, the decision may be made not to offer rehabilitation services, even though a younger individual with similar disabilities would receive them (Albert & Zarit, 1977).

The major expression of custodial philosophy in the care of elders is the emphasis on nursing home care. Nursing homes offer few services that could possibly restore or even maintain function. Although their value has frequently been demonstrated, programs such as physical or occupational therapy are rarely available. Whatever family work that is done is usually to help relatives accept having placed someone in the nursing home, rather than assessing whether home care might at some time become possible.

Public policies have supported the growth of nursing homes. Medicare provides some reimbursement for nursing homes, and once an older person has exhausted his or her financial resources, the federal Medicaid program will assume payments (although in some cases the patient will be moved to a less costly "Medicaid" bed, or to an entirely different facility, often with a lower level of care). In contrast, there is very little third-party payment available from Medicare or other insurance carriers for outpatient or home services. These are services that might allow a mentally or physically disabled older person to remain at home. The result has been that the percentage of the older population in nursing homes and similar institutions is increasing (Kahn, 1975). Since the number of aged in the population has been growing, that means that the actual numbers of older people in nursing homes has risen sharply in recent years.

Because nursing homes typically do not have a rehabilitation focus, they do not generally promote the maintenance of function. Kahn (1975) has formulated the concept of "excess disabilities," which means that a person functions at a lower level than would be expected based on physical problems. For instance, a stroke patient who has the capacity to walk, but who continues to use a wheelchair has an excess disability.

One factor contributing to excess disabilities in old age is how people react to their health problems. Individuals who give up or who become withdrawn do not usually make a good adaptation to physical disabilities (Zarit & Kahn, 1975) and may warrant psychological intervention.

The environment also affects successful adaptation to disabilities. If an environment encourages independence in activities such as dressing, walking, or bathing, then people will tend to function at or near optimum levels. When those activities are taken away, people may lose both the confidence and the physical ability to carry out those functions. With older persons having severe memory loss, overprotection hastens their decline. While they might in time lose the capacity for such activities such as dressing, taking those functions away from them prematurely will make them totally dependent sooner than they might otherwise be.

In addition to the inconsistent level of care in nursing homes, there are other problems associated with institutional settings. Relocation from community to nursing home is a traumatic event for many older people, and it may even be more catastrophic for dementia patients (Borup, Gallego, & Heffernan, 1979, 1980). Because of their deficits in new learning, dementia patients will have considerable difficulty learning routines in a new environment. Persons who make a poor adjustment are frequently tranquilized, and while psychoactive medications have their therapeutic uses with older people, they readily can become toxic or can have other negative effects. Dementia patients are particularly vulnerable, because of their sensitivity to the effects of medications (Lipowski, 1980). The bizarre behaviors of patients in nursing homes, including hallucination, agitation, and motor difficulties, are typical of medication reactions and are not usually observed in patients maintained at home on low or drug-free regimens.

Despite all these shortcomings, nursing homes would be appropriate placements if they relieved the family's burden and if families preferred not to be involved in care. But relocation to a nursing home often only shifts the type of burden families experience (Sainsbury & Grad de Alarcon, 1970). Families do not readily abandon their older relatives, and in fact will take on the burden of visiting them in nursing homes and interacting with the staff. Seeing their relative in an institution is itself stressful. Since the reimbursement from Medicare runs out after a few months, placement is likely to be a financial strain as well. Many dementia patients fail to qualify for any Medicare reimbursement, which makes the financial burden even greater.

Community Care for Older People

An alternative to nursing homes is to identify ways of relieving some of the burden from family caregivers, so that they can continue providing home care. It is often assumed that because there are no medical treatments for senile dementia, the problem is intractable and the only solution is nursing home care. But if senile dementia is viewed as a problem with many components, some of which can be solved, then it becomes reasonable to work with families to identify ways of lowering the strain on them. Kahn (1975) has proposed that dementia is a "bio-psycho-social" phenomenon, and while the biological may not currently be modified, the psychological and social aspects are often amenable to treatment.

Like any problem, senile dementia and the caregiver's burden seem insurmountable when viewed globally, but by working on the solvable problems in each area—the personality and behavior changes, the coping skills of the caregiver, social supports, and medication—it is possible to reduce the stress on the family. This will allow caregivers to delay, or prevent altogether, placing their relative in a nursing home.

Community Interventions with Families of Dementia Patients

A program of interventions will be described which is designed to delay or prevent institutionalization of dementia patients, through assisting family members to cope more effectively with the specific problems they are experiencing which lead to burden. The program has two phases: an assessment phase and a treatment phase. Interventions partly address controlling problem behaviors, and partly the ways families react to these changes. The goal is to relieve some of the immediate stresses on the family. This is the most viable alternative available for families who choose not to institutionalize their relative. It is not a perfect solution, because the destructive processes of the dementia are not controlled, but it is an alternative to more dehumanizing care.

This program has been developed at the Andrus Older Adult Center, a research and training site for mental health and aging, which is sponsored by the Andrus Gerontology Center of the University of Southern California. It has features similar to other new programs for dementia patients and their families (see Mace & Rabins, 1981). The program currently assists approximately 100 new dementia patients and their families a year. Family members have frequently reported that they have been unable to receive any assistance for themselves or their relative elsewhere.

Assessment

Because senile dementia is frequently misdiagnosed, assessment is a vital part of the intervention program. The most common problem is that family members have gotton only the most cursory explanation of medical diagnosis, or have been given incorrect information, such as the person's problem being due to old age or hardening of the arteries. In some instances, families are seeking help for the first time. Finally, treatable disorders are sometimes mistaken for senile dementia, with the result that proper interventions are not made (Butler & Lewis, 1982; Gurland, 1980; Zarit, 1980).

The most common treatable cases of apparent mental impairment are delirium and depression. Some physicians also refer to "pseudodementia" to denote treatable illnesses which present with dementialike symptoms (Libow, 1977). Delirium refers to disturbed behavior caused by a disruption of cerebral metabolism (Lipowski, 1980); it can be brought about by many different factors, including drug toxicity, common illnesses (bladder or kidney infections, pneumonia), electrolyte imbalances, and malnutrition. Clinical depression is often accompanied by withdrawal from activities and lack of energy. It is often mistaken for dementia because the patient's lack of responsiveness is taken as a sign of cognitive decline. A person with a retarded depression may seem disoriented because lack of attention has interfered with learning the information or responding to the interviewer's question. Most depressed older persons are capable of performing at normal levels on simple dementia screening tests such as those discussed below. When there is some question of diagnosis, Gurland (1980) suggests treating the patient for depression first to see whether there is any improvement in cognitive functioning.

Behavioral assessments are useful for differentiating senile dementia from other problems. Brief mental status testing combined with a careful history of the problem are reliable ways of identifying cases of dementia.

Mental Status Testing

Mental status testing usually includes questions of orientation to time, place, and person. Persons with severe memory loss associated with senile dementia will typically make errors on these tests, while depressed and normal older people do not score in the impaired range. While patients with dementia and delirium will both make errors on a mental status test, there is often a qualitative difference in their answers. For example, when asked where they are, a patient with dementia might answer, "I don't know," while one with delirium might make up an answer. For a more complete discussion of these differences refer to Kahn and Miller (1978) or Zarit (1980).

History of the Problem

Senile dementia usually has an insidious onset, with symptoms gradual and progressive. By the time families are aware that it is more than a passing problem, symptoms may date back several years. In contrast, the onset of delirium and depression can usually be dated to a specific time or event in the not too distant past. Often the event is the introduction of a new medication, or in the case of depression, it may follow a major life change. Normal older persons may have concerns about their memory, but there is no pattern of serious decline in memory performance or daily functioning. As a general rule, dementia patients are brought in to a clinic or physician by someone else who has become aware of their problems. Patients who present themselves complaining of loss of memory are likely *not* to have dementia (Kahn, Zarit, Hilbert, & Niederehe, 1975; Orr, Reever & Zarit, 1980; Zarit, Cole, & Guider, 1981).

Medical diagnosis of dementia is a problem, since there are no definitive tests. Diagnosis can be made only by excluding other causes of the mental changes (NIA Task Force, 1980). Even results from CAT scans, computerized x-rays of the brain, can be ambiguous. It should also be noted that a delirium can be superimposed on a dementia, which would be reported as a sudden worsening of symptoms in a dementia patient. The following case study exemplifies the problems in correct identification of dementia.

> Mr. and Mrs. B. were accompanied by their son and daughter. Mr. B., age seventy-four with an eighth-grade education, had retired from his job as a green-grocer two years earlier. Shortly after his retirement he had developed spurs on his heels and had seen an orthopedist, who had prescribed lifts for his shoes. He had difficulty walking with the lifts and when the pain from the spurs subsided, he stopped wearing the lifts. He continued to have an altered gait, dragging his feet and walking slowly. His family was also concerned because he was so inactive, having discontinued most of the activities that he had once enjoyed, like reading. They had consulted their physician, who ordered a neurological examination. The neurologist did a thorough examination, including a CAT scan, and found evidence of cerebral atrophy. The family reacted very strongly to this diagnosis and sought another opinion from our counseling center.
>
> Mr. B. was very cooperative during the intake assessment. He made one error on the ten-item Kahn MSQ questions. He was somewhat retarded in his response and depressed in affect. Further neuropsychological testing was done, but the results were ambiguous. However, in the process of testing, Mr. B. was given immediate feedback that he was performing within normal limits on many of the tests and that there was no reason to presume that he should limit his activities. Consequently, he started increasing his activities and when an opportunity to return to work part time arose, he did so. His family reported that his mood and even his walking improved, apparently because he was assured that he was not "senile."

It is possible that Mr. B. has an early, mild dementia. But in the absence of clear evidence, it is more useful to view his problem as related to inactivity and depression. Sometimes the diagnosis of senile dementia is so devastating to a person as to create many of the behavior problems associated with it. In follow-ups of Mr. B. six months and one year later, he was still improved and working.

Once other causes of disturbed behavior are ruled out and it is determined that someone has a dementing illness, a specific assessment is made of the problems the family is experiencing. The diagnosis of senile dementia does not denote a particular set of problems. Although some people speak of stages of the disease, our research has shown that the deficits in functioning vary considerably from one patient to another and cannot readily be conceptualized as following stages. Further, what families find distressing is highly individual (Zarit, 1982).

Typical kinds of questions and issues investigated during the assessment process include: what problem behaviors are present (e.g., restlessness, asking the same question over again, not sleeping at night), inability to carry out activities of daily living (e.g., bathing, dressing, cooking), the stress on the caregiver, and help that the caregiver might be receiving. This information forms the basis for the intervention.

Treatment Techniques

In the treatment program at the Andrus Older Adult Center, three treatment techniques have been found to be useful: information, problem-solving, and support. These techniques are used in three treatment modalities: counseling for the primary caregiver, family meetings, and support groups. Treatment usually begins with the primary caregiver, though the treatment modalities have been used in varying combinations.

1. *Information about Senile Dementia:* Families often have sketchy information about senile dementia, or may have no information at all. They frequently report that physicians have told them very little. As a result, they have a lot of questions about senile dementia. Answers to these questions help caregivers understand why their relative has changed so drastically. Areas they typically ask about include causes of the illness, medical treatments, and what the illness does to the patient's behavior.

Causes. Caregivers will ask questions about the causes of senile dementia. We respond that there currently is no answer, but research is being done to investigate possible causes.

Sometimes families will worry about inheritance of the disease, and we tell them that while there is some speculation about possible inheritance, having the disease in the family will, at most, increase someone else's chances of developing it only by a small degree. Less frequently, families will ask about communicability, and while there is some speculation that Alzheimer's disease is caused by a slow-acting virus, it does not appear to be communicable. Sometimes the first sign of the illness is that the person withdraws from activities (e.g., work, hobbies). Families later may ascribe inactivity as the cause. It is important to discuss with them that inactivity is more likely the result than the cause of the disease.

Cures. Families will, naturally, be concerned with the possibility of a cure for the illness. One of the most crucial parts of an intervention is to dissuade them from seeking out quack or ineffective cures, while still maintaining hope that something can be done.

Among the treatments which have been tried unsuccessfully are hyperbaric oxygen (Thompson, Davis, Obrist, & Heyman, 1976) and various vitamin and drug regimens (Funkenstein et al., 1981). Among the commonly prescribed medications are phenothiazines, amphetamines, vasodilators, and Hydergine (dihydroergotoxine). While some symptomatic relief is possible, none has been consistently effective, and phenothiazines and amphetamines can become toxic to the patient. More recently, Alzheimer's disease has been found to be associated with deficits in acetylcholine, and therapy involving ingestion of large amounts of choline, particularly through the substance lecithin, has been attempted. Unfortunately, the results have not been promising (Arehart-Treichel, 1981). Other miracle cures, such as nose sprays to improve memory, or the use of Gero-vitol, have not been found effective in controlled research. In general, families wishing to pursue "cures" are not dissuaded, especially as most of these substances (the psychoactive drugs are the exception) are apparently harmless, but they are also encouraged to view the drugs as an experiment and not to place too much hope on them.

Effects on Behavior. Important gains take place by explaining and relabeling to the family troubling behavior caused by the illness. As an example, caregivers generally report being upset by the repetitive questions that a dementia patient asks or feel that patients should be aware when they forget or repeat questions. These problems are explained to caregivers as manifestations of memory loss, that is, someone with severe memory loss *cannot* remember that he cannot remember. Similarly, it is explained that memory loss is not the result of the patient's lack of effort. Attempts to stimulate memory should be viewed as an experiment. If ineffective or frustrating either to the patient or caregiver, they should be discontinued. In one study, efforts to improve memory among dementia patients were found to have only small effects on the patients but had a depressing effect on caregivers, who saw how severely impaired their relative was (Zarit, Zarit, & Reever, 1982).

Caregivers also ask questions about whether the dementia patient should continue certain activities, or how much assistance they should provide. Because dementia results in severe memory loss, disruption of the patients' usual habits may result in their no longer being able to perform that activity. Hence, caregivers are advised to allow dementia patients to do as much for themselves as possible. They need to intervene only when there is obvious danger, such as leaving the stove on or driving dangerously. Some dementia patients, however, can perform even those complex tasks, and so the advice that is given is based on an assessment of the particular circumstances of the case.

Caregivers will also ask about the course of the illness. Both major types of dementia, Alzheimer's and Multi-infarct, are degenerative, although there can be some plateaus with the latter type. The diseases have been observed to last much longer than the four or five years usually cited. Rather than telling families that they face a certain downward course, however, we tell them that each patient is different, and that it is difficult to predict what will happen.

2. *Problem-solving*. Problem-solving involves teaching caregivers to manage disruptive or disturbing behavior more effectively, as well as modifying their own reactions, so that the strain on themselves is not too great. The first step in problem-solving is to have caregivers identify when a particular problem occurs and to record what happened before or after the problem. This is called a behavioral analysis (Goldfried & Davison, 1976; Kanfer & Saslow, 1965) and sometimes provides information that suggests the solution. A common example is observing that a patient who is up all night has spent the day taking naps. Often these patients are simply given sleeping pills, which are effective for only a short time (up to twenty-eight days) and may have a paradoxical effect. Behavioral analysis would suggest keeping the person up and active during the daytime, and this, in fact, frequently reduces problems of sleeping at night.

Often a behavioral analysis suggests ways in which caregivers might change their own response to the dementia patient. In some cases, they might need to change their expectations toward the dementia patient. When caregivers feel frustrated over behavior such as asking repetitive questions, it is because they expect the dementia patient to be able to limit himself, but if they understand that this is one aspect of the dementia and may be a way the dementia patient seeks reassurance, they can tolerate the problem more. Sometimes caregivers are upset, not because of the behavior itself, but because of how they evaluate it. As an example, one caregiver saw her husband staring off into space. When she asked him what he was doing, he said he was watching TV. At first, she began to get upset as she had in the past with similar events, but she caught herself, and thought instead, "At least he's happy." Finally, by observing the pattern of dementia patients' behavior, caregivers will also begin to see that they get upset at certain times and not at others. They sometimes can observe that it is the accumulation of stress, and not any one particular thing, that upsets them. At that point, caregivers can be encouraged to develop a plan to get some relief, before tension builds up too high.

Solutions have included going into a room by oneself, going for a walk, or getting someone into the house to stay with the patient while the caregiver goes out. Finding ways for caregivers to lower the stress on themselves is critical and is discussed in more detail below.

Caregivers vary in their problem-solving skills and ability to make changes. Some caregivers are effective problem-solvers and readily see how they can take steps to reduce the stress on themselves as well as to provide better care for the dementia patients. Others have more difficulty making behavioral and cognitive changes. For these persons, the counseling process resembles brief psychotherapy (e.g., Beck, Rush, Shaw, & Emery, 1979; Lewinsohn, Munoz, Youngren, & Zeiss, 1978).

3. *Support*. The problem-solving is one way of relieving some of the burden of care from caregivers. Caregivers also report feeling isolated and alone, and so the understanding of a counselor can be important.

Another sort of support is also critical. Caregivers often fall into a role of trying to provide around-the-clock care. Most people, however, need some relief from being continually in the caregiving role. Many caregivers believe initially that it is wrong for them to turn the care of their relative over to anyone else, or they feel guilty for having to ask for help. Spouses, particularly, feel that it is part of their responsibility to provide all of the care and that their children should not be expected to help. An examination of these beliefs often leads to an alternative rationale. One way of explaining that it is important to accept some help is impressing on them the need of taking care of themselves in order to continue providing assistance to the dementia patient.

Help may come from social service agencies or from within the family. Such things as housekeepers, someone to sit with the dementia patient, day care, and respite care would make the caregiver's task a lot easier. These services, however, are not consistently available or may be quite expensive in some communities.

When caregivers have available friends or relatives they are not utilizing, it is important to explore with them their reasons. They can be helped to find ways to ask for help, and also to test their belief that they would be overburdening friends or relatives. In most cases, it will turn out that there is more help available than they thought.

Treatment Modalities

1. *Individual Counseling*. Working with the primary caregiver on a one-to-one basis often proves to be a desirable step after the assessment phase. A trained counselor who is knowledgeable about senile dementia and psychotherapy can make this intervention. The counselor's role goes beyond just letting caregivers vent their feelings, or giving them an

understanding person to talk to. It involves taking an active role to help them relieve the most pressing stresses on themselves and overcoming difficulties they have in making changes. Counseling includes answering caregivers' questions about the causes and possible treatments for senile dementia. Furthermore, caregivers often ask for help at a point when they are feeling quite isolated and stressed. The individual sessions focus on reducing their stress and giving them emotional support. Another focus is management of problem behaviors. Finally, while the goal in most cases is to reach out to informal supports, usually other family members, caregivers are typically reluctant to share their problems with others. The individual counseling helps reframe the asking of help in a more positive way, as well as serving to identify people in the support network who should be invited to a family meeting.

2. *Family Meetings*. By far the most impressive changes have been brought about in family meetings. In many cases individual counseling goes quite well for a while and then reaches an impasse when the next goal in treatment is to reach out to family and friends. The timely calling of a family meeting may make the difference between stopping treatment with moderate gains and real success in ameliorating the problem.

As mentioned earlier, caregivers feel most burdened when they are receiving few visits from family and friends. If providing support to the caregiver is the focus of the intervention and visits from the family and friends are perceived as vital to reducing feelings of burden, then the family meeting is one natural way to proceed. The aims of the meeting are to bring the family's level of information up to that of the caregiver, to answer questions, to identify the caregiver's most pressing needs, to problem-solve with the family, and to strengthen or develop a family support system.

The people invited to the family meeting can include relatives, friends, or anyone else who visits or calls the caregiver. Often these people are willing and able to help, but have no idea how to do so, and caregivers are hesitant or embarrassed to ask. Sometimes all the caregiver wants or needs is a phone call. In one case, a husband was caregiver for his wife twenty-four hours a day. Most of his family did not realize how difficult that was for him, but the discussion of her problems at the family meeting made them aware of how demanding care for her was. Family members then readily volunteered to take turns sitting with their mother, so that their father could have some time away from her. Whether it is a phone call or actually sitting with the impaired person, the caregiver needs to know that his or her family understands what he or she is dealing with, and that their sympathy and support is there when it is really needed. Caregiving is a very lonely job, especially when friends no longer visit, which is usually the case.

3. *Support Groups*. An intervention that has come into wide use is support groups for caregivers. These groups allow caregivers to share information with one another and help them understand their own experience better. Caregivers have said in our groups that they felt they were going crazy until they learned that other caregivers experienced the same frustrations as they. Groups are especially critical for those caregivers who maintain that they cannot possibly ask for any help because no one else could take care of the impaired person. In the groups they will see other caregivers who seek help, both from families and service programs such as day care or homemakers, and will be more willing to try the same for themselves.

Support groups have been started in many parts of the country in the last few years. Often, they are not professionally led, and the caregiver goes into them without any other preparation. We recommend a different approach. First, we want to see caregivers individually before placing them in a group. This is important, because at first the caregiver will have a lot of questions and asking them in an ongoing group will be repetitious to other group members. Some caregivers are under a great deal of stress when they first seek help, and we believe they can get more immediate relief from individual counseling than in a group. Second, our groups are professionally led. This is done because the group process can become untherapeutic without some informed leadership. One so-called leaderless support group was dominated by a woman who had institutionalized her husband. Consequently, the group's time and energy were spent discussing costs of nursing homes, how to deal with staff, and so on. The members with spouses or parents at home tended to drop out, but unfortunately, not before the idea that institutionalization is inevitable had been planted.

The problem-solving process takes on new dimensions in the group. Caregivers make suggestions to one another based on their own experience of what has been successful. The group leaders find that participants' problem-solving alternatives are sometimes quite creative. Caregivers will often try something new when proposed by another caregiver even though they might not follow a counselor's suggestion. Caregivers also model after one another, learning new strategies of responding to the dementia patient by observing what the other participants did. Modeling is an important source of new learning, in particular in areas where caregivers had previously had trouble making changes. In one group, some of the women caregivers had been reluctant to bring help into the household to care for their husbands. They felt that they should be able to do everything their husbands needed, despite being overwhelmed by the demands for constant attention. The example set by the men of the group who used household help was instrumental in overcoming the womens' belief that they should be able to manage by themselves.

Summary

Families usually assume the care of an older person with serious physical or mental disabilities. Senile dementia, which is a progressive and devastating impairment, can place tremendous strain on family caregivers. They frequently find themselves torn between their desire to keep their relative out of a nursing home, and the burden caregiving causes on their physical and emotional health. Interventions which identify modifiable aspects of the problem can be effective in lowering the burden on caregivers. Interventions include education, problem-solving, and support for caregivers. These interventions can be made in counseling sessions, family meetings, or support groups for caregivers. By providing an alternative to nursing home care, these interventions serve both the dementia patient and the family.

References

Adams, M., Caston, M. A., & Danis, B. C. A neglected dimension in home care of elderly disabled persons: Effect on responsible family members. Paper presented at the meeting of the Gerontological Society, Washington, D.C., 1979.

Albert, W. C., & Zarit, S. H. Income and health care of the aging. In S. H. Zarit, (Ed.), *Readings in aging and death: Contemporary perspectives*. New York: Harper & Row, 1977.

Arehart-Treichel, J. Senility: The acetylcholine connection. *Science News*, 1981, *120*, 387–389.

Beck, A., Rush, A. J., Shaw, B., & Emery, G. *Cognitive therapy of depression*. New York: Guilford, 1979.

Bergmann, K., Foster, E. M., Justice, A. W., & Mathews, V. Management of the demented elderly patient in the community. *British Journal of Psychiatry*, 1979, *132*, 441–449.

Borup, J. H., Gallego, D., & Heffernan, P. Relocation and its effect on mortality. *Gerontologist*, 1979, *19*, 135–140.

Borup, J. H., Gallego, D., & Heffernan, P. Relocation: Its effect on health functioning and mortality. *Gerontologist*, 1980, *20*, 468–479.

Bouvier, L., Atlee, E., & McVeigh, F. The elderly in America. *Population Bulletin*, 1975.

Brody, E. Aged parents and aging children. In P. K. Ragan (Ed.), *Aging parents*. Los Angeles: University of Southern California Press, 1979.

Butler, R. N., & Lewis, M. I. *Aging and mental health* (3rd ed.). St. Louis: Mosby, 1982.

Funkenstein, H. H., Hicks, R., Dysken, M. W., & Davis, J. M. Drug treatment of cognitive impairment in Alzheimer's disease and the late life dementias. In N. E. Miller & G. D. Cohen (Eds.), *Clinical aspects of Alzheimer's disease and senile dementia*. New York: Raven Press, 1981.

Goldfried, M. R., & Davison, G. C. *Clinical behavior therapy*. New York: Holt, Rinehart & Winston, 1976.
Gurland, B. J. The assessment of the mental status of older adults. In J. E. Birren & R. B. Sloane (Eds.), *Handbook of mental health and aging*. Englewood Cliffs, N.J.: Prentice-Hall, 1980.
Hachinski, V., Lassen, N., & Marshall, J. Multi-infarct dementia: A cause of mental deterioration in the elderly. *Lancet*, 1974, *2*, 207–210.
Hoening, J., & Hamilton, M. W. *The desegregation of the mentally ill*. London: Routledge & Kegan Paul, 1969.
Kahn, R. L. The mental health system and the future aged. *Gerontologist*, 1975, *15*(1), 24–31.
Kahn, R. L., & Miller, N. E. Assessment of altered brain function in the aged. In M. Storandt, I. C. Siegler, & M. Elias (Eds.), *The clinical psychology of aging*. New York: Plenum Press, 1978.
Kahn, R. L., Zarit, S. H., Hilbert, N. M., & Niederehe, G. Memory complaint and impairment in the aged. *Archives of General Psychiatry*, 1975, *32*, 1569–1573.
Kanfer, F. H., & Saslow, G. Behavioral analysis: An alternative to diagnostic classification. *Archives of General Psychiatry*, 1965, *12*, 529–538.
Kay, D. W. K., Beamish, P., & Roth, M. Old age mental disorders in Newcastle upon Tyne. Part I. A study of prevalence. *British Journal of Psychiatry*, 1964, *10*, 146–158
Kleban, M. M., Brody, E. M., & Lawton, M. P. Personality traits in the mentally impaired aged and their relationship to improvements in current functioning. *Gerontologist*, 1971, *11*, 143–150.
Kovar, G. Health of the elderly and use of health services. *Public Health Reports*, 1977, *29*, 9–19.
Kramer, M., Taube, A., & Redick, R. W. Patterns of use of psychiatric facilities by the aged: Past, present and future. In C. Eisdorfer & M. P. Lawton (Eds.), *The psychology of adult development and aging*. Washington, D.C.: American Psychological Association, 1973.
Larson, R. Thirty years of research on the subjective well-being of older Americans. *Journal of Gerontology*, 1978, *33*, 109–129.
Lewinsohn, P. M., Munoz, R. F., Youngren, M. A., & Zeiss, A. M. *Control your depression*. Englewood Cliffs, N.J.: Prentice-Hall, 1978.
Libow, L. S. Senile dementia and "pseudosenility": Clinical diagnosis. In C. Eisdorfer & R. O. Friedel (Eds.), *Cognitive and emotional disturbances in the elderly*. Chicago: Year Book Medical Publishers, 1977.
Lipowski, Z. J. *Delirium*. Springfield, Ill.: Charles C. Thomas, 1980.
Lowenthal, M. F. *Lives in Distress*. New York: Basic Books, 1964.
Lowenthal, M. F., & Robinson, B. Social networks and isolation. In R. H. Binstock & E. Shanas (Eds.), *Handbook of aging and the social sciences*. New York: Van Nostrand Reinhold, 1976.
Lowenthal, M. F., Berkman, P., & Associates. *Aging and Mental Disorder in San Francisco*. San Francisco: Jossey-Bass, 1967.
Mace, N. L., & Rabins, P. V. *The 36-hour day*. Baltimore: Johns Hopkins University Press, 1981.
Macmillan, D. *Hospital-community relationships. An approach to the prevention*

of disability from chronic psychoses: The open mental hospital within the community. New York: Millbank Memorial Fund, 1958.

Miller, N. E., & Cohen, G. D. (Eds.), *Clincal aspects of Alzheimer's disease senile dementia*. New York: Raven Press, 1981.

NIA Task Force. Senility reconsidered. *Journal of the American Medical Association*, 1980, *244*(3), 259–263.

Orr, N. K., Reever, K. E., & Zarit, S. H. Longitudinal change in memory performance and self-report of memory problems. Paper presented at the meeting of the Gerontological Society, San Diego, Calif. 1980.

Pfeiffer, E. Psychopathology and social pathology. In J. E. Birren & K. W. Schaie (Eds.), *Handbook of psychology and aging*. New York: Van Nostrand Reinehold, 1977.

Reever, K. E., & Bach-Peterson, J. The older person with senile dementia in the community and their primary caregiver. Unpublished Master's thesis. Los Angeles: University of Southern California, 1979.

Ross, H. E., & Kedward, H. B. Psychogeriatric hospital admissions from the community and institutions. *Journal of Gerontology*, 1977, *32*, 420–427.

Sainsbury, P., & Grad de Alarcon, J. Mental illness and the family. *The Lancet*, 1963, *i*, 544–547. (a)

Sainsbury, P., & Grad de Alarcon, J. Evaluating a community care service. In H. L. Freeman & J. Barndale (Eds.), *Trends in mental health services: A symposium of original and reported papers*. Oxford, U.K.: Pergamon Press, 1963. (b)

Sainsbury, P., & Grad de Alarcon, J. The psychiatrist and the geriatric patient: The effects of community care on the family of the geriatric patient. *Journal of Geriatric Psychiatry*, 1970, *1*, 23–41.

Sanford, J. F. A. Tolerance of debility in elderly dependents by supporters at home: Its significance for hospital practice. *British Medical Journal*, 1975, *3*, 471–473.

Shanas, E. The family as a social support system in old age. *Gerontologist*, 1979, *19*(2), 169–174. (a)

Shanas, E. Social myth as hypothesis: The case of the family relations of old people. *Gerontologist*, 1979, *19*(1), 3–9. (b)

Silverstone, B. An overview of research on informal supports: Implications for policy and practice. Paper presented at the meeting of the Gerontological Society, Dallas, Tex., 1978.

Sussman, M. B. The family life of old people. In R. H. Binstock & E. Shanas (Eds.), *Handbook of aging and the social sciences*. New York: Van Nostrand Reinhold, 1976.

Thompson, L. W., Davis, G. C., Obrist, W. D., & Heyman, A. Effects of hyperbaric oxygen on behavioral and physiological measures in elderly demented patients. *Journal of Gerontology*, 1976, *31*, 23–28.

Wilder, C. S. *Limitations of activity due to chronic conditions: United States, 1969 to 1970*. Vital and Health Statistics, 1973. Series 10, No. 80, Department of Health, Education and Welfare.

Zarit, S. H. *Aging and mental disorders: psychological approaches to assessment and treatment*. New York: The Free Press, 1980.

Zarit, J. M. Predictors of burden and distress for caregivers of senile dementia patients. Unpublished doctoral dissertation. University of Southern California, 1982.

Zarit, S. H., Cole, K. D., & Guider, R. L. Memory training strategies and subjective complaints of memory in the aged. *Gerontologist,* 1981, *21,* 158–164.

Zarit, S. H., & Kahn, R. L. Aging and adaptation to illness. *Journal of Gerontology,* 1975, *30,* 67–72.

Zarit, S. H., Reever, K. E., & Bach-Peterson, J. Relatives of the impaired elderly: Correlates of feelings of burden. *Gerontologist,* 1980, *20,* 649–655.

Zarit, S. H., & Zarit, J. M. Families under stress: Interventions for caregivers of senile dementia patients. *Psychotherapy: Theory, Research and Practice,* 1982, *19*(4), 461–471.

Zarit, S. H., Zarit, J. M., & Reever, K. E. Memory training for severe memory loss: Effects on senile dementia patients and their families. *Gerontologist,* 1982, *22,* 373–377.

Index